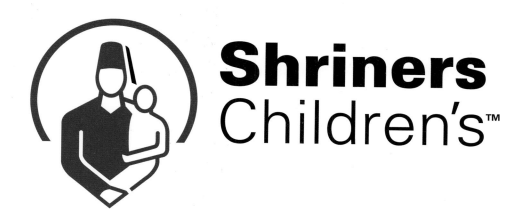

SHRINERS CHILDREN'S: 100 YEARS
PROVIDING THE GIFT OF HOPE AND HEALING

COPYRIGHT © 2023 SHRINERS HOSPITALS FOR CHILDREN
2900 N Rocky Point Dr, Tampa, FL 33607

ON THE COVER:
The earliest photograph of a Shriners Children's hospital, Shreveport, Louisiana, 1922.

ISBN 979-8-9869725-1-0

CREDITS

Produced by The Winthrop Group, Inc.
Designed by Anne Marie Mascia.

The author expresses his thanks to the many people at Shriners Children's and elsewhere who have helped compile materials for this book. This book is dedicated to the medical staff, support personnel, volunteers, and donors who have given their love to the children of Shriners Children's for over 100 years.

All images are from the Shriners Children's archives with the exception of the following, printed by kind permission. *Page 3:* Photograph of Bob Hudson courtesy of Kansas Business Hall of Fame. *Page 6:* Oil Painting by Giovanni A. Scarinci, 1939. Shriners Children's Philadelphia. *Page 7:* Photograph by Carol M. Highsmith, Library of Congress. *Page 8:* Kismet Temple: Library of Congress. *Page 10:* Islam Temple Divan courtesy of Asiya Shrine Center, San Mateo, California. *Pages 11-13, 25, 27, 32, 33:* Images from *The Crescent* and *The Shrine* courtesy of John Wilder, Aleppo Temple Archives. *Page 14:* Odd Fellows seal from Wikimedia Commons. *Page 14:* Photograph of Workmen's Circle rally courtesy of the YIVO Institute for Jewish Research, New York. *Page 15:* International Order of Foresters certificate from the University of Newcastle Special Collections. Licensed under CC BY-NC-ND 4.0. *Page 18-19:* Photograph of signpost and Polio Precautions poster courtesy of March of Dimes. *Courage* magazine courtesy of the Sangamon Valley Collection at the Lincoln Library, Springfield, IL. *Page 20:* Photograph of Michael Hoke from the *Yackety Yack*, 32 (1922), p. [27]. *Page 22:* Photograph of Forrest Adair courtesy of Georgia Archives, Vanishing Georgia Collection, dek035. *Page 26:* Photograph of trumpeter from John M. Holmes, *"Unto the least of these"* (Greenville, SC, 1948). *Page 28:* Wikimedia Commons. *Page 34:* Photograph of Florence J. Potts courtesy of Hospital Archives, The Hospital for Sick Children, Toronto. *Page 45:* Photograph of Dr. Donald R. Lannin by William Seaman, Copyright 1956 Star Tribune. *Page 49:* Photographs of Boy Scouts and patient pouring water both courtesy of San Francisco History Center, San Francisco Public Library. *Page 54:* Photograph of Santa courtesy of the Southeast Portland chapter of ABATE of Oregon, Inc. *Pages 64-65:* Photograph of boys in kitchen used by permission, Utah State Historical Society. *Page 68:* Photograph of Dr. Alexander Mackenzie Forbes by Wm. Notman & Son Ltd, 1920. II-235232. McCord Stewart Museum. *Page 74:* Photograph of Elliot and Clarissa courtesy of Rachel Louis. *Pages 88-89:* black and white photographs from John M. Holmes, *"Unto the least of these"* (Greenville, SC, 1948). *Page 92:* Portrait of Frida Kahlo and Dr. Juan Farill by Gisèle Freund © IMEC, Fonds MCC, Dist., RMN – Grand Palais / Gisèle Freund / Art Resource, NY / © 2022 Banco de México Diego Rivera Frida Kahlo Museums Trust, Mexico, D.F. / Artists Rights Society (ARS), New York. *Page 102:* Photograph of cheering patients from the Herald Examiner Collection / Los Angeles Public Library. *Pages 102, 138:* Photographs of Bonnie St. John courtesy of Bonnie St. John. *Page 123:* Photograph of Shriners Northern California orthopedic team by Pico van Houtryve. *Page 130:* Photograph of Pat Morita courtesy of Evelyn Morita. *Page 145:* Photograph of Darla Hansen today courtesy of Darla Hansen. *Page 153:* Photograph of Hannah Brammer courtesy of Hannah Brammer. *Page 155:* Photograph of Colton courtesy of Demi Porter. *Page 172:* Photograph of J. Albert Key from *Barnes Hospital Record*, vol. 10, no. 2 (February 1956). *Page 177:* Figure of normal gait cycle from "A Practical Guide to Gait Analysis," *J Acad. Orthop. Surg.* (2002). *Page 179:* Figure of microfibroblast from *Nat. Rev. Rheumatol.* 10 (2014). *Page 180:* Photograph of Dr. Howard Green by Barbara Steiner courtesy of the Boston Medical Library. *Page 181:* Photograph of Dr. Michael P. Whyte by Daniel Dubois / Vanderbilt University. *Page 189:* Figure from "Skeletal muscle apoptosis after burns is associated with activation of proapoptotic signals," *Am J Physiol. Encocrinol. Metab.* 279 (2000). *Page 191:* Figure from "NMDA Receptor signaling is important for neural tube formation and for preventing antiepileptic drug-induced neural tube defects," *J Neuroscience* 38 (2018). *Page 192:* Voluntary permanent subscriber certificate issued by Shriners' Hospital to Union Lodge, No. 31, about 1925. Shriners Hospitals for Children. Scottish Rite Masonic Museum & Library, A2000/078/005. *Page 193:* Photograph of RYG Foundation gala courtesy of Adam Yenish.

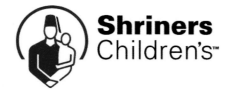

For additional information about Shriners Children's visit **www.shrinerschildrens.org**

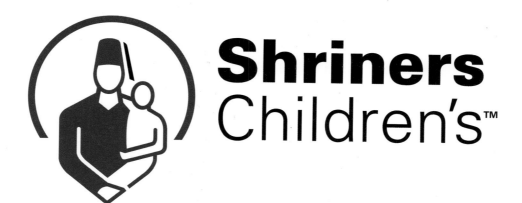

Shriners Children's™

100 YEARS

PROVIDING THE GIFT OF HOPE AND HEALING

BRADFORD VERTER
The Winthrop Group, Inc.

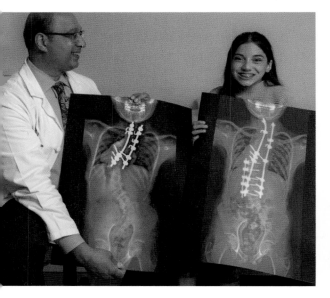
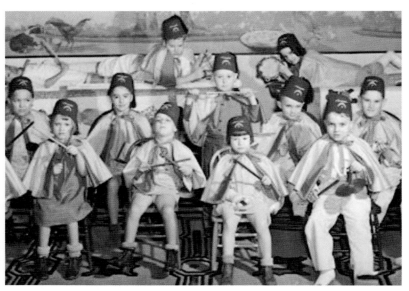
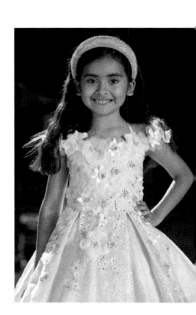
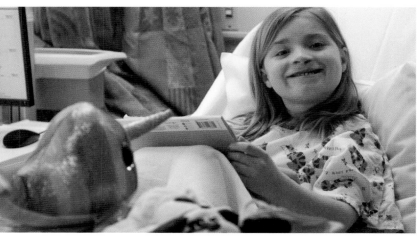
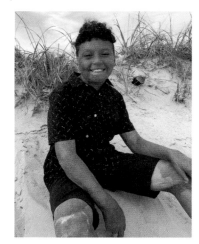
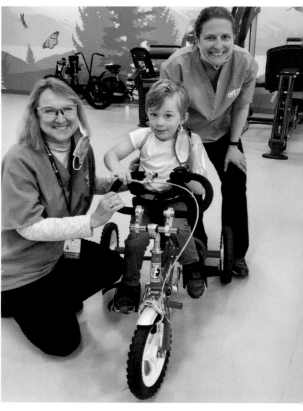
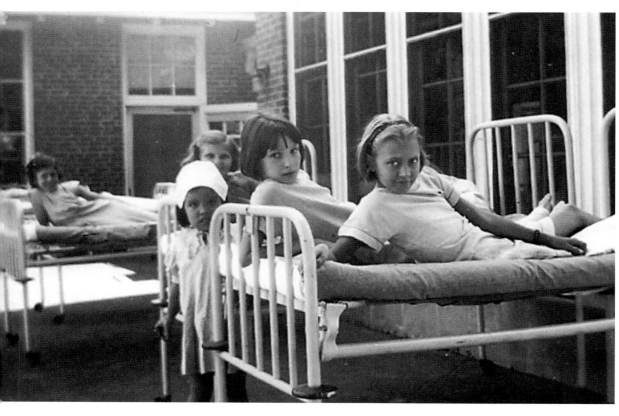
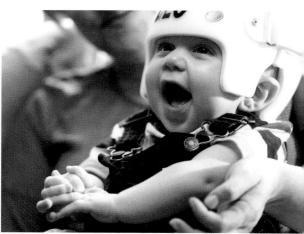

FROM THE BOARD OF DIRECTORS

Shriners Children's has been a place of hope and healing for more than 1.5 million children over the last 100 years. When our first hospital opened in 1922 to help children with polio, the founding location was committed to improving the lives of children. They surely had no idea, however, the magnitude and reach that we would have around the world. We are proud of the institution that our brothers started a century ago, and we are excited for the future as we continue to care for children, regardless of their families' ability to pay.

While the name, service lines and locations of Shriners Children's have adapted over time, one thing has remained the same: our experienced, innovative and dedicated medical professionals have worked together to provide the most amazing care anywhere. Today's patients experience the same individualized care that our first patients received 100 years ago.

It has been an honor to serve Shriners Children's during the 100-year celebration, and we are especially grateful for the ongoing support from all those who hold Shriners Children's near their heart. This peek into our history is only a glance at the amazing accomplishments we've had. It's a robust history full of wonder, excitement and growth. It is 100 years of transformations only made possible by you.

Sincerely,

William S. "Bill" Bailey
Chairman of the Board 2021-2022

Kenneth G. "Kenny" Craven
Chairman of the Board 2022-2023

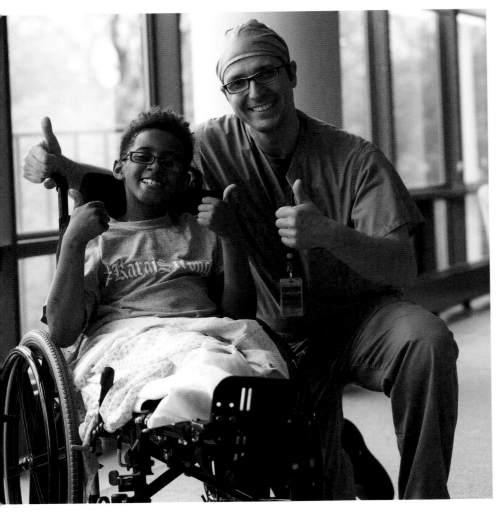

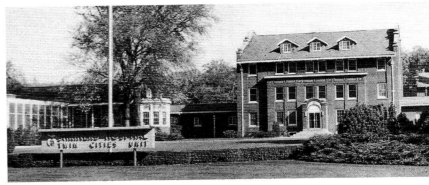

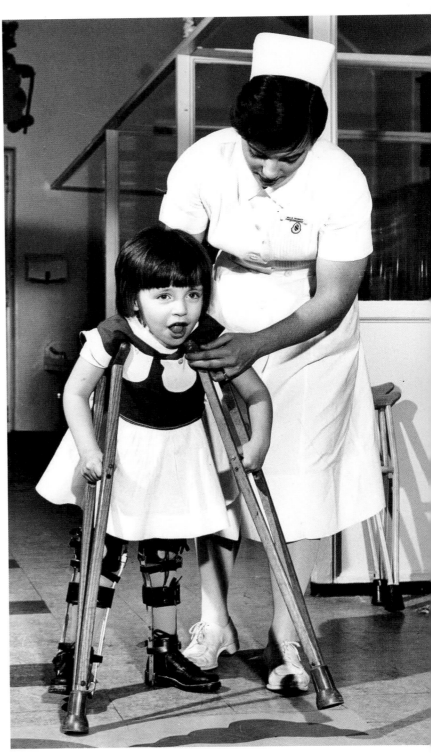

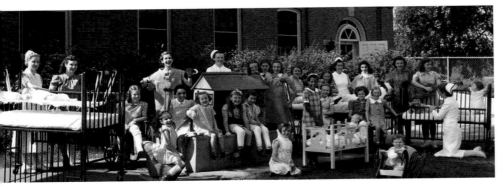

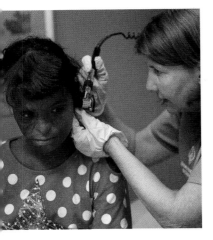

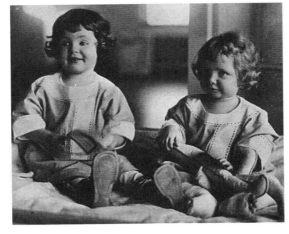

INSIDE THIS BOOK

100 YEARS OF SHRINERS CHILDREN'S
pgs 2-3

A NATIONAL NETWORK
pgs 4-5

THE WORLD'S GREATEST PHILANTHROPY
pgs 6-33

BRICKS AND MORTAR: THE SHRINERS HOSPITALS
pgs 34-119

BRINGING OUR EXPERTISE TO THE WORLD
pgs 120-123

THE FINEST HOURS IN SPORTS
pgs 124-127

EVERYDAY MIRACLES
pgs 128-161

THE MIRACLE WORKERS
pgs 162-165

CELEBRITY ENCOUNTERS
pgs 166-169

FURTHERING MEDICAL SCIENCE
pgs 170-191

LOVE TO THE RESCUE
pgs 192-193

THE NEXT HUNDRED YEARS
pg 194

1920
Forrest Adair delivers Bubbles Speech

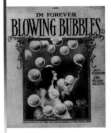

1919
William Freeland Kendrick first proposes to establish Shriners Hospitals for Crippled Children (now known as Shriners Children's)

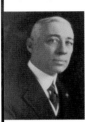

1945
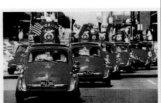

After a dip during the Great Depression and World War II, Shriners membership begins to boom

1932
Afflicted with polio, President Franklin Delano Roosevelt raises disability awareness

1945
New hospital opens in Mexico City

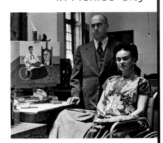

1952
New hospitals open in Houston, Texas; Los Angeles, California; and Winnipeg, Manitoba

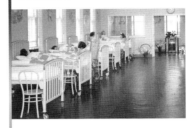

1951
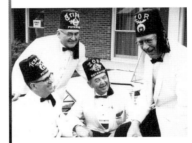

Dues to the hospital fund from each Shriner raised from $2 to $5 per year

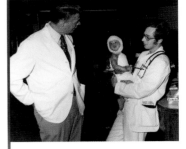

1963
First burns unit opens in Galveston, Texas

1960
Under the leadership of Harvey A. Beffa, Shriners Children's begins to expand its mission to burn care

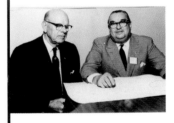

1922   1932   1942   1952   1962   19

1922
First Shriners Hospital opens in Shreveport, Louisiana

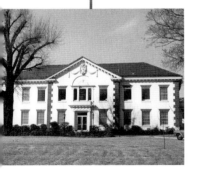

1925
First East-West Shrine Bowl held in San Francisco

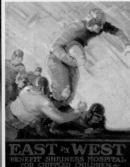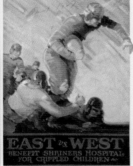

1927
Over five years, Shriners Hospitals open in 15 cities across North America

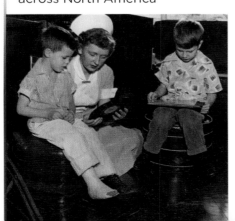

1947
Celebrity Shriners patient Jimmie Carrick makes national headlines after taking his first step

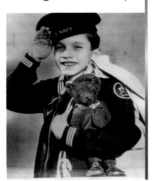

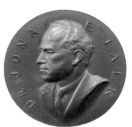

1955
Dr. Jonas Salk discovers a vaccine for polio

1967
New hospital opens in Erie, Pennsylvania

1968
New hospitals open in Cincinnati and Boston

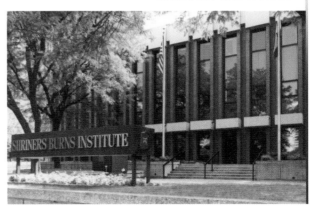

1973

Shriners Children's first department devoted to research opens in Montreal

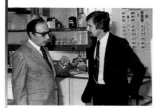

1970

Randy Dieter takes "Editorial Without Words" photograph

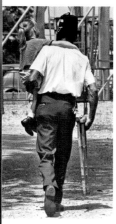

1987

New hospital opens in Tampa, Florida

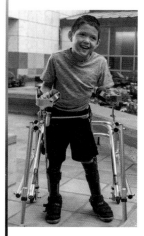

1986

Hospitals expand mission to treat spina bifida

1997

Northern California facility moves from San Francisco to Sacramento

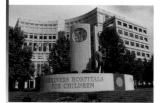

1996

Recognizing its broader mission, Shriners Children's removes the term "crippled" from its corporate name

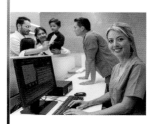

Shriners Hospitals for Children®

2011

A.B."Bob" Hudson bequeaths $60 million, the largest single donation in the organization's history

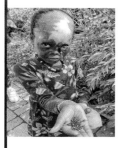

2010

Entirely self-funded up to this point, the first third-party payment was received

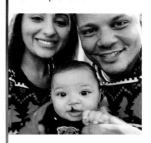

2021

Ohio location moves from Cincinnati to Dayton

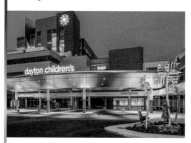

2017

Shriners Children's begins to offer global outreach clinics in locations worldwide

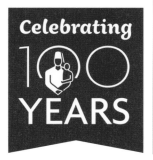

72 1982 1992 2002 2012 2022

1977

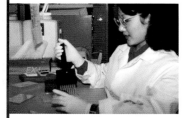

First advanced research center established in Montreal

1980

Spinal cord injury unit established within Shriners Children's Philadelphia

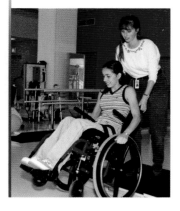

1992

Ohio Hospital inaugurates the first air ambulance for burn patients

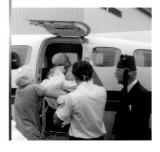

2005

Hospitals expand operations to treatments for cleft lip and palate

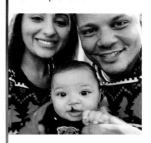

2006

New hospital opens in Mexico City

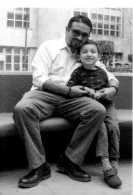

2022

Shriners Children's celebrates its 100-year history of providing medical treatment to over 1.5 million children worldwide, regardless of their ability to pay

Celebrating 100 YEARS

FOR 100 YEARS, SHRINERS Children's has been committed to reaching as many children as possible, wherever they may live, and offering them unique patient-centered, wrap-around care. Areas of specialization include orthopedics, burn injuries, spinal cord injuries, craniofacial disorders, rheumatic diseases, pediatric surgery and sports injuries. Shriners Children's medical research centers develop new knowledge that can lead to new or improved treatments and therapies for our patients.

From modest beginnings, Shriners Children's has grown to a network of hospitals and clinics in the United States, Mexico and Canada. Together, the healthcare system has treated more than 1.5 million patients. Long committed to providing care for children worldwide, Shriners Children's both responds to natural disasters and also provides planned outreach clinics. In this way, Shriners Children's is able to reach children and families from over 170 countries around the world. Outreach clinics in Central and South America, the Pacific Islands, and Eastern Europe, and training programs in specialized pediatric care for physicians and medical students around the globe have made Shriners Children's impact truly international.

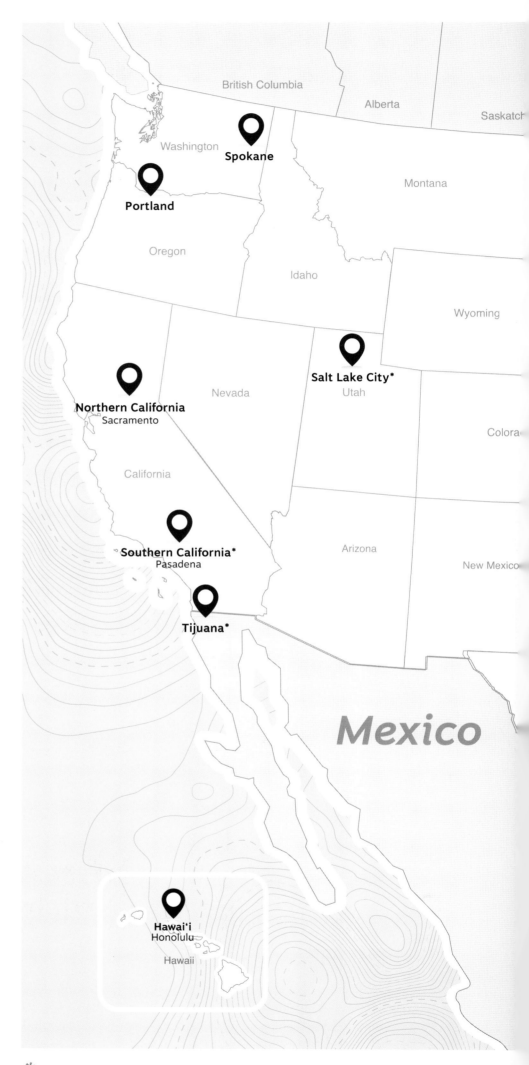

* Outpatient care only: necessary inpatient care provided at an affiliated facility

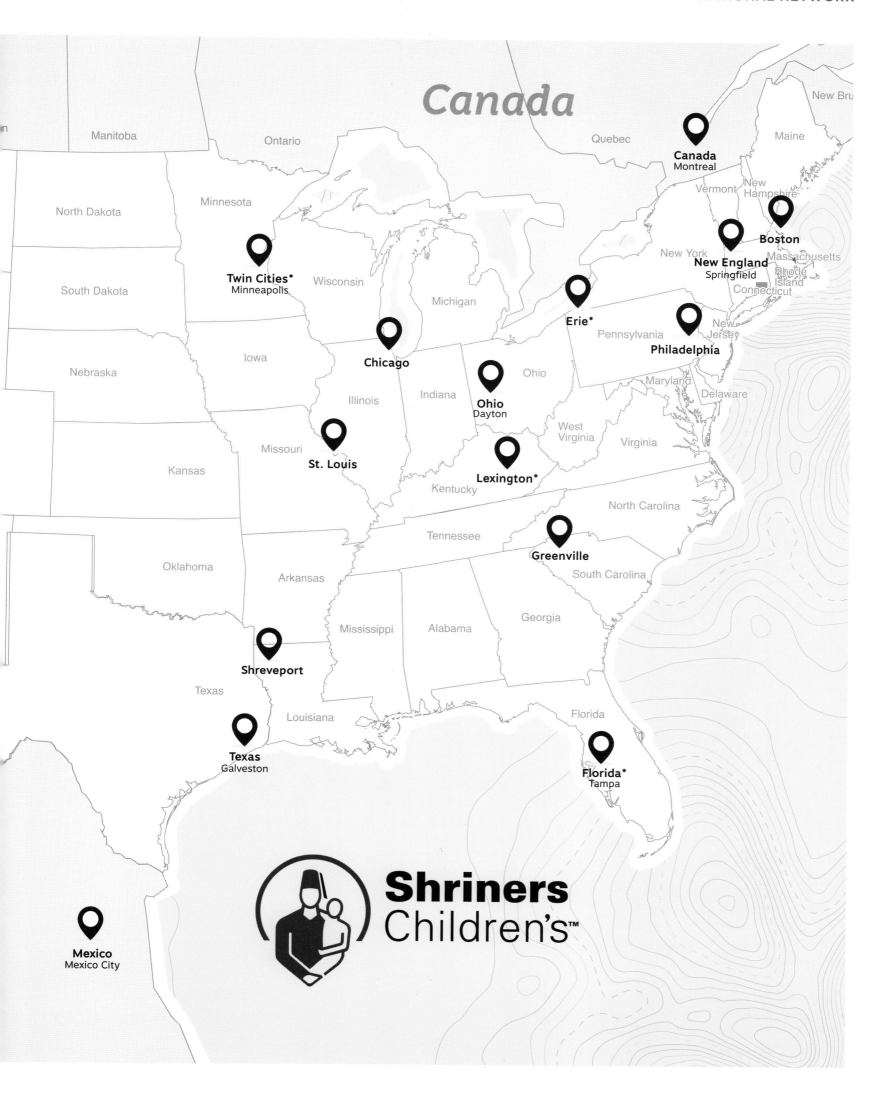

Canada

Canada
Montreal

Boston

New England
Springfield

Twin Cities*
Minneapolis

Erie*

Philadelphia

Chicago

Ohio
Dayton

St. Louis

Lexington*

Greenville

Shreveport

Texas
Galveston

Florida*
Tampa

Mexico
Mexico City

Shriners
Children's™

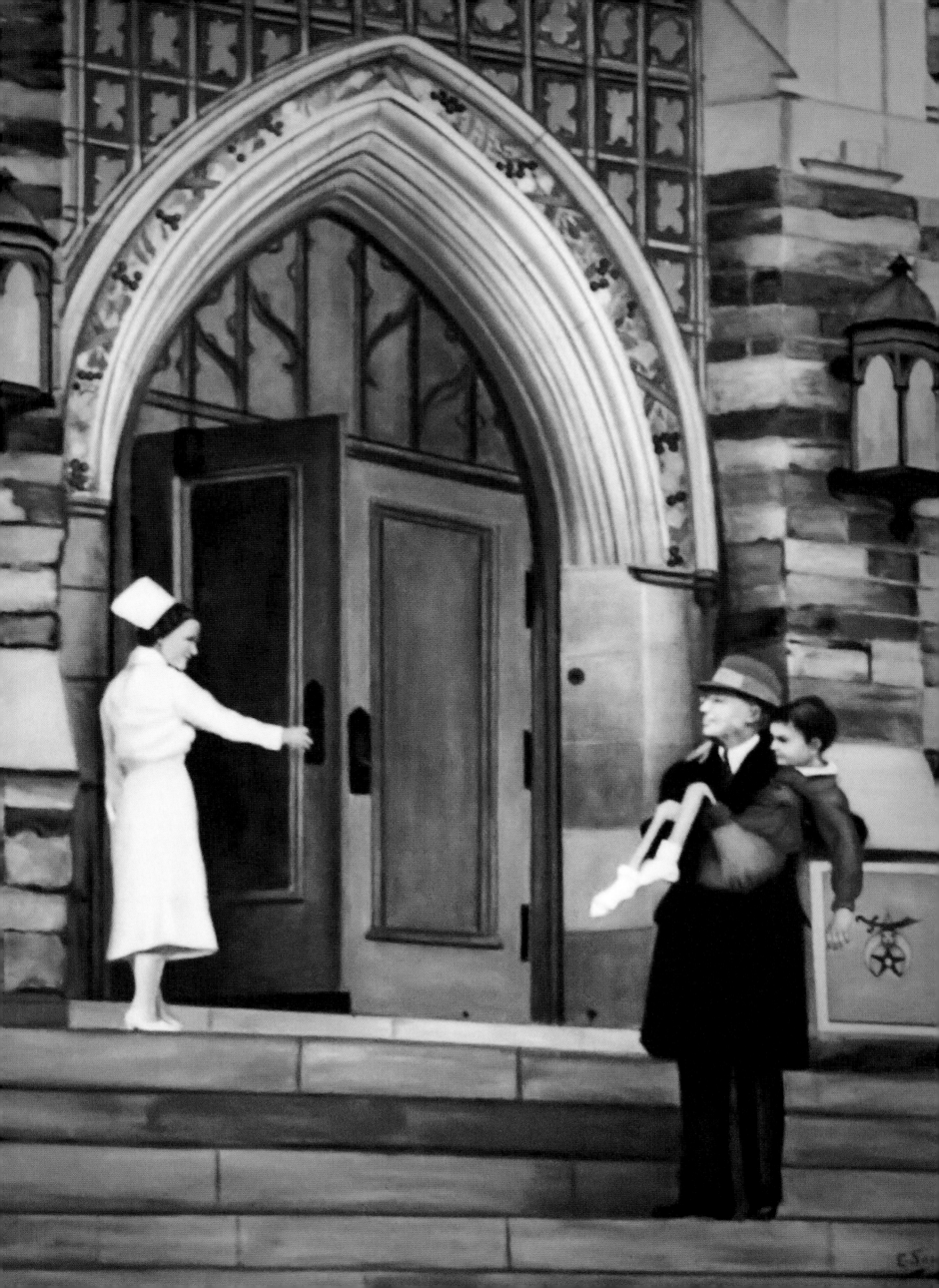

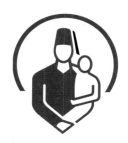

THE WORLD'S GREATEST PHILANTHROPY

SHRINERS HOSPITALS FOR Children, long celebrated as "the world's greatest philanthropy," has its origins in an organization devoted not to medicine but to fun and fellowship. Founded in 1872, the Ancient Arabic Order of the Nobles of the Mystic Shrine (A.A.O.N.M.S.) was one of the many hundreds of fraternities that flourished nationwide in the nineteenth and twentieth centuries. Envisioned as a playful alternative to the stuffy ritualism of other groups, the Shriners offered flamboyant costumes, zany antics, roguish pranks and luxurious displays. As leaders in their communities, many Shriners also shared a sense of civic responsibility. Desiring an official philanthropy, they channeled their good humor and remarkable energy to a higher purpose. Together, they built a charitable network that, during the past 100 years, has provided vital medical care for more than 1.5 million children.

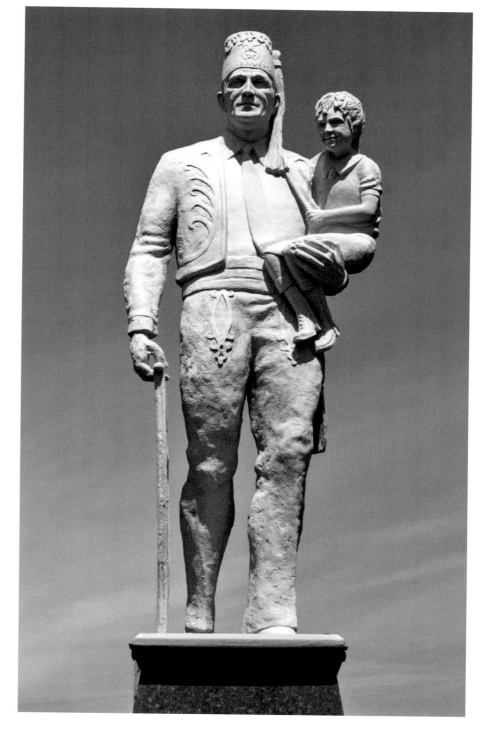

The Silent Messenger, Tripoli Shrine Temple, Milwaukee, Wisconsin.

Facing page:
Freeland Kendrick carrying 8-year-old Jacobo to the portals of the original Shriners Children's hospital in Philadelphia.

7

FELLOWSHIP AND FUN

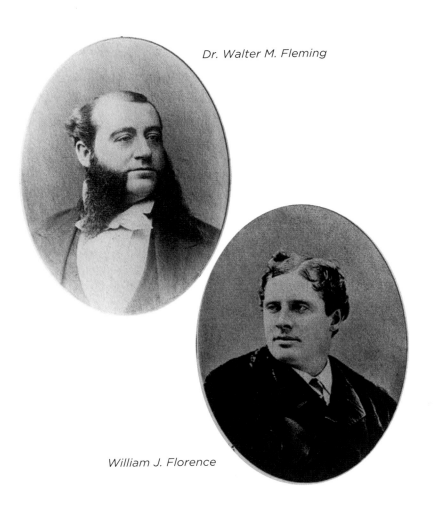

Dr. Walter M. Fleming

William J. Florence

F IN 1910 YOU WERE TAKING BETS ON WHICH men's club was most likely to found the world's greatest philanthropy, no one would have put money on the Shriners. The organization was established by Freemasons Dr. Walter M. Fleming and William J. Florence. One was a doctor, the other a stage comedian. Both were fascinated by the cultures of the Middle East, and they borrowed titles, costumes, designs and vocabulary culled from the Arabian Nights to lend their fraternity an air of exotic adventure.

Membership in the "Blue Lodges" of Freemasonry was, and remains, a prerequisite for being a Shriner (A.A.O.N.M.S. is an anagram of "A Mason"); but in this spin-off, the emphasis was on good fellowship and fun. Organized in chapters they called "temples" with exotic names like Karnak, Al Malaikah, Za-Ga-Zig and Lu Lu, the fraternity grew quickly. Mecca Shriners, the first temple, was organized with a membership of 13 "nobles." By 1895, there were more than 70 temples in 43 states with a combined membership of over 37,000 nobles. Between 1900 and 1910, membership nearly tripled, from 55,000 to 149,000. By 1922, over half a million fun-loving Masons had joined the Shriners fraternity.

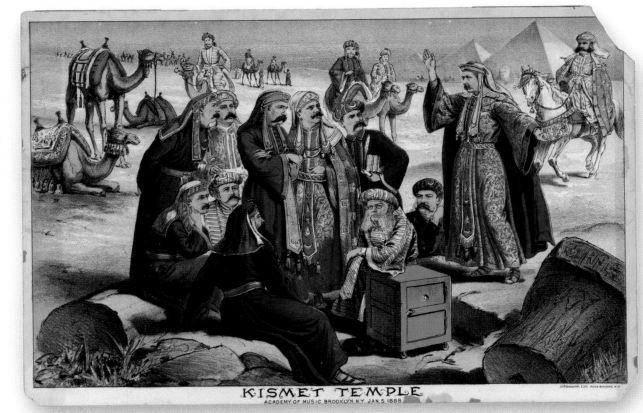

A lithograph depicting Nobles of Kismet Temple, Oasis of Brooklyn, 1888. The men depicted in the foreground, impressively whiskered and sumptuously dressed, are all recognizable as leading figures in New York society during the Gilded Age.

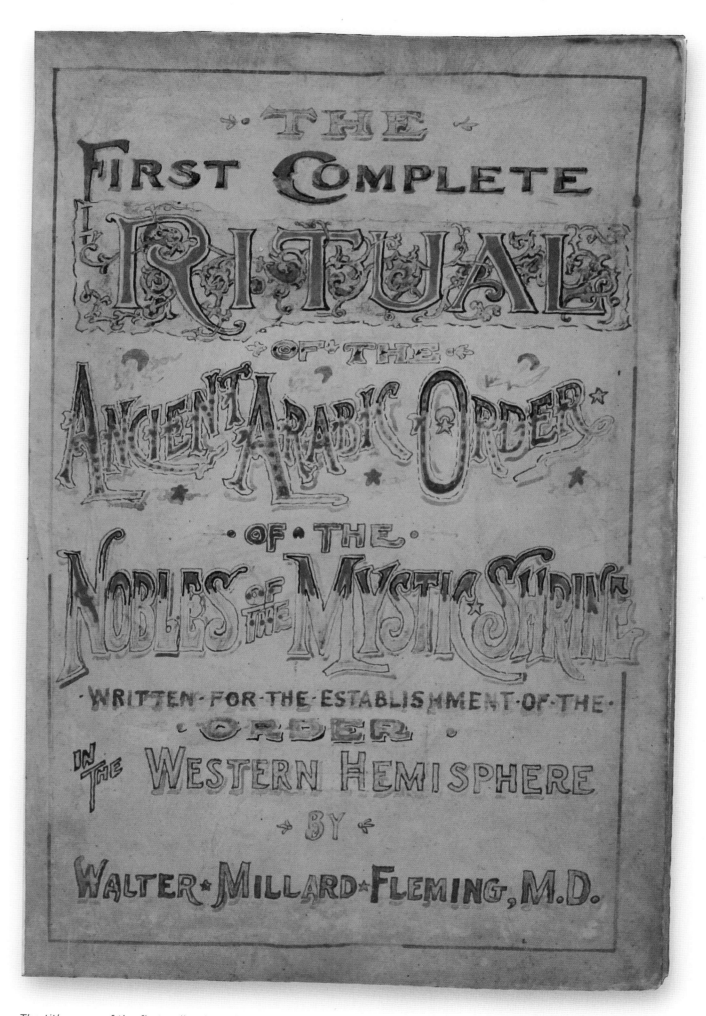

The title page of the first collection of Shriner ceremonies. Entirely handwritten by Walter M. Fleming, the volume includes initiation rituals and invocations for opening and closing business meetings.

THE FRATERNITY GROWS

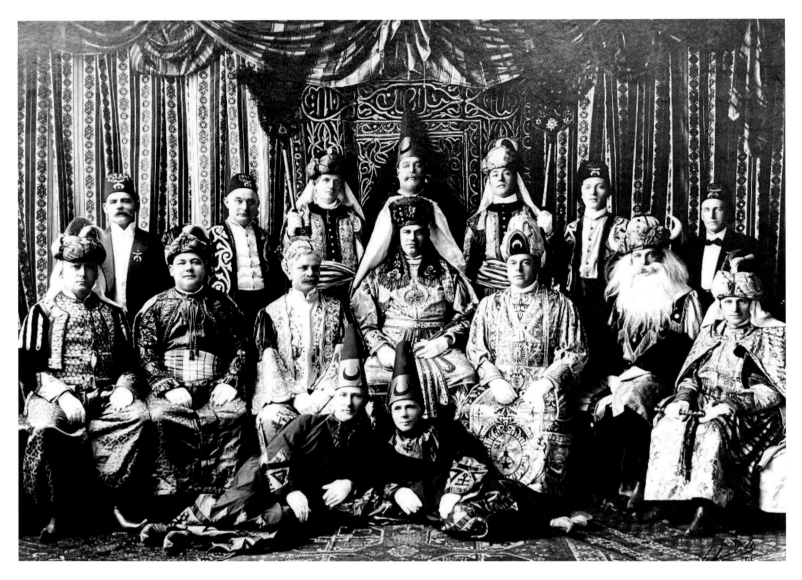

A Shriners temple Divan, 1921. Note the wide range of fanciful regalia, including fezzes, turbans and a Viking helmet with fake beard.

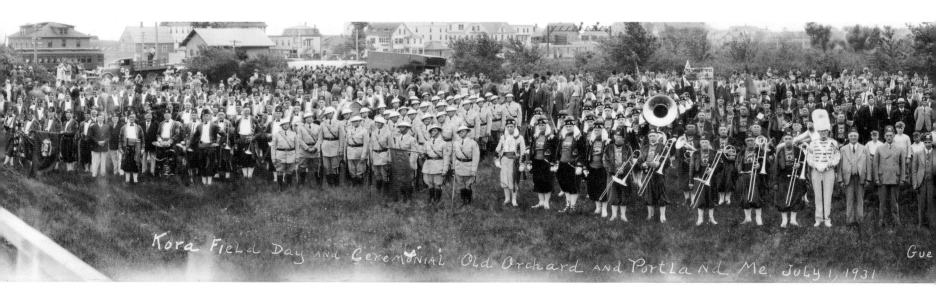

Kora Field Day and Ceremonial Old Orchard and Portland Me. July 1, 1931

Shriners from several temples prepare to march in a parade, Portland, Maine, 1931.

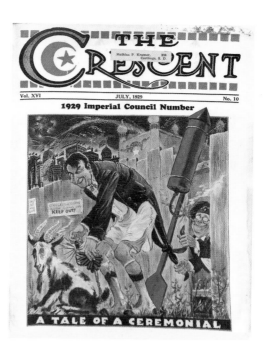

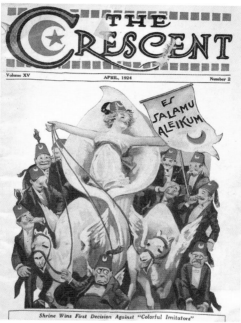

The Crescent, *distributed to nationwide in the 1910s and 1920s, featured stories, poems, editorials, and news of the Shriners fraternity.*

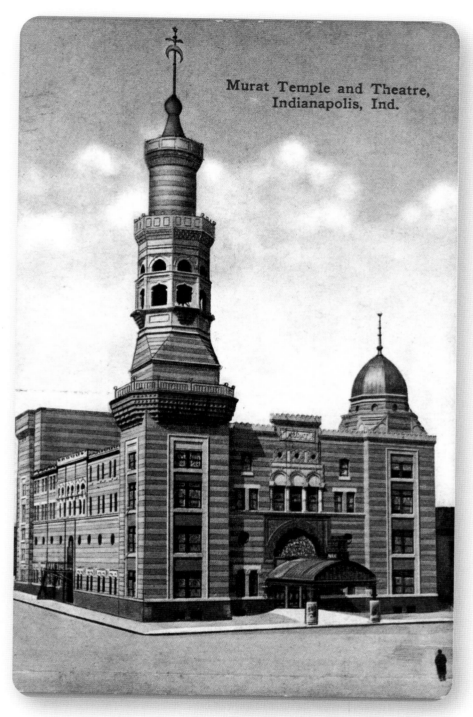

Shriners erected extravagant edifices for their meetings, many featuring architectural motifs from the Near East.

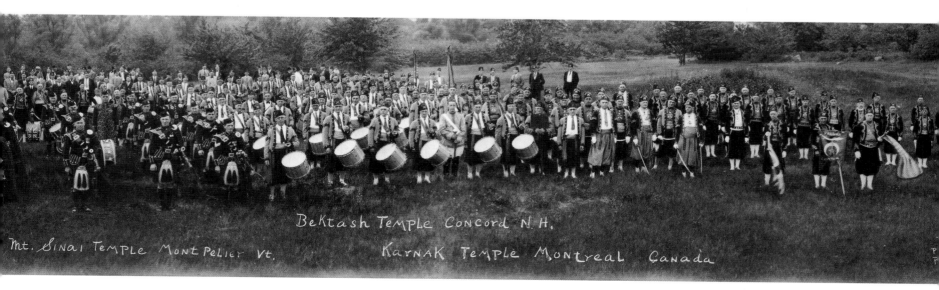

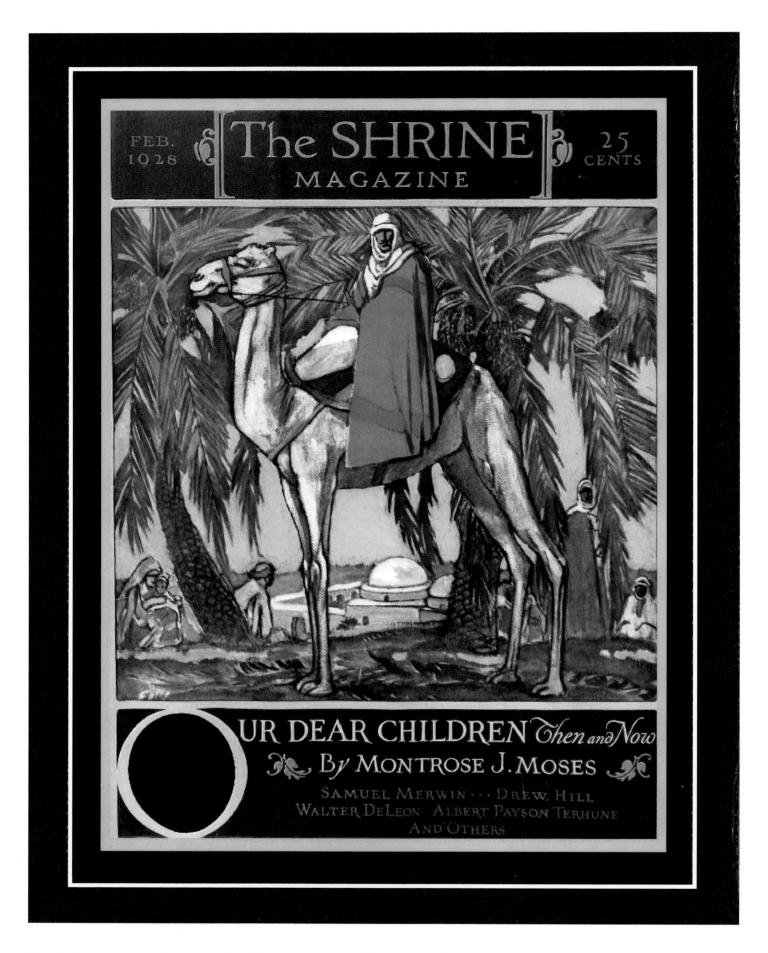

The Shrine *was a sumptuous but short-lived magazine published by Shriners International for a wide readership. Each issue featured stories, poems, and articles by such leading writers as George Bernard Shaw (best known for* Pygmalion, *adapted as the musical* My Fair Lady*), J. M. Barrie (*Peter Pan*) and Albert Payson Terhune (*Lad: A Dog*). The paintings for these two covers were by Charles Buckles Falls, a renowned graphic artist who designed patriotic posters during World War I. The desert motifs, central to the early iconography of Shriners International, draw from the same well of imagination that catapulted Rudolph Valentino (*The Sheik*) and Lawrence of Arabia to worldwide fame.*

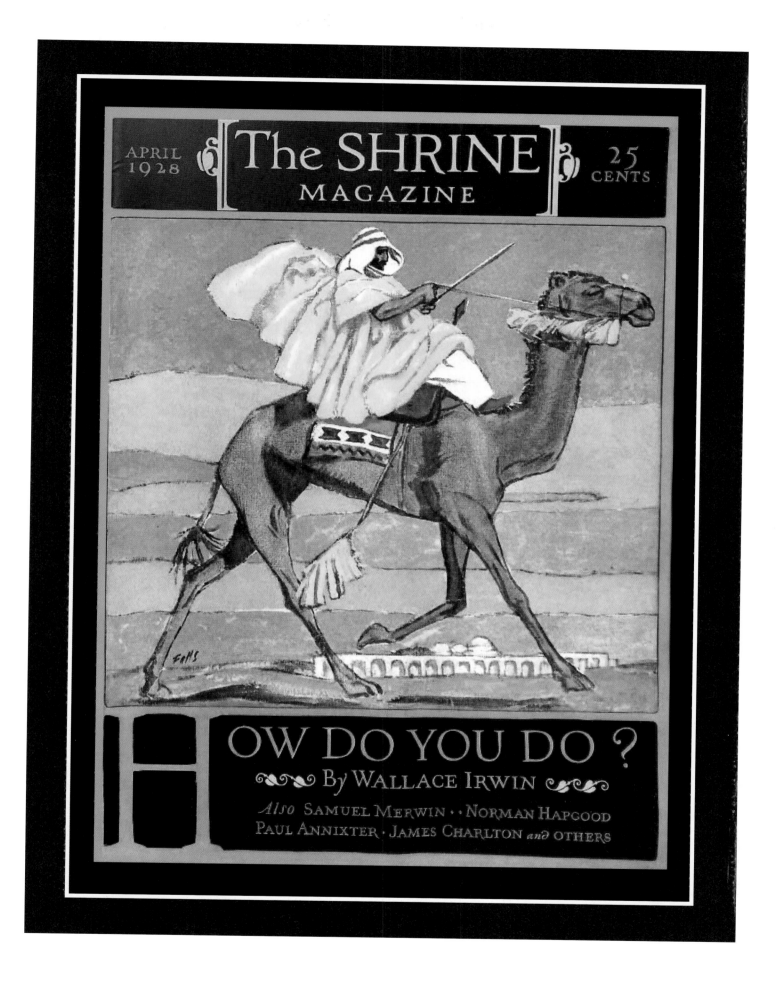

FRATERNAL PHILANTHROPY

ONE REASON fraternal organizations were so popular in the nineteenth century is that many of them offered support to the families of members in need. Public hospitals were scarce, and in the absence of public welfare programs (which were not established until the 1930s), most care for children and the elderly was provided by religious groups and private charities. In his Second Inaugural Address, President Abraham Lincoln called for his fellow countrymen "to care for him who shall have borne the battle and for his widow, and his orphan." Masons and other fraternal organizations responded.

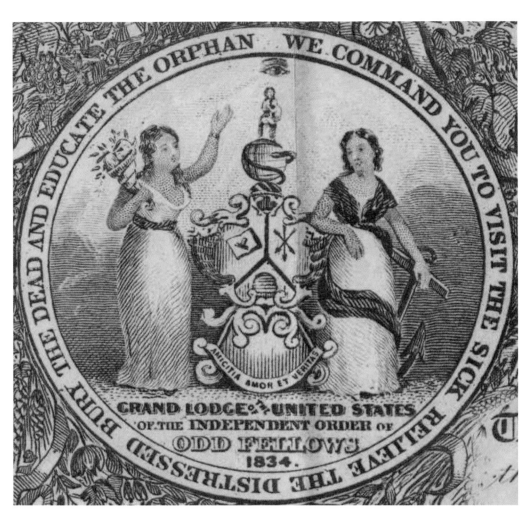

The seal of the Independent Order of Odd Fellows emphasized its charitable works.

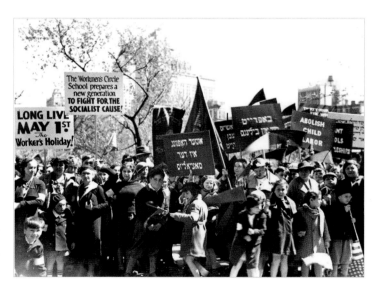

Many immigrant groups formed mutual aid societies founded on ethnic or religious identity, including the Knights of Columbus, the Ancient Order of Hibernians, the Sons of Italy, and the Workmen's Circle, pictured here at a May Day rally in New York City, 1934.

An invitation to a ball hosted by the Ancient Order of United Workmen in Utica, New York, in 1883. Founded in 1868, this was the first society founded on mutual social and financial support. The North Dakota branch would evolve into the Pioneer Mutual Life Insurance Company.

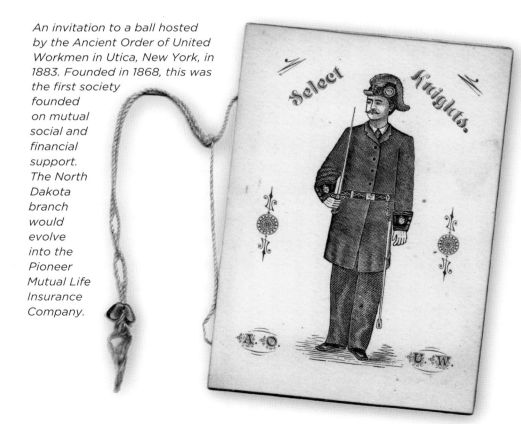

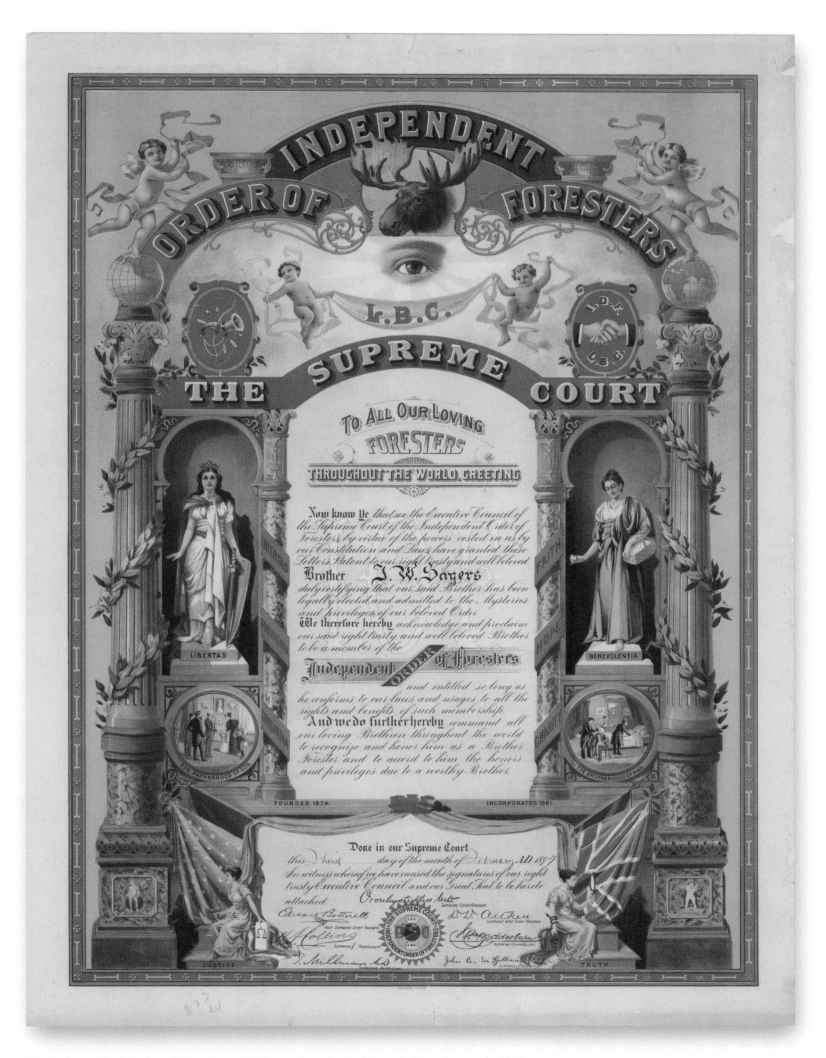

The Independent Order of Foresters (IOF) was founded in Newark, New Jersey, in 1874 as a separate North American branch of the Ancient Order of Foresters, a British fraternal society. Today, the IOF is an insurance company: Foresters Financial.

CARING FOR CHILDREN

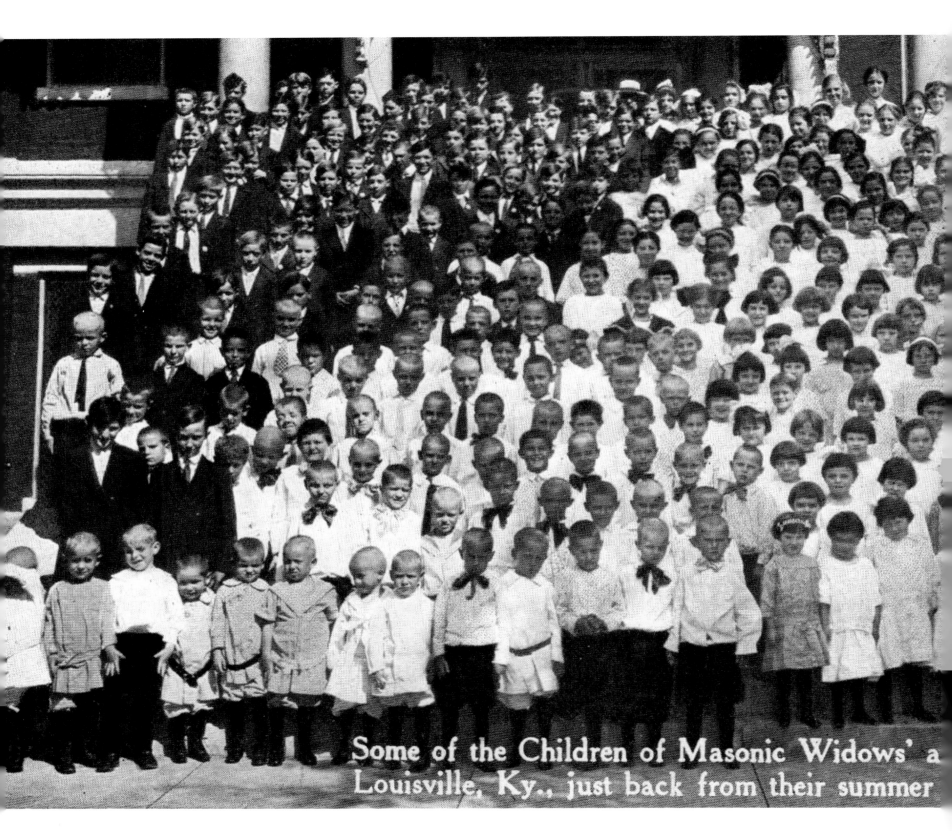

Some of the Children of Masonic Widows' a
Louisville, Ky., just back from their summer

After the Civil War, Freemasons and other fraternal orders established orphanages and homes for children with disabilities.

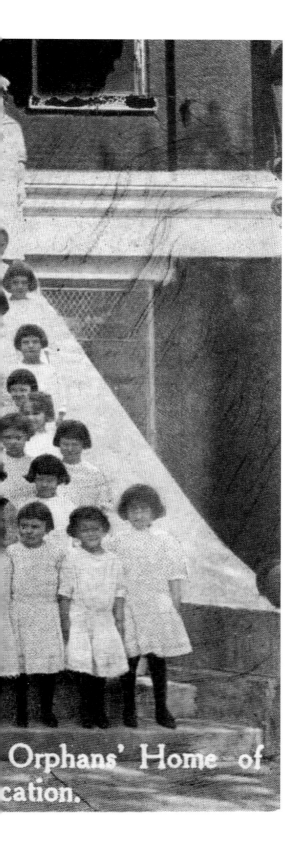

Orphans' Home of
cation.

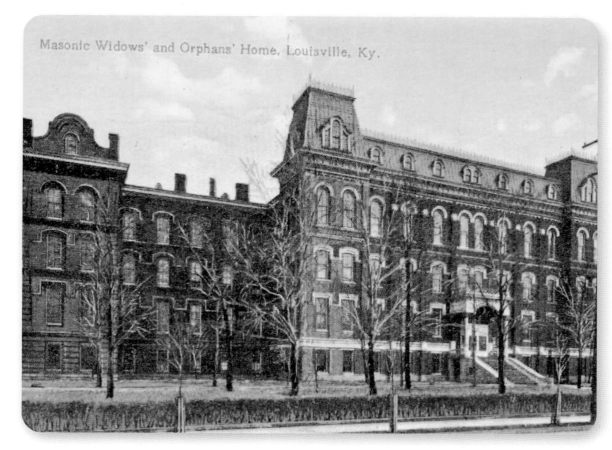

The Masonic Widows and Orphans Home in Louisville, Kentucky,
was the first fraternal institution devoted to social welfare.

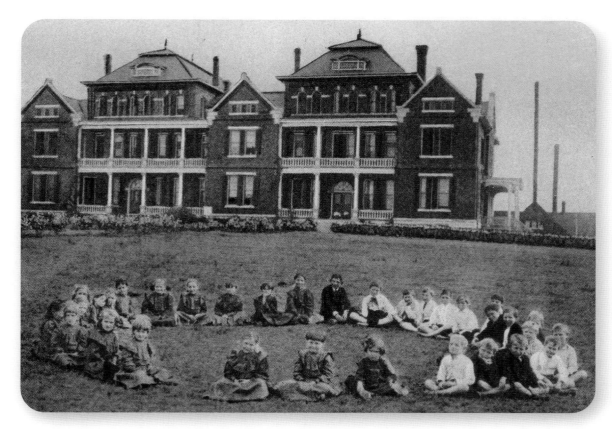

Children on the lawn of the Masonic Home for Widows and Orphans,
Fort Worth, Texas, circa. 1910.

A HEALTH CRISIS

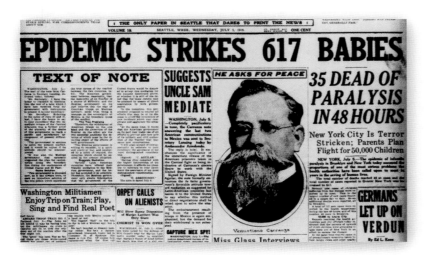

A polio outbreak in Brooklyn on June 17, 1916 spread quickly, terrifying the nation.

POLIO SEEMED TO COME OUT OF nowhere. A highly contagious virus, the disease had catastrophic effects. Some adults suffered from the paralytic effects of polio — President Franklin D. Roosevelt, afflicted at age 39, is the most famous example. But the virus targeted young children most devastatingly, seizing toddlers just as they were learning to walk. In 1916, an epidemic broke out with a vengeance. Between June and October, 6,000 people died from polio and 27,000 were paralyzed, 80% of whom were under the age of 5. For 40 years, the disease would rage across North America, crippling hundreds of thousands of children. Recovery from polio was at best a slow and painful process, but for many children the devastations of the disease left them without the prospect of ever being able to walk again. The Shriners moved to give them hope.

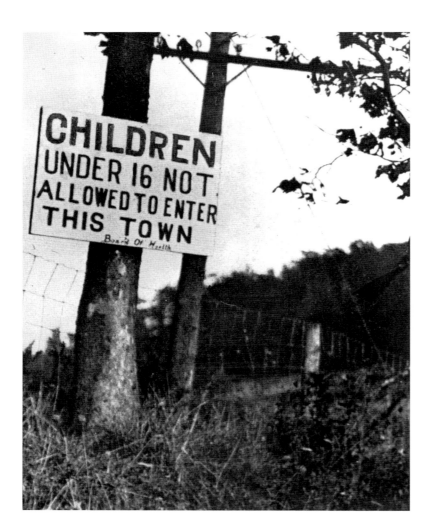

Uncertain how to cope with the new disease, communities resorted to desperate measures.

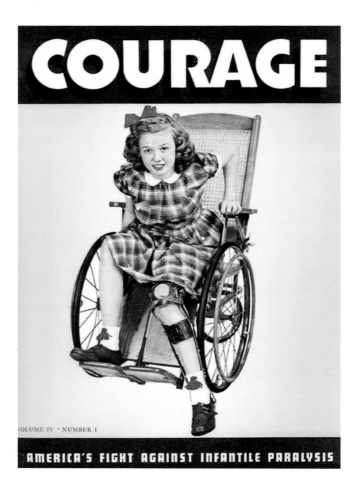

Cover of a 1943 publication of the National Foundation for Infantile Paralysis, founded by President Franklin Delano Roosevelt in 1938.

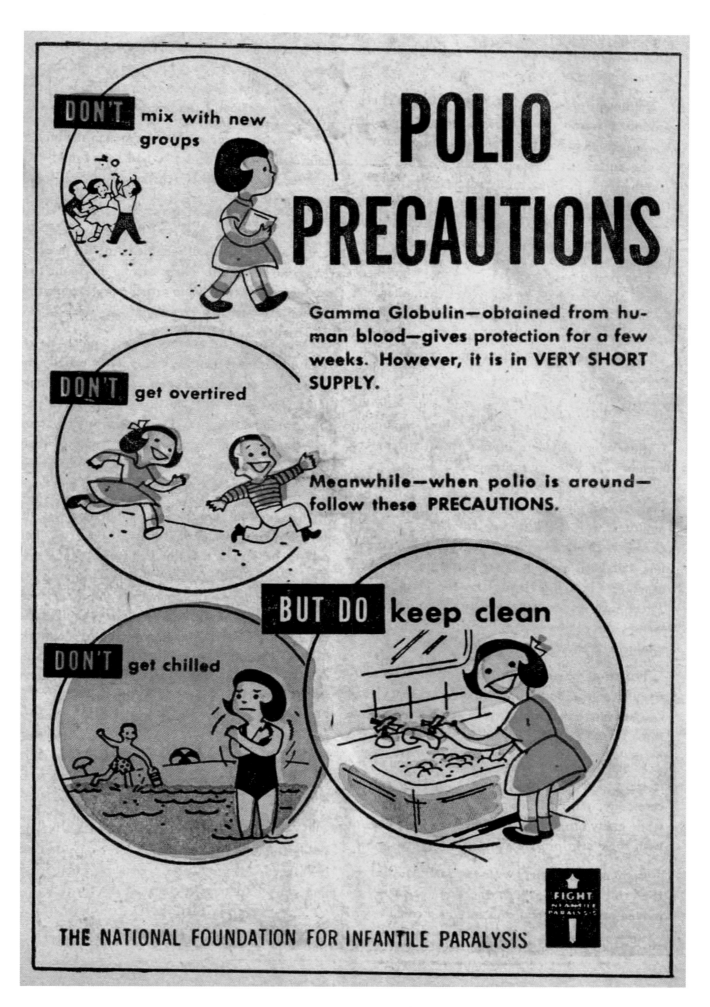

This 1953 ad urged elementary precautions, but the incidence of polio kept rising throughout the 1940s and early 1950s. The National Foundation for Infantile Paralysis would later reorganize as the March of Dimes.

MICHAEL HOKE FOUNDS A CLINIC

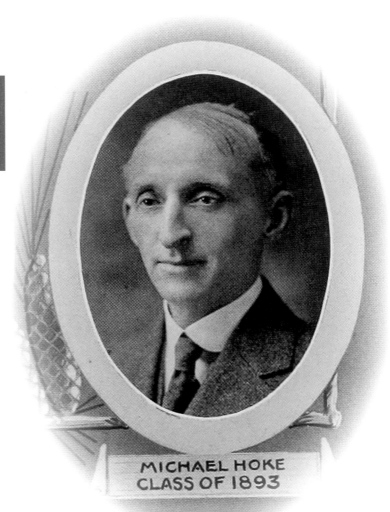

MICHAEL HOKE
CLASS OF 1893

Michael Hoke in 1922.

ORTHOPEDIC SURGERY WAS IN ITS infancy when Dr. Michael Hoke (1874–1944) decided to focus his efforts on the needs of children. A former football star at the University of North Carolina, Hoke opened one of the first orthopedic clinics in the country in Atlanta, Georgia, offering free services to children in need. Offering to donate his skills for free, he agitated for a charitable hospital for children with orthopedic conditions. "I can only give them my technical skill," he said. "I haven't the means to supply beds and nursing for the weeks and weeks it takes to straighten twisted limbs and spines."

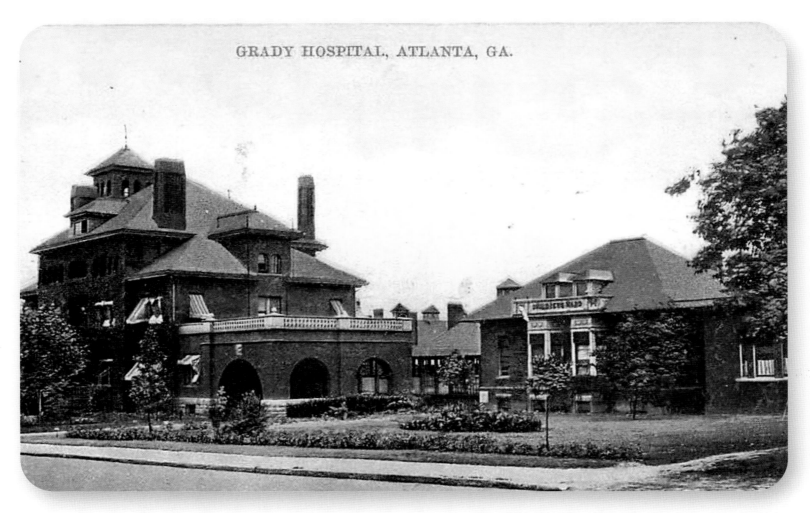

GRADY HOSPITAL, ATLANTA, GA.

The Children's Ward at Grady Hospital, where Dr. Hoke established a free clinic for crippled children around 1912.

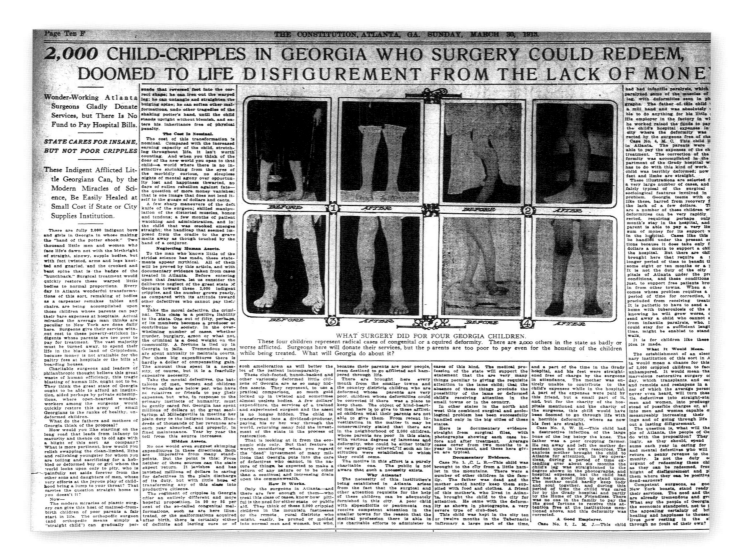

Above: Hoke published the cures that he accomplished through surgery.

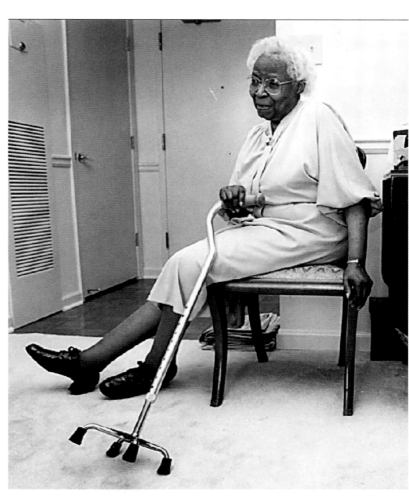

Right: Nell Henry, treated in 1906, was one of Dr. Hoke's first patients. She lived to 101.

21

FORREST ADAIR BUILDS A HOSPITAL

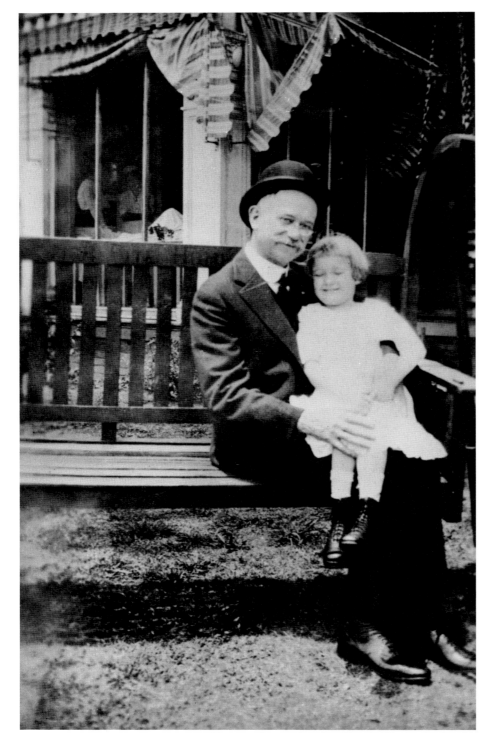

Forrest Adair with a patient at the hospital he established in Atlanta, Georgia.

DR. HOKE'S STORY touched Forrest Adair (1864–1936), head of the real estate firm that had rebuilt the city from scratch after the Civil War. A prominent Freemason, Adair secured the funding to establish the Scottish Rite Home for Crippled Children in 1915, with Dr. Hoke as its chief surgeon. Adair was also an active Shriner. In 1917, he hosted a visit to Atlanta from a fraternal delegation. All were impressed with his children's hospital, but none more than W. Freeland Kendrick.

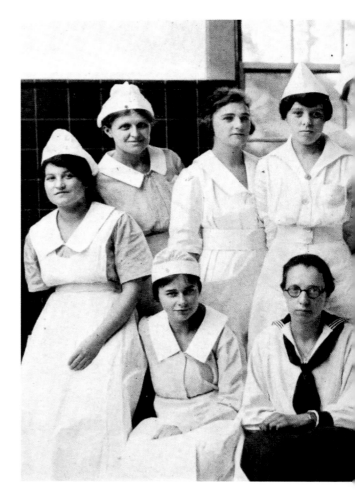

Nurses from the Scottish Rite Hospital for Crippled Children, Atlanta, Georgia, 1920.

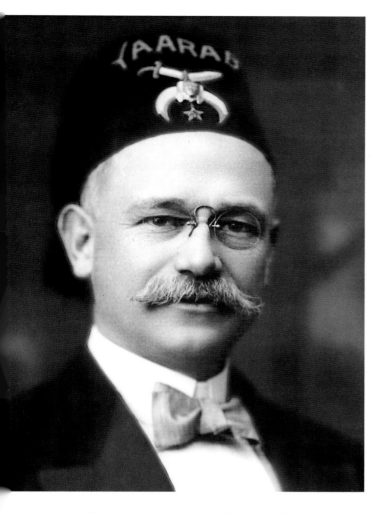

Forrest Adair was a leader in the Shriners fraternity both locally and nationally.

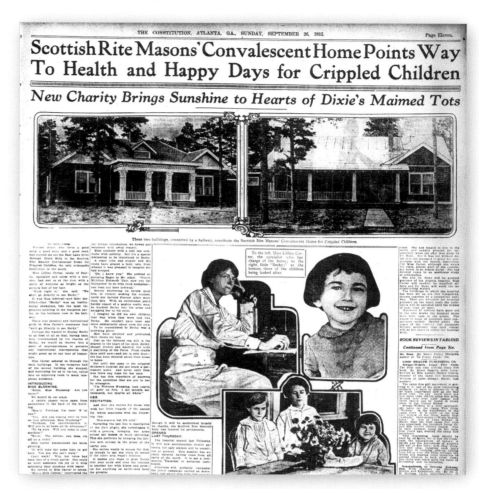

With Dr. Hoke serving as Chief Surgeon, the Scottish Rite Hospital was widely recognized as a model for pediatric care.

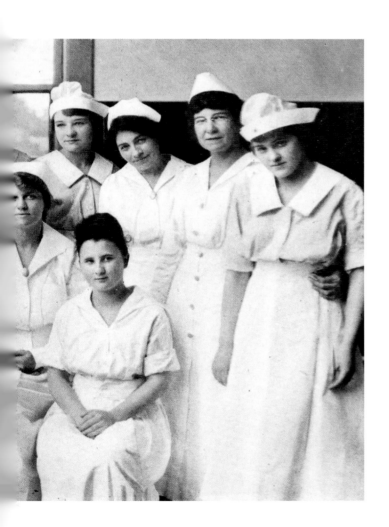

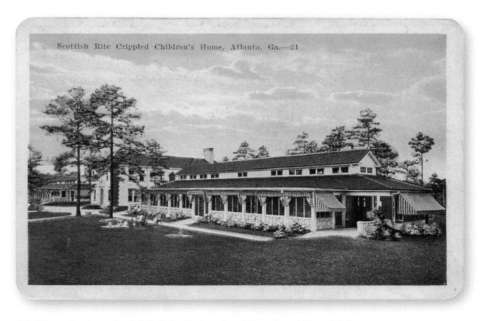

Visiting the hospital Adair built inspired Freeland Kendrick to propose a new mission for the Shriners.

FREELAND KENDRICK
ESTABLISHES AN INSTITUTION

A CONSUMMATE POLITICIAN, W. Freeland Kendrick (1876–1953) would serve as mayor of Philadelphia in the mid-1920s. Kendrick's greatest achievement, however, was helping to found the Shriners' nationwide network of "little miracle shops." During the annual convention in July 1919, Kendrick was elected leader for the coming year. At the end of the convention, he announced that building a hospital for children was his top priority. By the time the Shriners met for their annual convention in 1920, Freeland Kendrick had visited more than half of the 147 local chapters of the fraternity to lobby the nobility to support his vision.

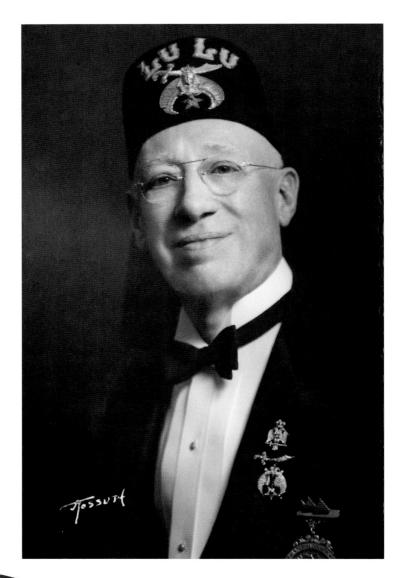

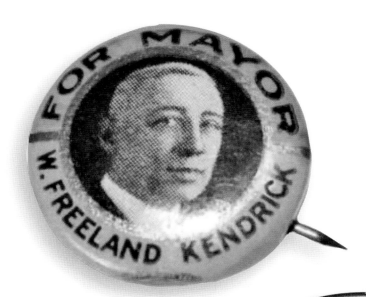

W. Freeland Kendrick, one of the most widely beloved Shriners of his day, served as Imperial Potentate from 1919 to 1920 and Mayor of Philadelphia from 1924 to 1928.

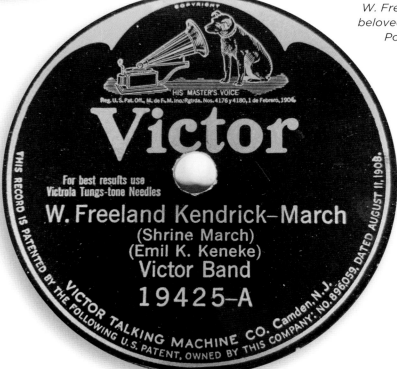

The W. Freeland Kendrick March was written for his inauguration in 1924.

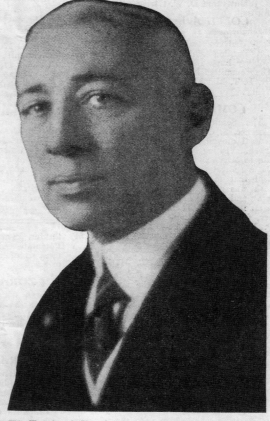
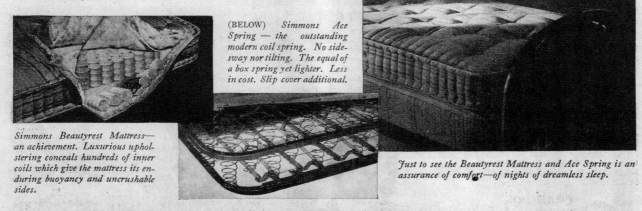
Kendrick's fame grew even further after he established Shriners Children's.
In 1928, a mattress company turned to him to secure a celebrity endorsement.

THE BUBBLES SPEECH

AT THE 1920 ANNUAL SESSION, Freeland Kendrick set forth his formal proposal for a hospital to be funded by a one-time assessment of $2 from each member. One of the most venerable members of the order rose up in opposition to the hasty ratification of an "enormous undertaking." The matter may have been dropped had Forrest Adair not risen to speak. "Let us stop building these temples of stone and marble, and polish up some of our unfortunate human beings," he thundered. It was time for the Shriners to concentrate their energy and wealth toward the cause of humanity. Adair's address would move the Shiners fraternal council to pass the proposal unanimously:

> "
>
> I was lying in bed yesterday morning about four o'clock … and some poor fellow who had strayed away from the rest of the band stood down there under the window for 25 minutes playing "I'm Forever Blowing Bubbles." . . . and I wondered if there were not a deep significance in the tune that he was playing for the Shriners – "I'm Forever Blowing Bubbles.". . . That fellow told us what we are doing. . . . I want to see this thing started. For God's sake, let us lay aside the soap and water and stop blowing bubbles and get down to brass tacks. . . . And if there is a Shriner in North America [who], after he sees your first crippled child has been treated … objects to having paid the two dollars, I will give him a check for it myself.
>
> "

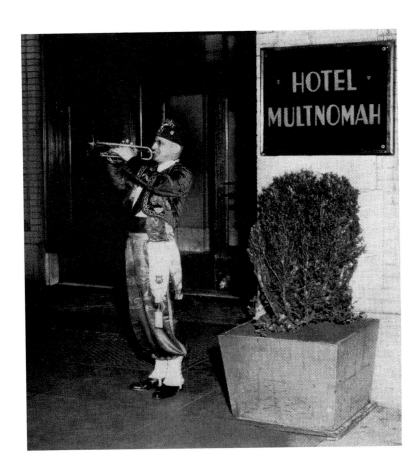

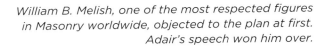

A member of Al Kader Shriners plays the song.

William B. Melish, one of the most respected figures in Masonry worldwide, objected to the plan at first. Adair's speech won him over.

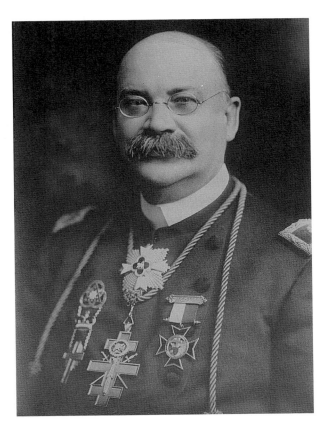

Released in late 1919, the song that Forrest Adair referenced in the Bubbles Speech quickly rose to the top of the charts.

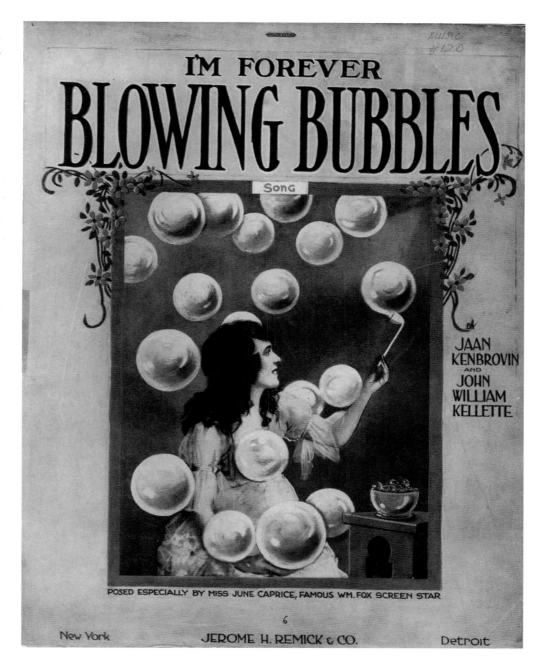

The Bubble Speech was recognized immediately as a canonical moment. It was first reported in the August 1920 issue of The Crescent.

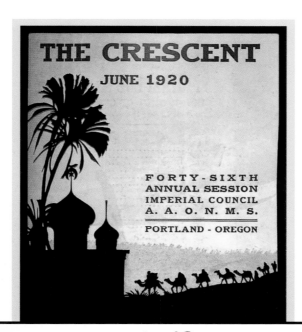

Noble Forest Adair, Yaarab, Atlanta, preached a most appealing sermon on "Blowing Bubbles," when the Crippled Children's Home matter was under discussion.

27

FROM A HOSPITAL TO A NETWORK

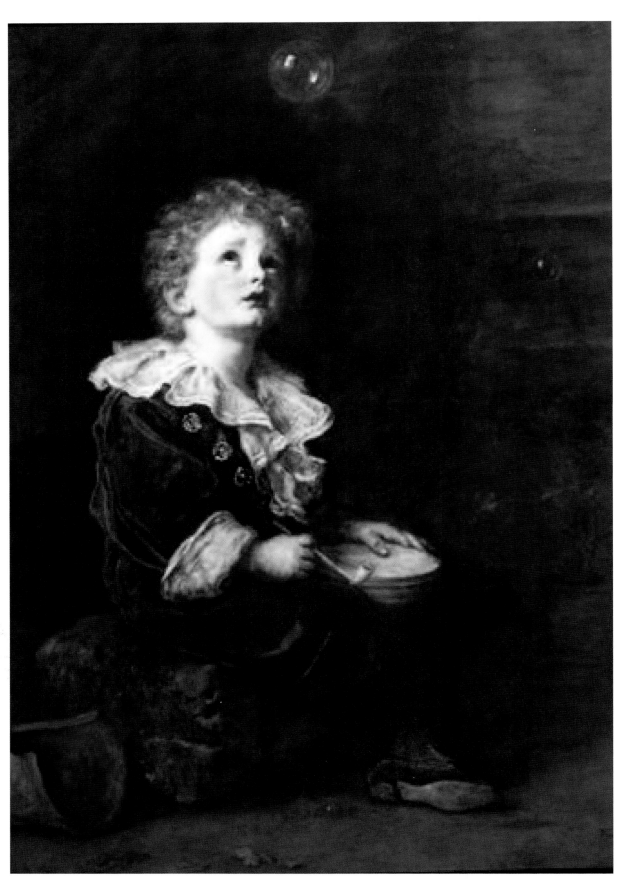

Originally titled A Child's World, *this 1886 painting by John Everett Millais is better known as "Bubbles." Copies of the painting once hung at virtually every Shriners Children's hospital.*

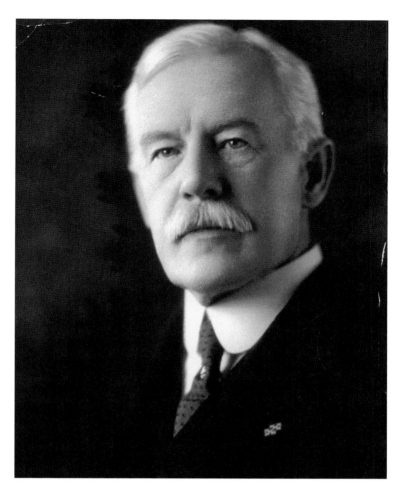

Sam P. Cochran of Hella Temple in Dallas helmed the committee to organize Shriners Children's. He would serve as the Chairman of the hospital's Board of Trustees until his death in 1934.

O N JUNE 24, 1920, THE DAY AFTER the Bubbles Speech, the mayor of Portland, Oregon, presented Freeland Kendrick with a check to inaugurate the hospital fund. Later that morning, the fraternity council appropriated an additional $100,000 ($1.4 million in 2022 dollars) for the work. It was Kendrick's 46th birthday, and he celebrated with the satisfaction that he and his brothers had begun what he anticipated would be "the most worthy, the most respected, and the biggest charity the world has ever known."

But what precisely would that charity look like? Kendrick's initial proposal called for a single Shriners Hospital to be funded by a one-time assessment of the members of the order. The board appointed at the convention decided to go even further. The Shriners should build not one hospital, but a nationwide network of hospitals and support them through annual contributions from the membership. "The cost to each Noble of our Order will be trifling in comparison with the good to be accomplished," wrote one member of the board, "and less than the average Shriner would spend in a day for cigars or other personal enjoyment." The recommendation of the board was accepted, and Shriners Children's was born.

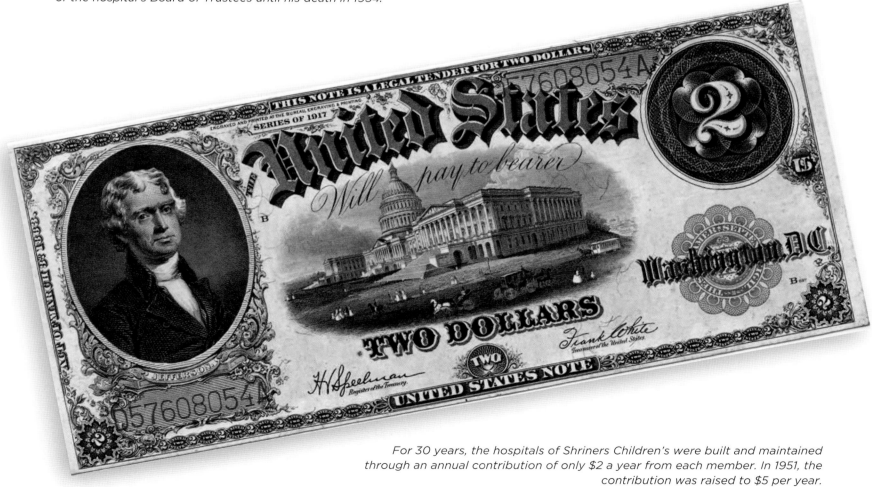

For 30 years, the hospitals of Shriners Children's were built and maintained through an annual contribution of only $2 a year from each member. In 1951, the contribution was raised to $5 per year.

THE FOUNDERS

In January 1923, the founders of Shriners Children's met in Dallas, Texas.

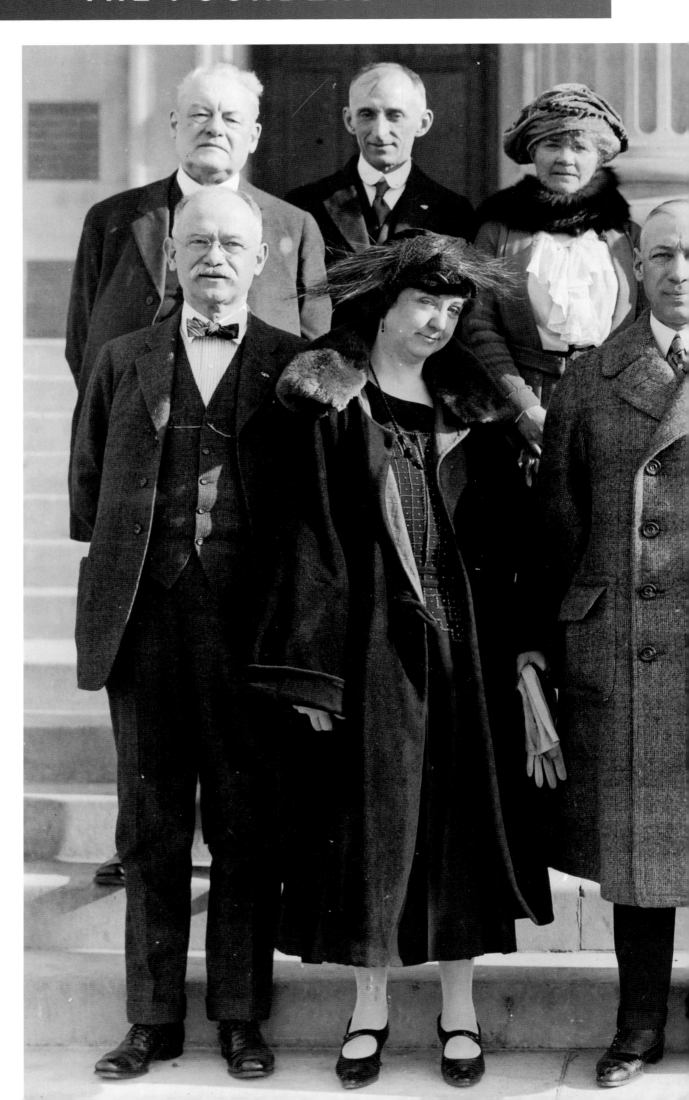

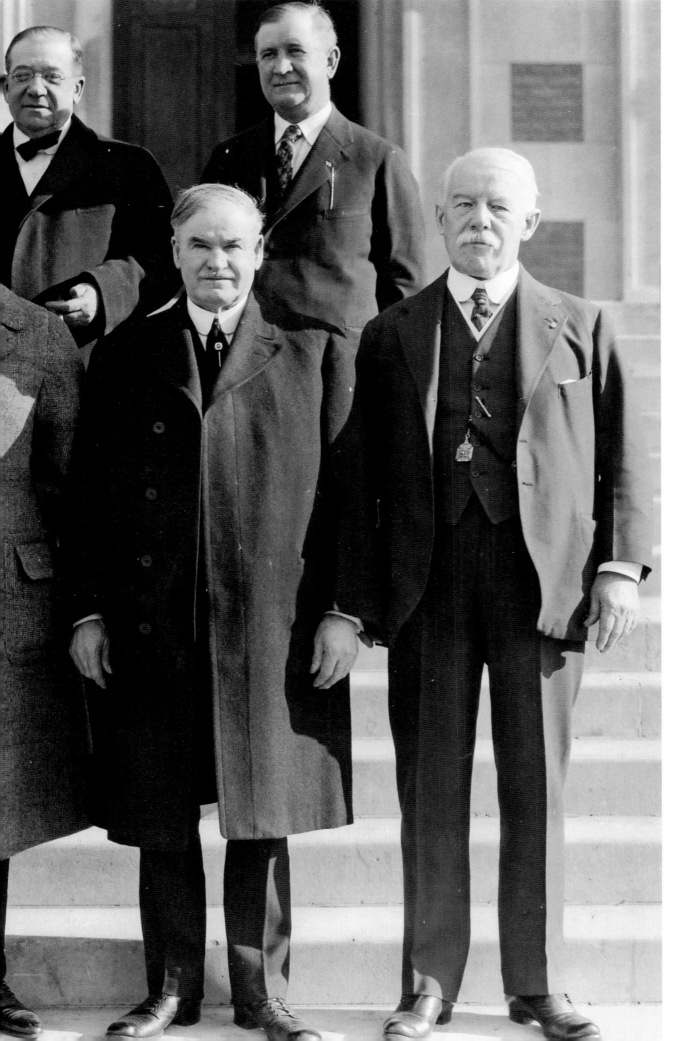

From left to right,
front row:
Forrest Adair,
Mabel B. Kendrick,
W. Freeland Kendrick,
James S. McCandless,
Sam P. Cochran.

Back row:
Bishop Frederick W.
Keator,
Dr. Michael Hoke,
Florence J. Potts,
Dr. Oscar M. Lanstrum,
John D. McGilvray.

Missing is
Philip D. Gordon,
who passed away
during the meeting.

THE NOBILITY STEPS UP

NOT EVERY SHRINER LOVED THE IDEA of sponsoring a new hospital system. Some were cautious about rushing into such an enormous project. Others resented even the nominal tax of two dollars a year, just on principle. But remarkably, the vast majority of the Ancient Arabic Order of the Nobles of the Mystic Shrine — whose membership numbered over half a million by 1923 — committed themselves wholeheartedly. Even before the first hospital had opened, Nobles swelled with pride at the good they were doing. For 50 years, the Shriners had the reputation

of being "the playground of Masonry." Now, its members had found a cause. Over the years to come, the Shriners would become increasingly identified with their mission. What had started as a side project would take root at the very core of the fraternity. Shriners would never lose their sense of humor, but now, the fun and fellowship were channeled to a higher purpose. Henceforth, they would devote everything to care for the most vulnerable people in the world: children in need of specialized medical care. Together, they would build what has been widely acknowledged as the world's greatest philanthropy..

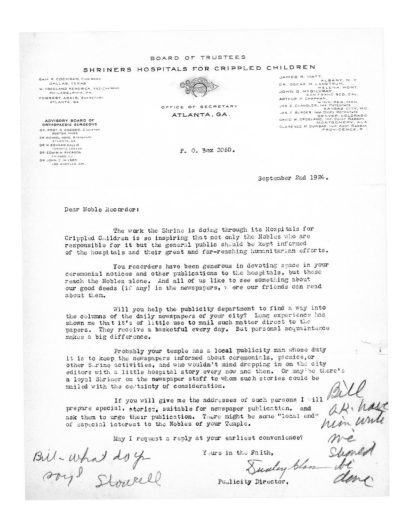

This circular letter from the Board of Trustees urges members of the fraternity to spread news of the new Shriners Children's hospitals.

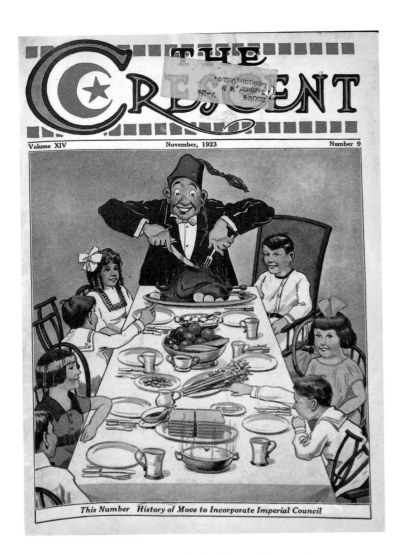

The November 1923 cover of the Shriners' magazine, featuring young Thanksgiving guests with crutches and wheelchairs, celebrated both the spirit of jollity and the ethos of giving.

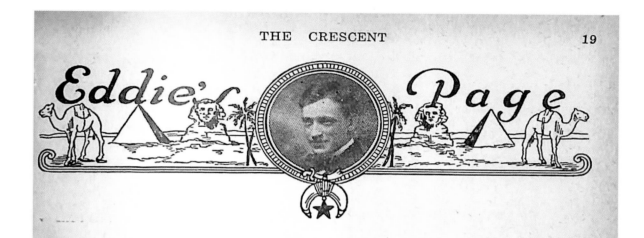

THE CRESCENT 19

Eddie's Page

A Shriner's Real Work

By NOBLE EDGAR A. GUEST

Written for the Crescent

———

Oh it's fun to be a Shriner,
   And it's good to laugh and sing,
And nothing can be finer
   Than a Shriner's caroling,
But when all the jests have faded,
   And the laughs have died away,
It is finer if a Shriner
   Can look back across the day
And discover that another
   Sees the sun begin to shine
And knows he has a brother
   In a man that's joined the Shrine.

Oh I know a sight that's bigger
   Than a Shriner's jeweled pin;
It's a crippled little figure
   Who has found the way to grin.
It's a little back made stronger
   Than it ever was before,
And a lighter heart and brighter
   Face a-gleaming at the door.
It's a spine that once was twisted
   Being made a real spine,
And the surgeons there assisted
   By the members of the Shrine!

Oh I'm strong for Mecca's laughter
   And I'm keen for Mecca's fun,
But some real work must come after
   All the jesting has been done;
And I wouldn't give a nickel
   For a chap's perpetual smile,
If his money wasn't sunny
   And as cheerful as his style.
If to him the helpless pleaded
   Without any answering sign,
If he failed where he was needed,
   I should say he'd failed the Shrine.

We are all down here to labor
   To make earth a better place,
To be more and more the neighbor
   As we share life's common race;
And our laughter shall be sweeter
   And our fun more worth our while
By the ripples of the cripples
   We are helping now to smile.
Let me say it loud and louder;
   By each strengthened hip and spine
I am just a little prouder
   Of my fez and of my Shrine.
        —Edgar A. Guest.

Once the most popular poet in America, Edgar A. Guest was also a Shriner.
His poem expresses the deep pride the nobility took in their new mission.

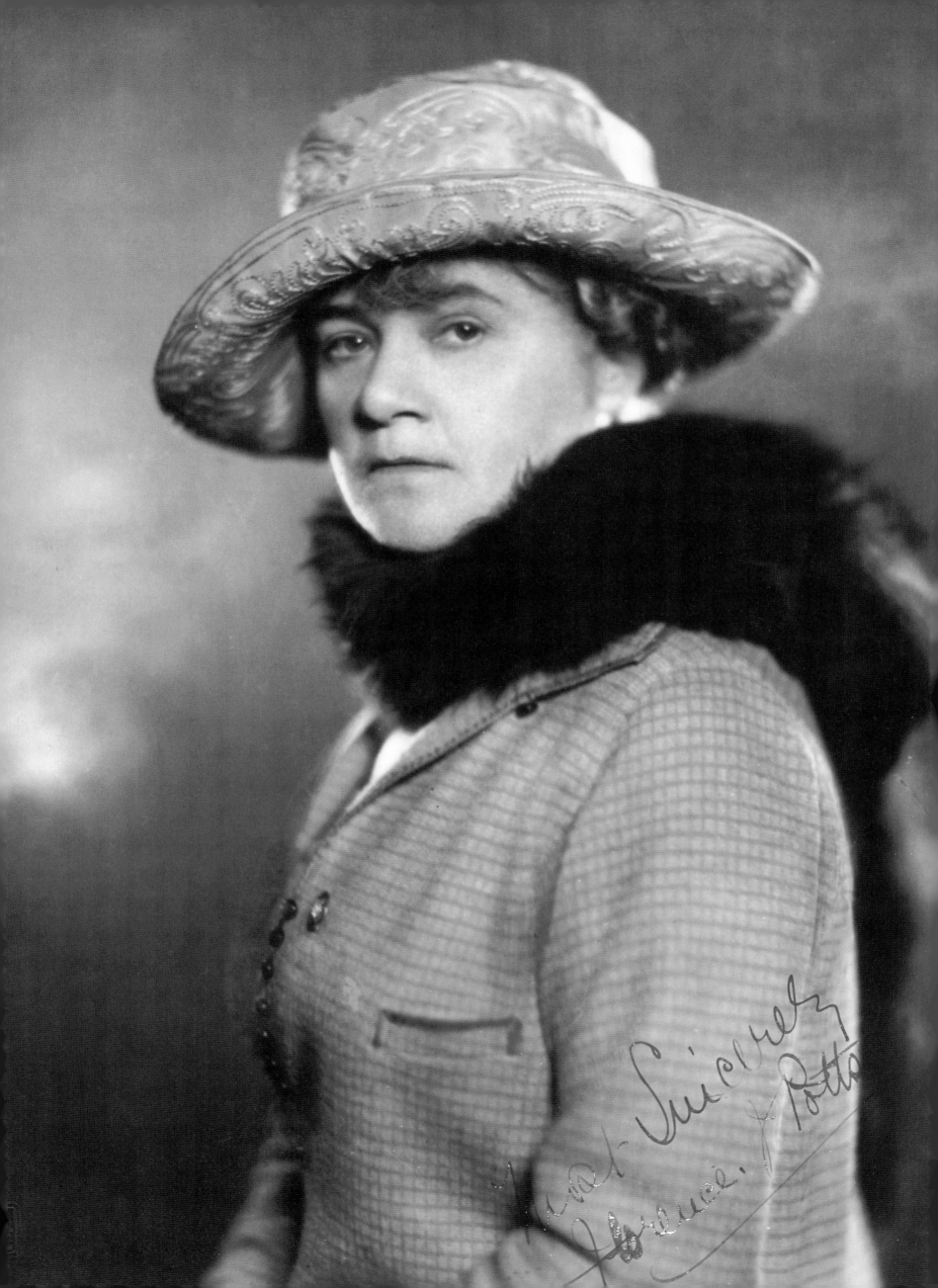

Most Sincerely
Florence Potter

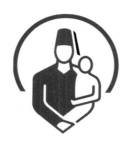

BRICKS AND MORTAR: THE SHRINERS HOSPITALS

ONCE THE NOBLES HAD decided upon a course of action, they moved with extraordinary speed. Within two years of the decision to establish a network of hospitals, the first Shriners Hospital opened in Shreveport, Louisiana. By the end of 1924, there were seven hospitals, and by the end of 1927, there were 15. The Shriners Children's healthcare system would continue to grow over the course of the century, but nothing matched the pace of the first years.

The extraordinary dedication of the board of directors had much to do with it. By 1922, they had amassed a hospital fund of almost $875,000 — over $15 million in today's money. This would grow swiftly over the coming decades. The board enlisted an advisory committee of leading orthopedists to identify chief surgeons for each location. Perhaps their most brilliant move, however, was to hire Florence Potts (1871–1941). Potts had risen through the nursing ranks of the Toronto Hospital for Sick Children when she was called to serve as director of nursing at Shriners Children's. From 1922 until her retirement, she supervised operations with a holistic vision, ensuring that patients across the network had not only the medical care they needed, but also a warm bed, healthy meals and access to education.

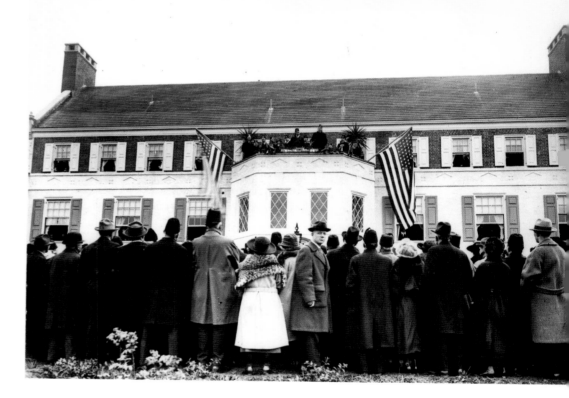

Members of Al Kader Temple and other supporters attend the dedication of Shriners Children's Portland, January 15, 1924. Standing at the center of the balcony behind a scale model of the facility is George Luis Baker. In addition to acting as the hospital's first chairman, Baker served as mayor of Portland from 1917 to 1933. The tall figure to his side is Frederick W. Keator, bishop of the Episcopal Diocese of Olympia and a charter member of Shriners Children's Board of Trustees.

Facing page:
As the first Director of Nursing at Shriners Children's, Florence Potts supervised operations at each of the first 15 hospitals until her retirement in 1934.

SHREVEPORT, LOUISIANA
SEPTEMBER 16, 1922

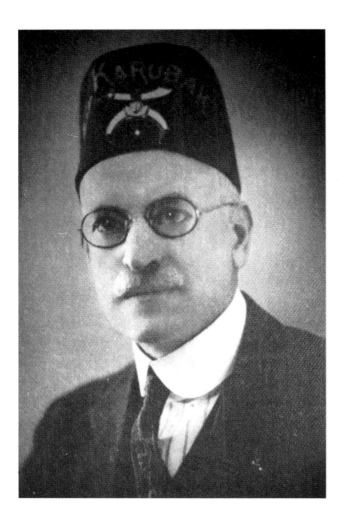

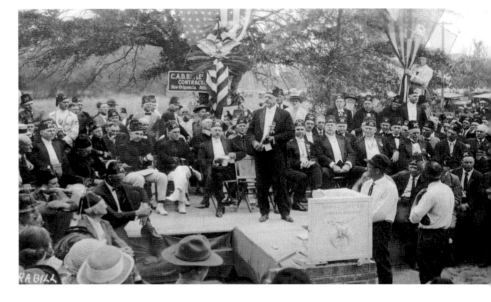

Laying the cornerstone for the first Shriners hospital, May 12, 1922.

The Shriners hospital in Shreveport was the first to open due to the extraordinary vision and dedication of J. H. Rowland and the Nobles of the El Karubah Shriners, who took about 18 months to raise funds to buy a plot and build a hospital that cost $300,000 (about $5 million today).

One of the first patients was Aileen, a 7-year-old girl from Gibsland, Louisiana, afflicted with clubfoot. She was unable to walk properly until her treatment at Shriners.

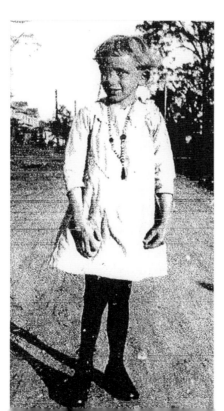

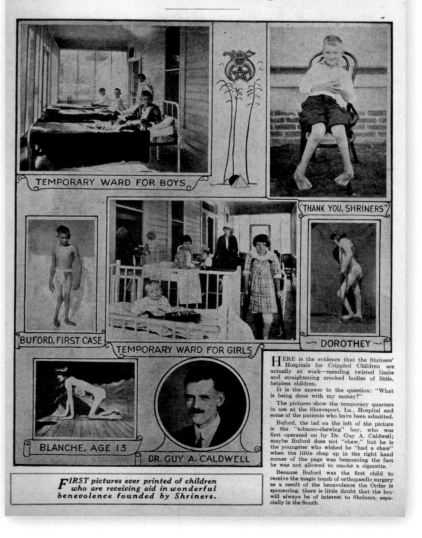

First Cases Treated by Shriners

TEMPORARY WARD FOR BOYS

"THANK YOU, SHRINERS"

BUFORD, FIRST CASE

TEMPORARY WARD FOR GIRLS

DOROTHEY

BLANCHE, AGE 13

DR. GUY A. CALDWELL

HERE is the evidence that the Shriners' Hospitals for Crippled Children are actually at work—mending twisted limbs and straightening crooked bodies of little, helpless children.

It is the answer to the question: "What is being done with my money?"

The pictures show the temporary quarters in use at the Shreveport, La., Hospital and some of the patients who have been admitted.

Buford, the lad on the left of the picture is the "tobacco-chewing" boy, who was first operated on by Dr. Guy A. Caldwell; maybe Buford does not "chew," but he is the youngster who wished he "had a chaw" when the little chap up in the right hand corner of the page was bemoaning the fact he was not allowed to smoke a cigarette.

Because Buford was the first child to receive the magic touch of orthopaedic surgery as a result of the benevolence the Order is sponsoring, there is little doubt that the boy will always be of interest to Shriners, especially in the South.

FIRST pictures ever printed of children who are receiving aid in wonderful benevolence founded by Shriners.

The Crescent *regularly featured articles on the progress of the hospitals and their patients.*

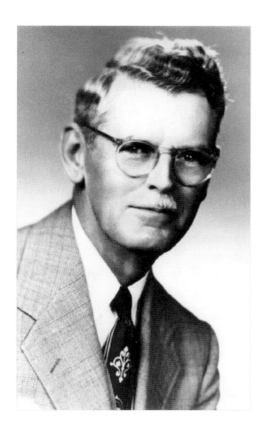

After one year and 175 operations, the hospital's first surgeon, Dr. Guy A. Caldwell, returned to private practice. He would continue to serve on the medical advisory board for the hospitals.

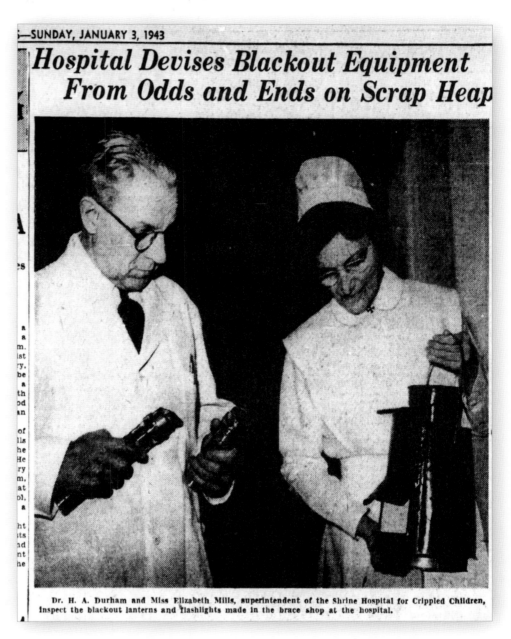

—SUNDAY, JANUARY 3, 1943

Hospital Devises Blackout Equipment From Odds and Ends on Scrap Heap

Dr. H. A. Durham and Miss Elizabeth Mills, superintendent of the Shrine Hospital for Crippled Children, inspect the blackout lanterns and flashlights made in the brace shop at the hospital.

Dr. Caldwell was replaced in 1923 by Dr. Herbert A. Durham, a veteran of World War I, who served the Shreveport hospital until his death in 1946. He appears here with Elizabeth Mills, long-time superintendent of the hospital.

A group of Shriners visit the Shreveport girls' ward in 1954.

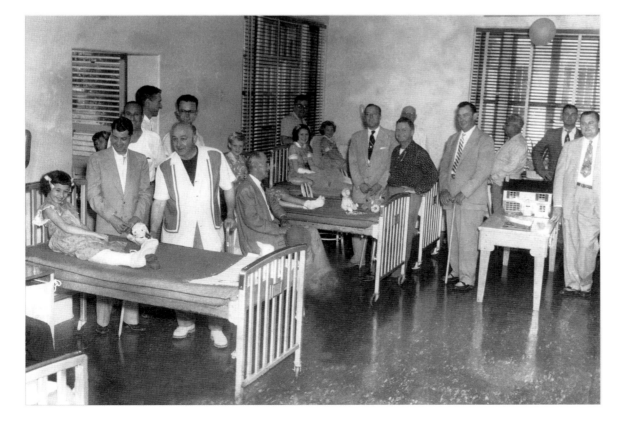

37

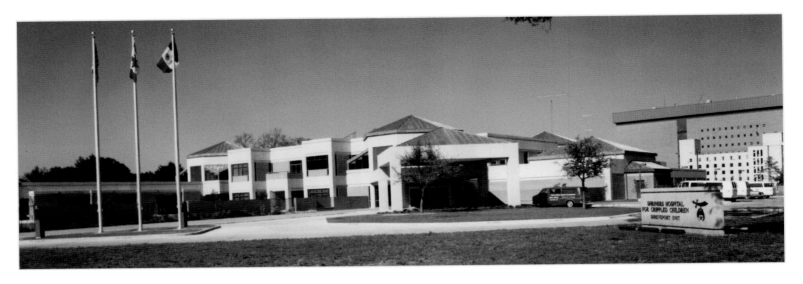

*Sixty years of Louisiana weather took its toll on the original Shreveport hospital.
In 1983, construction began on a new facility, which opened in 1986.*

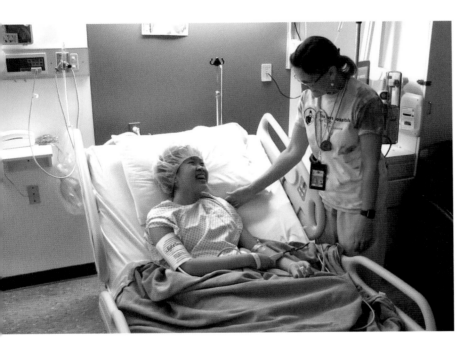

*In later years, the hospital would expand its range of services,
offering treatments for sports injuries, juvenile idiopathic
arthritis, cleft lip and palate and orthopedic injuries.*

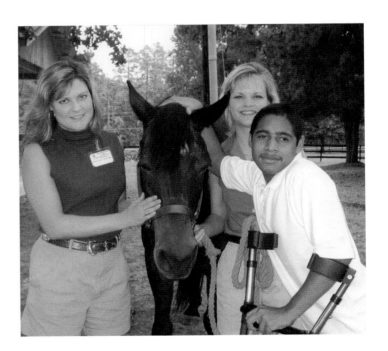

*The horses at Lickskillet Ranch near Shreveport are
specially trained to work with children with disabilities,
like 15-year-old Josue, who visited in 2001 with staff
members Kim Creghan and Ashley McMillan.*

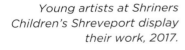

*Young artists at Shriners
Children's Shreveport display
their work, 2017.*

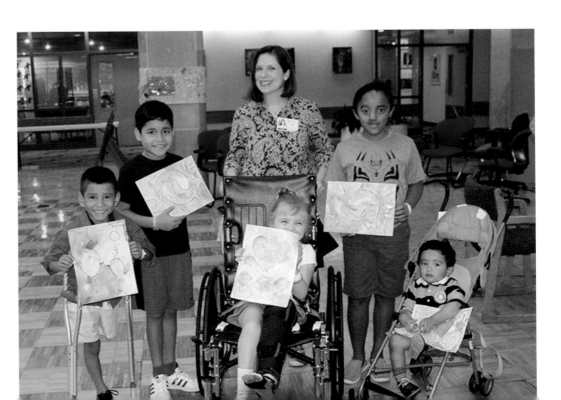

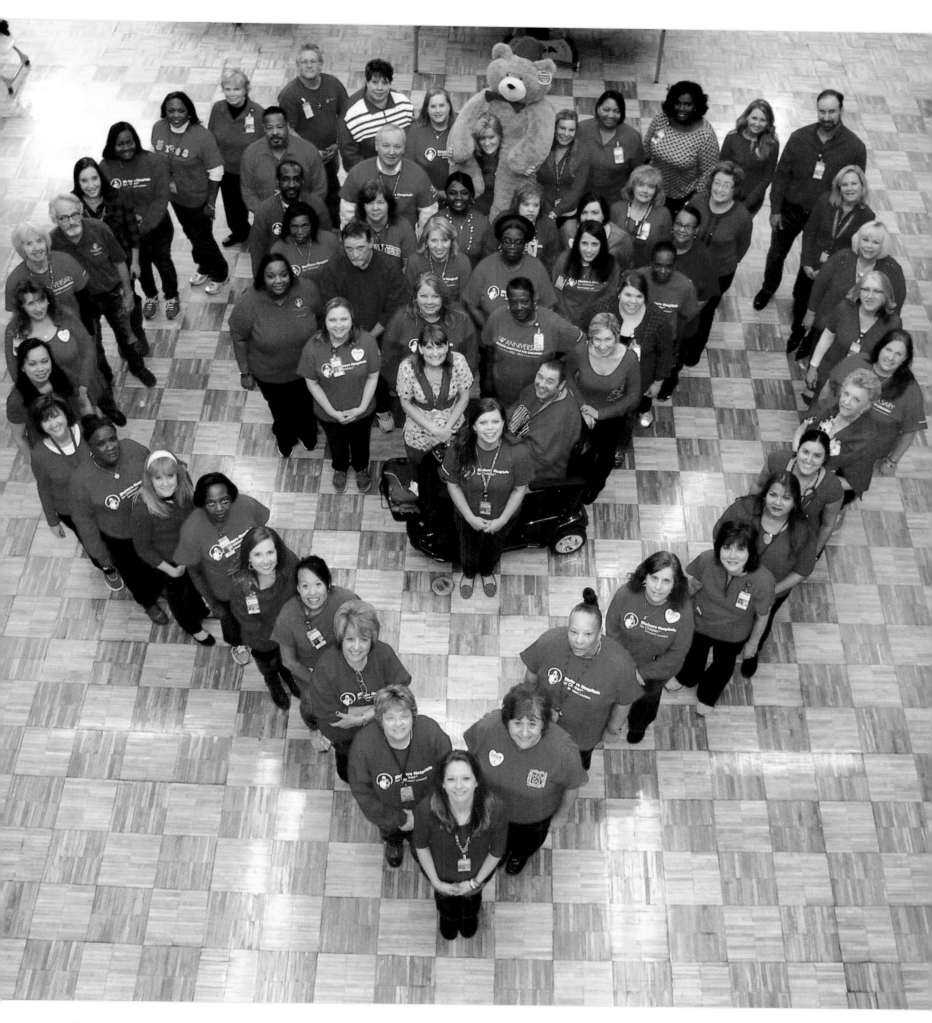

The team at Shriners Children's Shreveport, 2014.

HONOLULU, HAWAII
JANUARY 2 , 1923

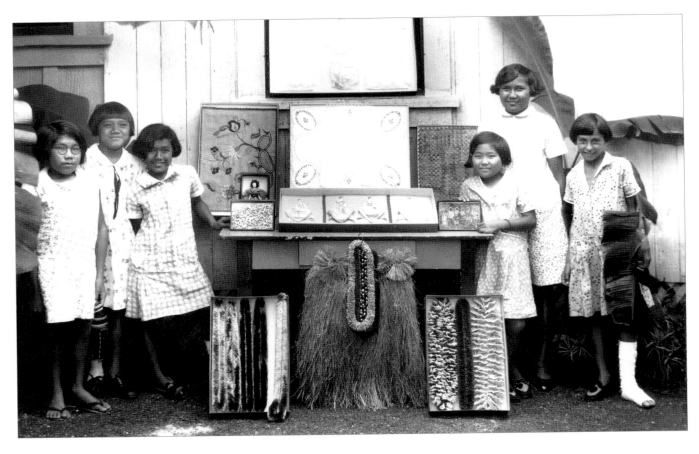

Patients at Shriners Children's Hawaii with their handicrafts, 1930s.

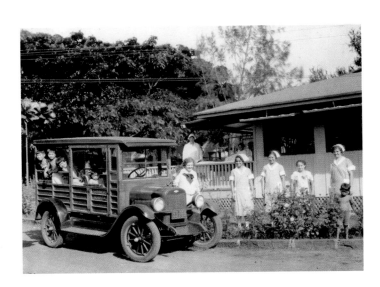

The second Shriners Hospital was conceived originally as a mobile unit, with doctors traveling to provide specialized orthopedic care for keiki (children) throughout the Hawaiian islands. The hospital's geographic service area encompasses the Pacific Basin, an area larger than the continental United States.

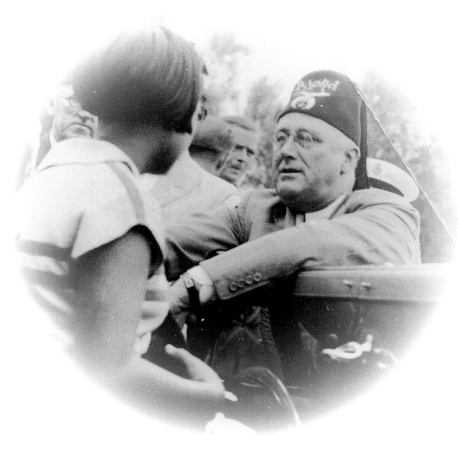

U.S. President Franklin Delano Roosevelt visited Shriners Children's in 1934 during the first trip to Hawaii ever made by a sitting president.

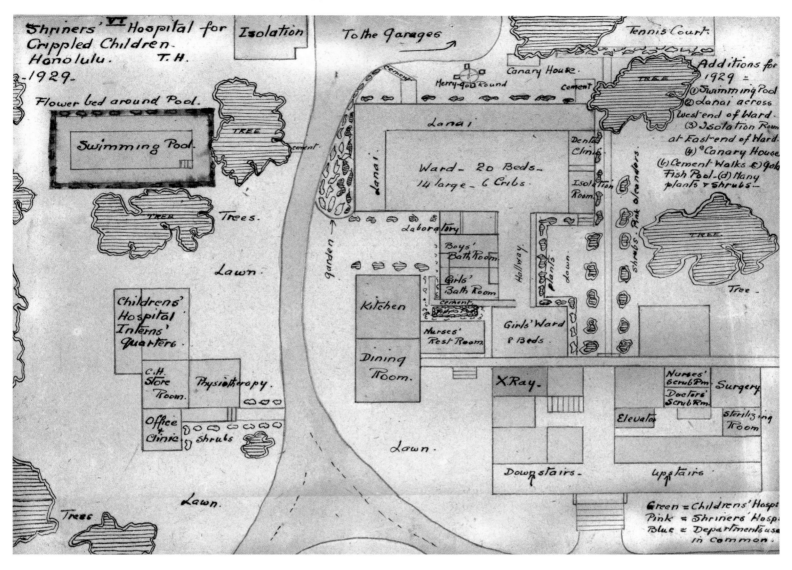

Shriners Children's Hawaii was first housed in a wing at the rear of Kauikeolani Children's Hospital on Kuakini Street in Liliha. In 1930, it moved into an independent facility on Punahou Street.

2 New Hospital Units Are Being Completed Here

Two new hospital units under the emergency medical program of the office of civilian defense are nearing completion and are prepared to go into immediate service, according to the office of civilian defense.

In addition to the units, the office of civilian defense also pointed out that it had augmented facilities of established hospitals.

One hundred beds have been added to the Shriners hospital on Punahou St., and a great deal of equipment has been stored there.

Officials pointed out that the new hospital units are for the protection of civilians on Oahu and that they are prepared to go into immediate service, although not entirely completed.

Thanks to its proximity to the Pacific Theater, the hospital became part of the emergency medical reserve during World War II. This news item is from The Honolulu Star-Bulletin, *March 16, 1942.*

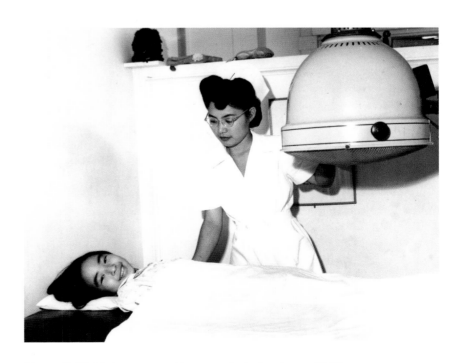

Nurse Faith Nakano operating a cast-drying lamp, 1947. Joining Shriners Children's Hawaii in 1942, she would work at the hospital for more than 65 years.

41

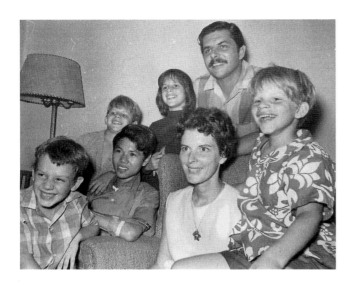

During the Vietnam War, the hospital became a primary care facility for children injured during the conflict. Tran, third from left, lost his arm to a hand grenade in Vietnam. After over a year of treatment at Shriners Children's, he was adopted by a family in Waialua.

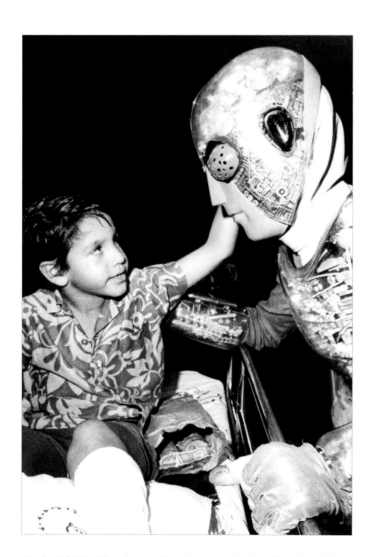

Android Kikaider, hero of a Japanese tokusatsu television program popular in Hawaii in the 1970s, visits a patient at Shriners Children's.

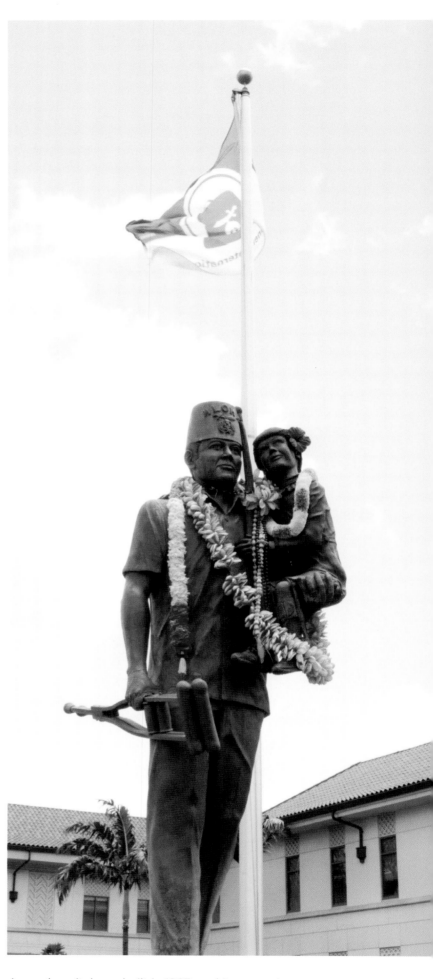

A new hospital was built in 1967, and its current state-of-the-art facility opened in 2009.

Right: Elijah, seated on the right with his family, was born with traumatic brain injury. Thanks to care at Shriners Children's, he has been able to lead a happy, healthy life.

Below: A partnership with the Adaptive Freedom Foundation allows patients at Shriners Children's Hawaii to experience the thrill of ocean paddling.

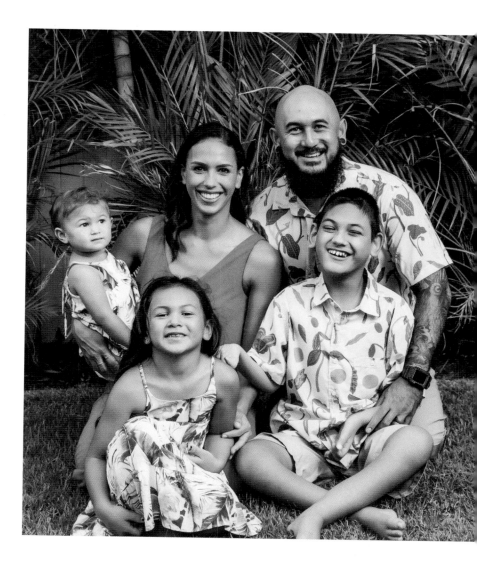

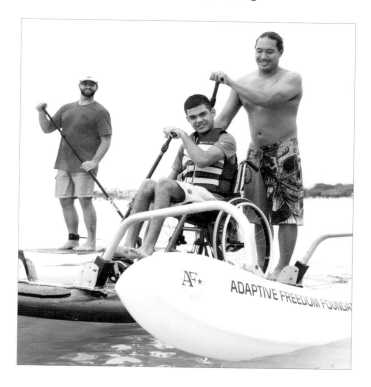

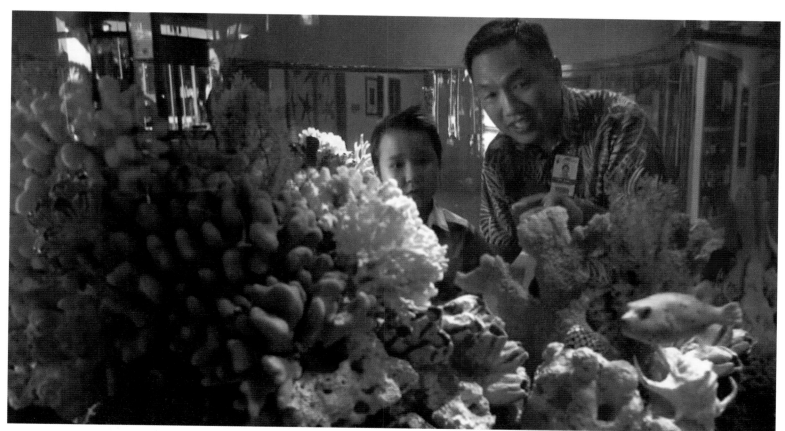

An 850-gallon C-shaped saltwater aquarium was specially designed to give an immersive experience to keiki of all abilities.

TWIN CITIES, MINNESOTA
MARCH 12, 1923

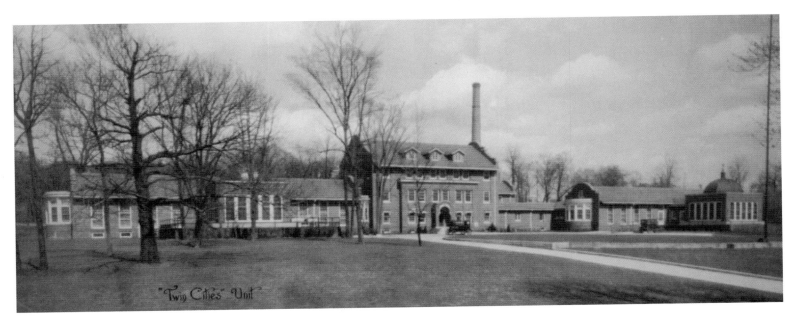

Shriners Children's Twin Cities was planned as the flagship of the hospital system.

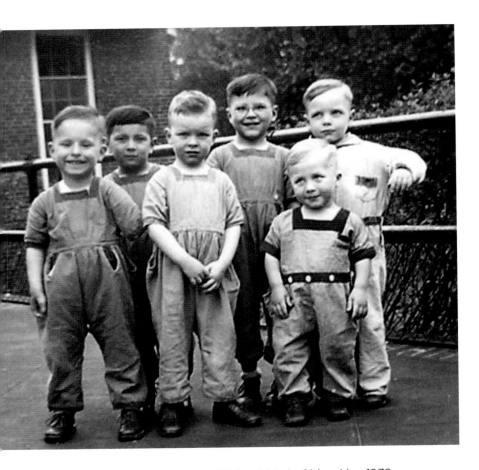

Toddlers at Shriners Children's Twin Cities, May 1939.

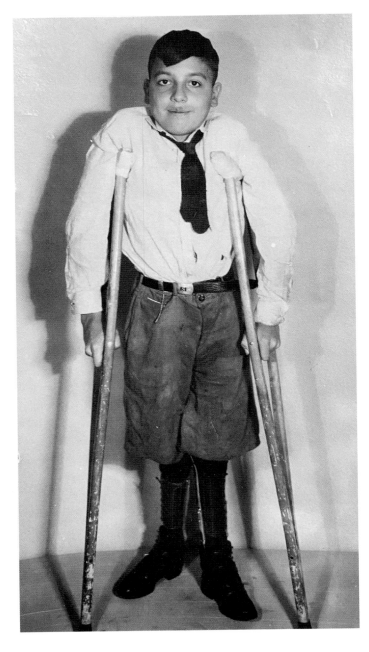

The first patient treated at Shriners Children's Twin Cities was a 13-year-old polio victim from the Blackfeet Indian Reservation in Browning, Montana. John P. Sharp would later become chief judge for the Blackfeet Nation, and the author of the tribe's new legal code.

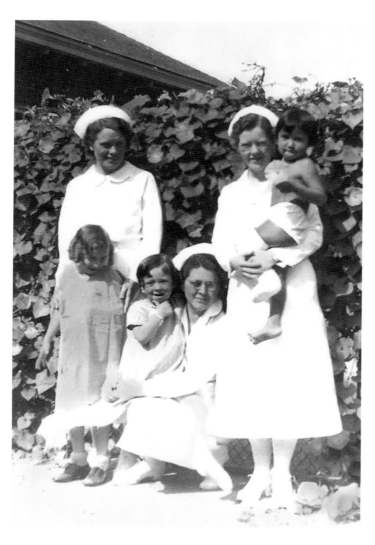

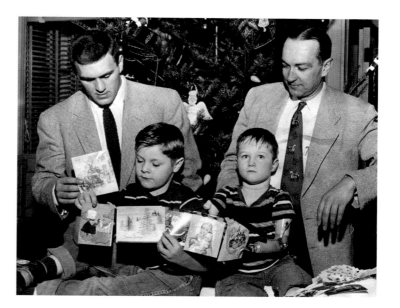

Until the late 1970s, most physicians in the Shriners Children's network worked for little or no pay, relying on private practice for their income. Dr. Donald R. Lannin, who served as chief surgeon at Twin Cities from 1952 to 1979, also worked as the team physician for the Minnesota Vikings. In this 1956 photograph he visits patients in the company of Bob Hobert, tackle for the Minnesota Golden Gophers.

Nurses at Shriners Children's Twin Cities take their patients for some fresh air, 1939.

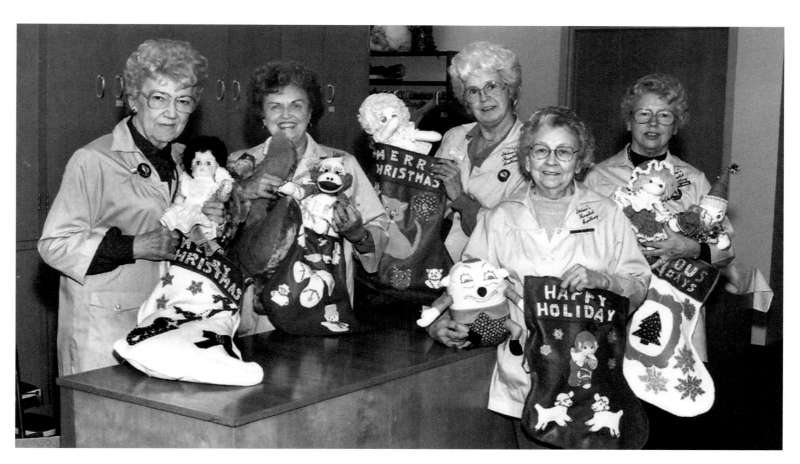

During the Great Depression, the hospital relied on volunteers from the ladies' auxiliary of Zuhrah Shriners. The tradition has endured.

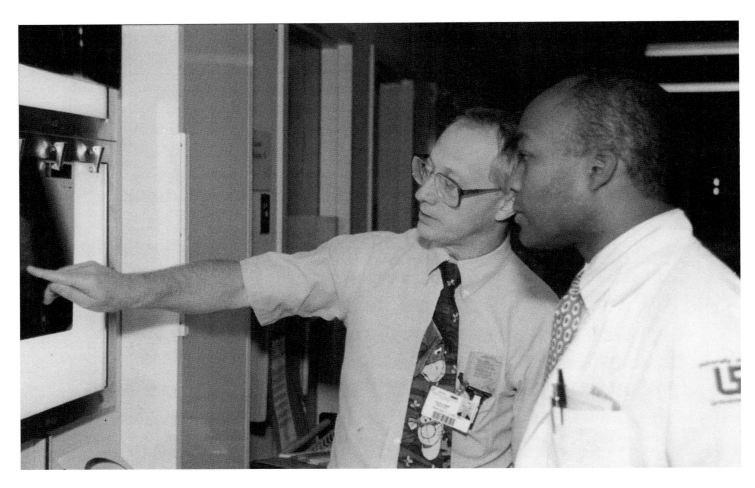

During an outpatient clinic in 1999, Chief of Staff Dr. Randall Loder reviews an X-ray with Dr. Jim Phillips, an orthopedic resident.

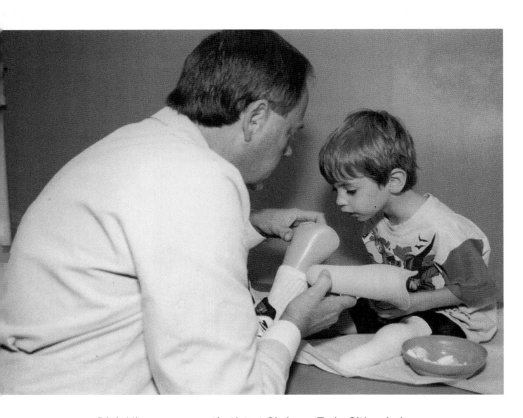

Dick Niessen, a prosthetist at Shriners Twin Cities, helps three-year-old Sam examine his new artificial limb.

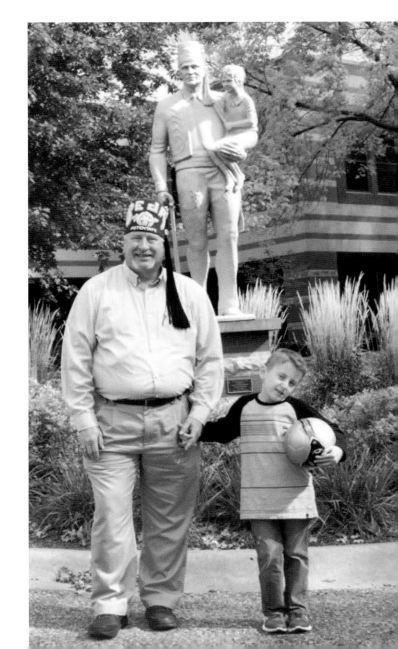

Gene Reece, Potentate of the Beja Shriners of Green Bay, Wisconsin, visits Carter at Shriners Twin Cities, 2016. Carter, who lives with brittle bone disease, raised $66,000 for the Shriners hospital building fund.

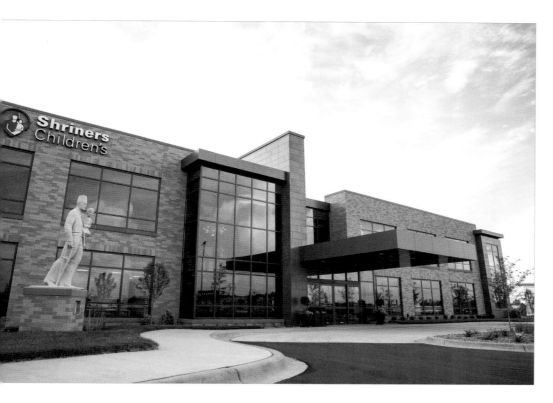

The hospital moved into a new building in 1990, and in 2020, left the downtown area for a new facility in Woodbury, Minnesota.

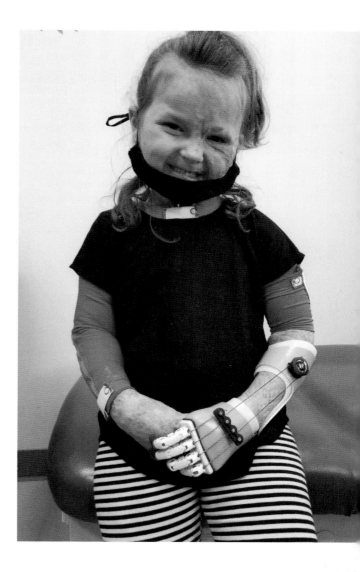

Peyton, a patient at Shriners Twin Cities, is delighted with her first prosthetic.

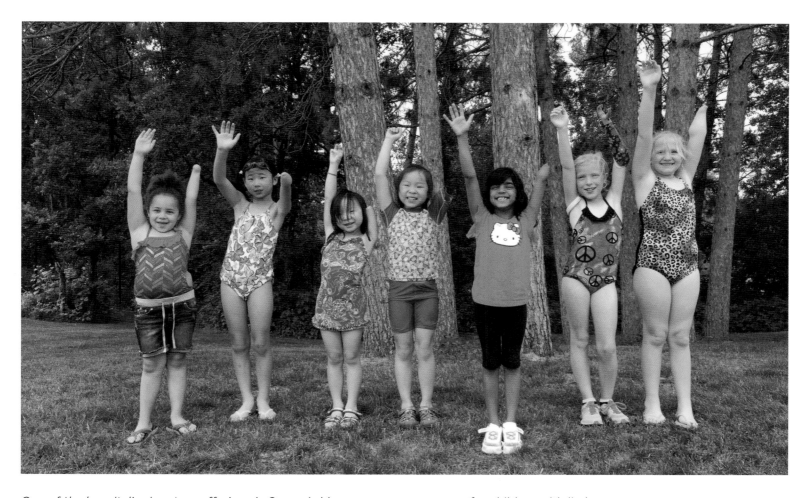

One of the hospital's signature offerings is Camp Achieve, a summer program for children with limb differences that gives kids an opportunity to be with other children who share similar conditions.

47

SACRAMENTO, CALIFORNIA
JUNE 16, 1923

The force behind the original Shriners Children's hospital in Northern California was John D. McGilvray, the principal of a stone and masonry contracting firm that had built many of the area's most impressive structures, including City Hall, the public library, and Stanford University.

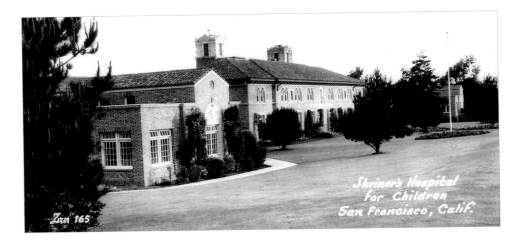

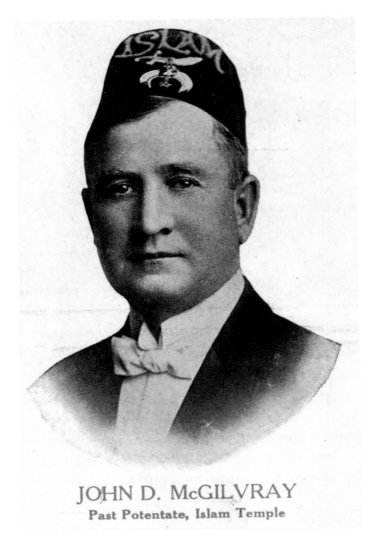

JOHN D. McGILVRAY
Past Potentate, Islam Temple

The hospital McGilvray built was architecturally splendid, in an Italian Renaissance style. Today, it is designated as a San Francisco landmark.

SHRINERS' HOSPITAL
FOR
CRIPPLED CHILDREN

Solicits submission of a site for erection of hospital buildings. Must be full size city block, within easy access to car lines. State definite price.

ISLAM TEMPLE   650 Geary St.

Gertrude R. Folendorf, who served as the hospital's first supervisor, assumed responsibility for the entire Shriners Children's network in 1936. A leading figure in nursing education, Folendorf received the profession's highest accolades before her retirement in 1955.

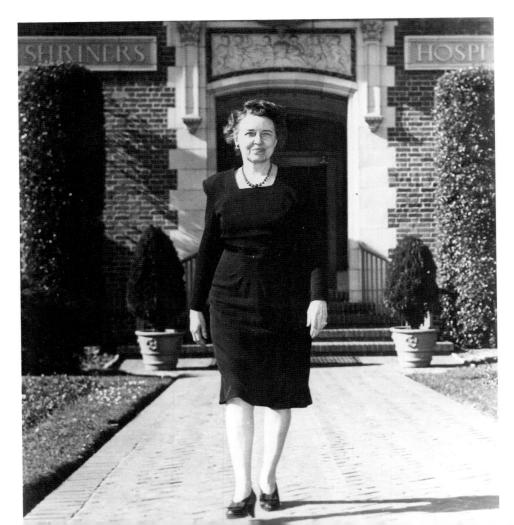

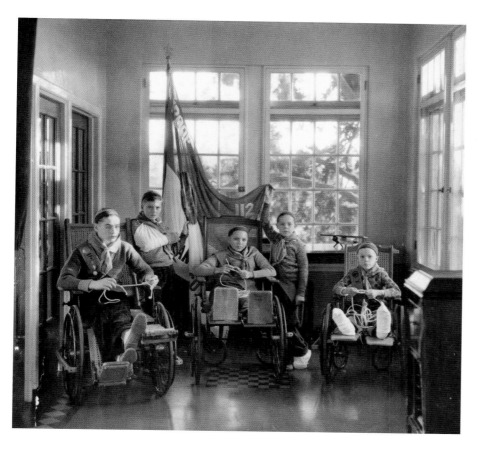

A group of Boy Scouts at Shriners Children's San Francisco, 1928.

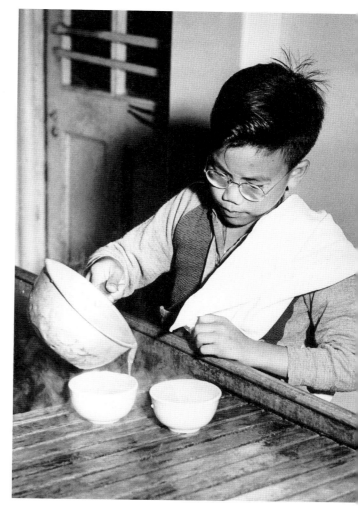

A patient practices pouring water into bowls as a means of developing his coordination.

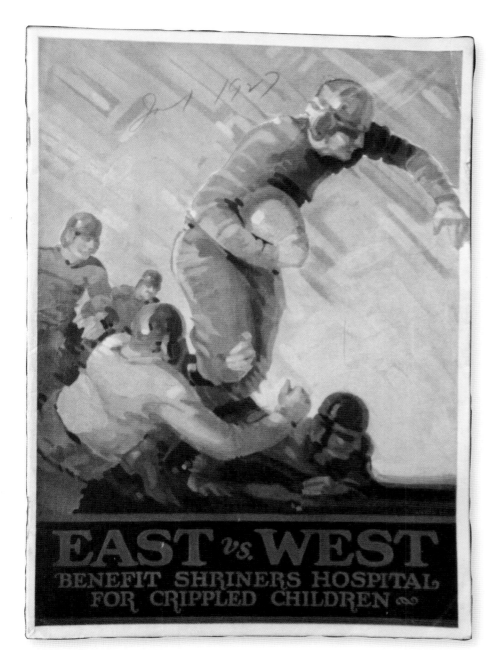

To raise funds for the hospital, the local Shriners founded the East-West Shrine Bowl. An annual event since 1925, this college all-star game, held for many years in San Francisco, has long been recognized as "football's finest hour."

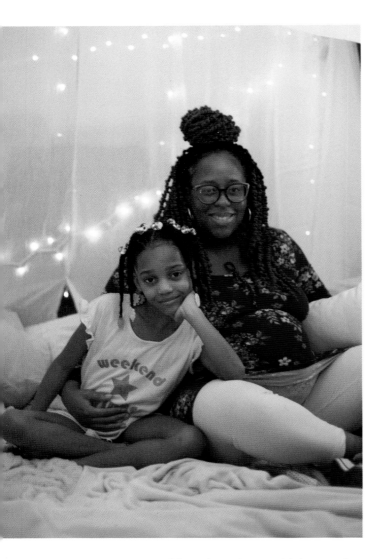

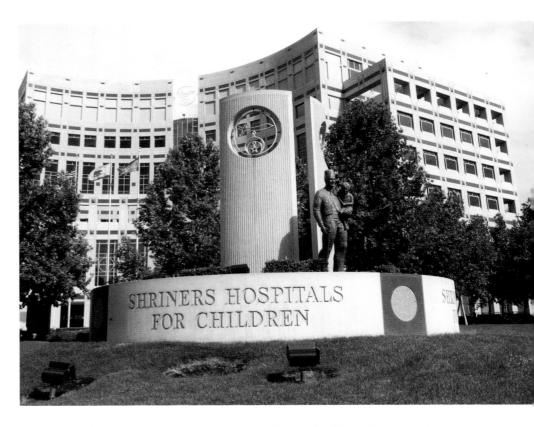

In 1997, the hospital relocated to a state-of-the-art facility in Sacramento. It is the only hospital in the system that addresses all four major areas of treatment — burns, orthopedics, spinal cord injuries and cleft lip and palate.

Seven-year-old Jordyn relaxes with her mother at Shriners Children's Northern California after a life-saving surgery for a serious bowel condition.

Orthopedist Dr. Preston James volunteered at Shriners Children's until 1991, when he retired from private practice and began a second career at the hospital as Assistant Chief of Staff. His daughter, Dr. Michelle James, followed in his footsteps, working alongside her father for over 20 years until his second retirement in 2013.

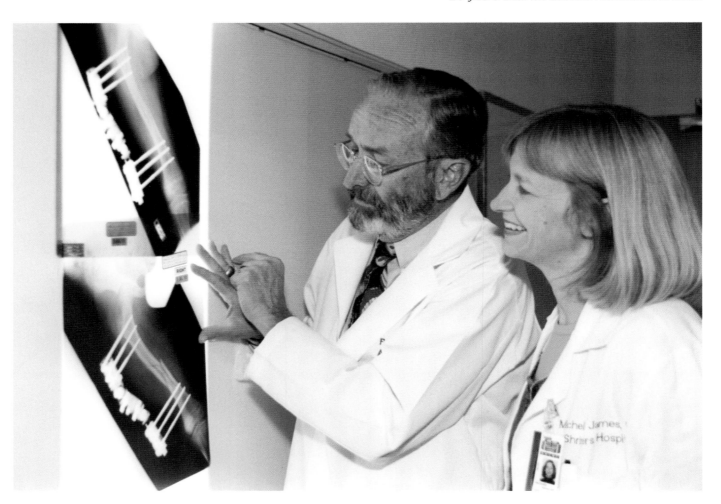

Left: Emma, a patient at Shriners Children's Northern California, enjoys pet therapy with chickens.

Below: Matteo, born with cerebral palsy, takes his first steps after surgery at Shriners Children's Northern California, 2021.

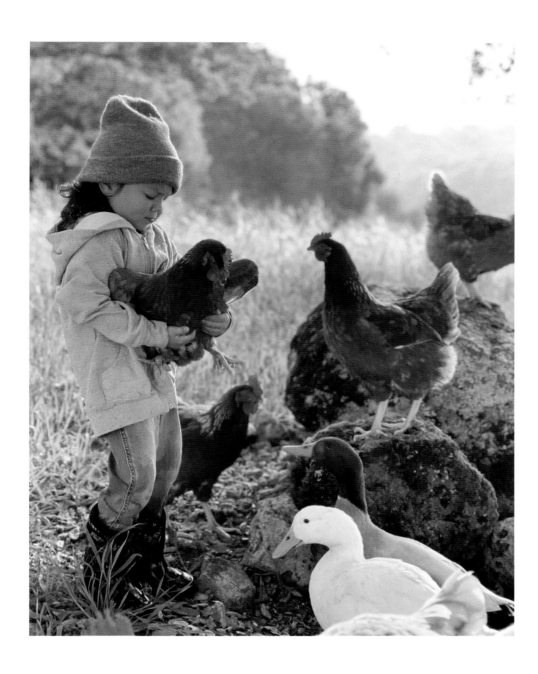

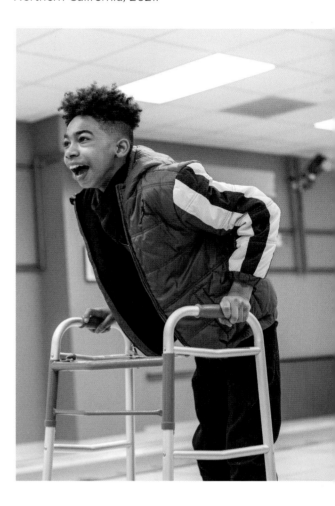

Dr. Jon Davids and one of his patients, 2021.

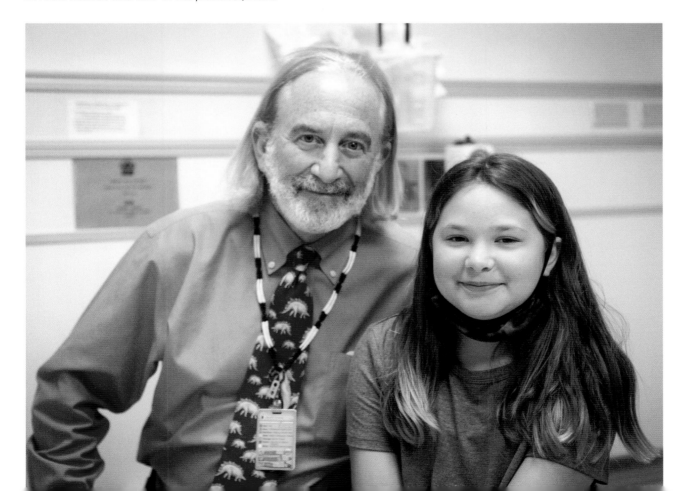

PORTLAND, OREGON
JANUARY 15, 1924

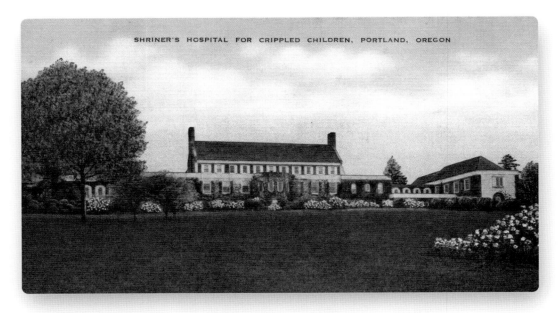

Portland has a special place in the history of Shriners Children's as the site where Forrest Adair delivered the Bubbles Speech that convinced the fraternity to fund the hospitals.

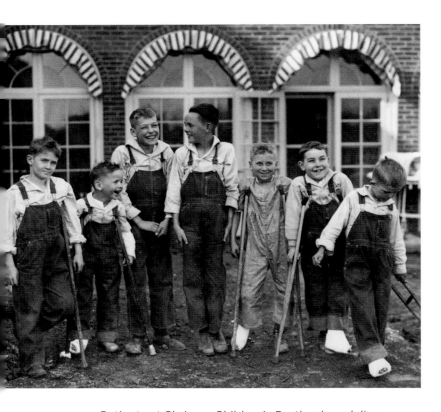

Patients at Shriners Children's Portland modeling their new overalls, 1920s.

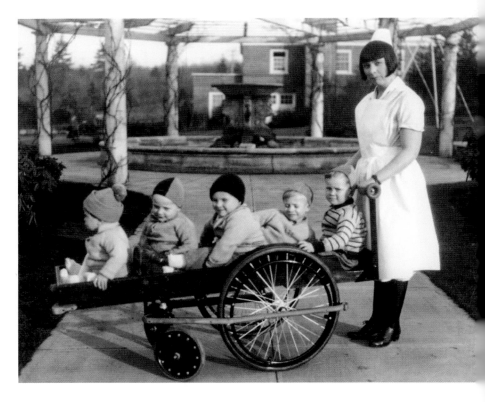

Young patients at Shriners Children's Portland out for a stroll, 1920s.

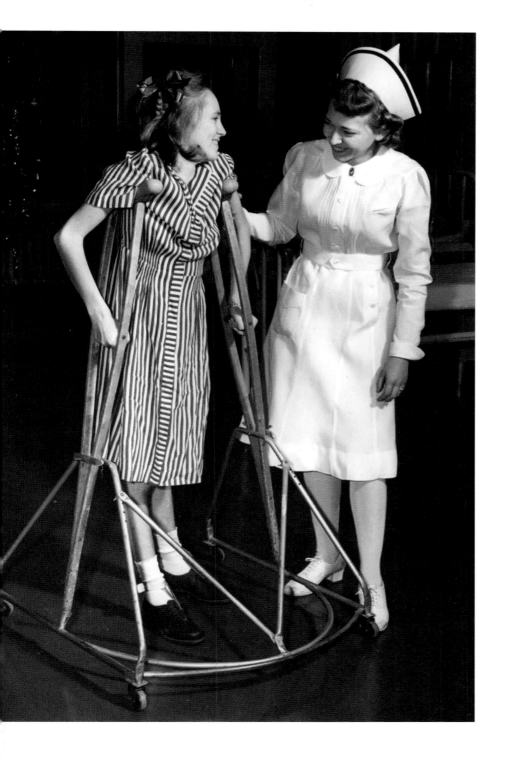

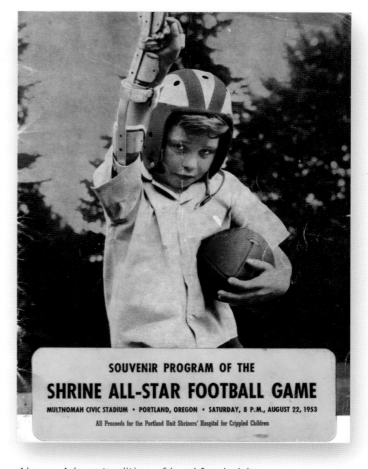

SOUVENIR PROGRAM OF THE
SHRINE ALL-STAR FOOTBALL GAME
MULTNOMAH CIVIC STADIUM • PORTLAND, OREGON • SATURDAY, 8 P.M., AUGUST 22, 1953
All Proceeds for the Portland Unit Shriners' Hospital for Crippled Children

Above: A long tradition of local fundraising for the hospital includes the annual Oregon East-West Shrine Game, first organized in 1952. The Food Caravan, a tradition since 1954, joins the efforts of Shriners from Al Kader, El Korah, Hillah and Afifi Temples across three states to collect food and cash donations for the hospital, presented at a grand evening social.

Left: A new walker introduced in the 1940s was designed to help patients transition from wheelchairs to crutches.

Below: The nursing staff at Shriners Children's Portland, 1930s.

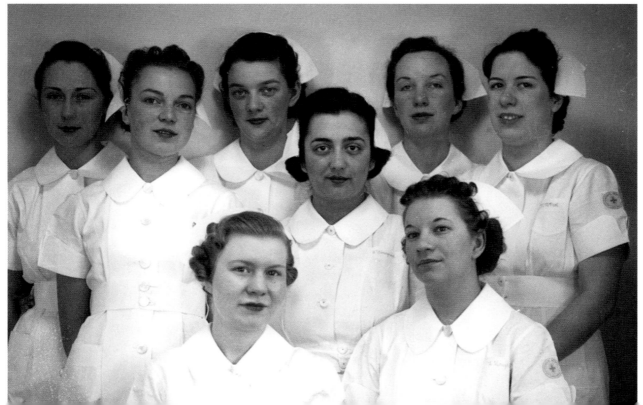

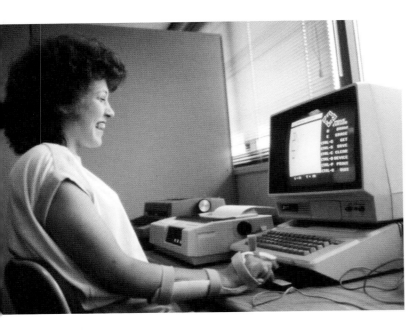

Anticipating the tech boom, a patient at Shriners Children's Portland takes a course on a cutting-edge computer, 1980s.

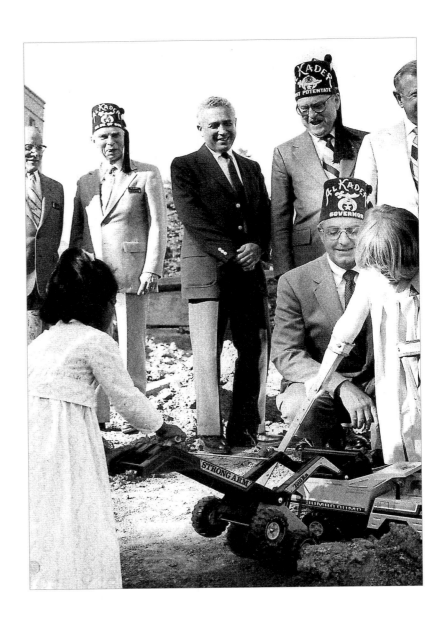

Right: In the early 1980s, the hospital moved from its original location in northeast Portland to its present location on Marquam Hill. Here, Oregon Governor Victor Atiyeh (kneeling) and other dignitaries look on as two patients break ground for the new building.

Since 1979, the Portland chapter of American Bikers Aiming Towards Education (ABATE) has sponsored an annual toy run to benefit Shriners Children's. Here Donnie Stephens, in a Santa suit, leads the pack.

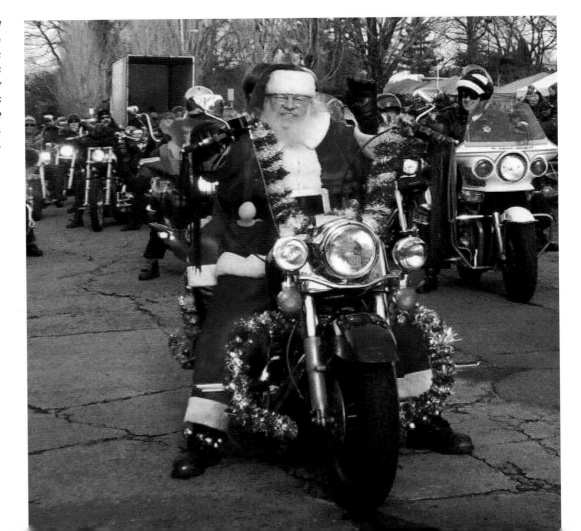

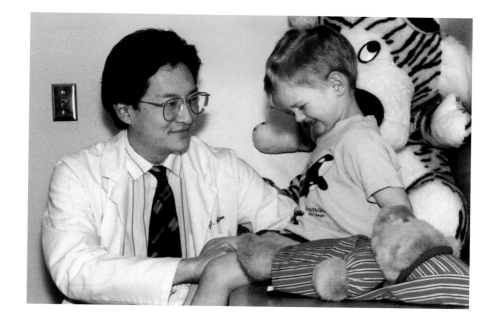

Left: Dr. Michael Aiona with one of the thousands of children he has treated since 1984.

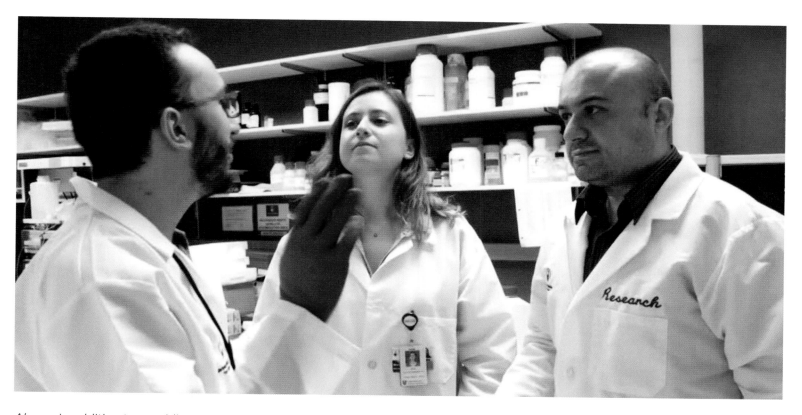

Above: In addition to providing state-of-the-art treatment for thousands of patients each year, the facility hosts the Portland Research Center, established in 1997 to focus on skeletal and limb development.

Below: Quinn, a young patient at the Portland unit, with her braces.

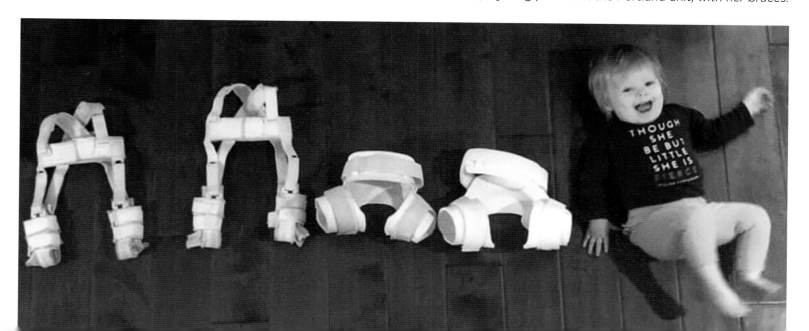

ST. LOUIS, MISSOURI
APRIL 8, 1924

When Shriners Children's St. Louis opened, it was the largest facility within the Shriners Children's system and the first free hospital for children with disabilities in Missouri.

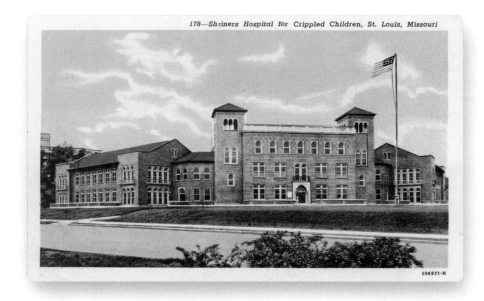

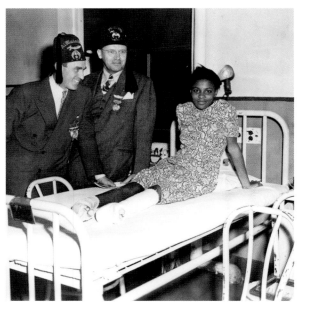

The first hospital in the system with a research budget, Shriners Children's St. Louis was the site of one of the first successful operations to lengthen a leg (1924) and was among the earliest facilities to use skeletal traction to fix a congenital hip dislocation (1930).

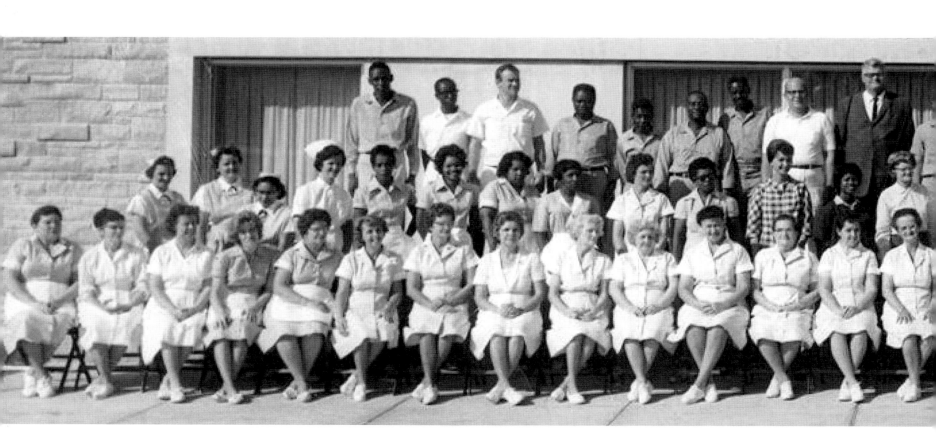

The staff at Shriners Children's St. Louis, 1967.

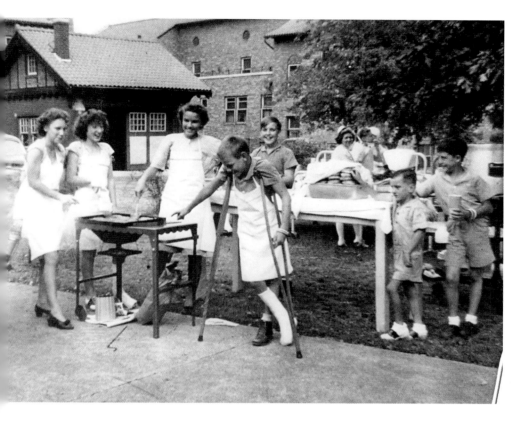

Patients at Shriners Children's St. Louis tend the grill at a summer barbecue, 1947.

In 1963, the hospital relocated to a large complex in suburban Frontenac, Missouri, where it operated for 52 years.

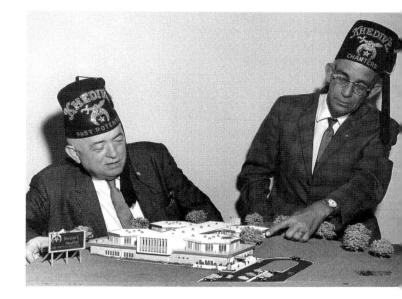

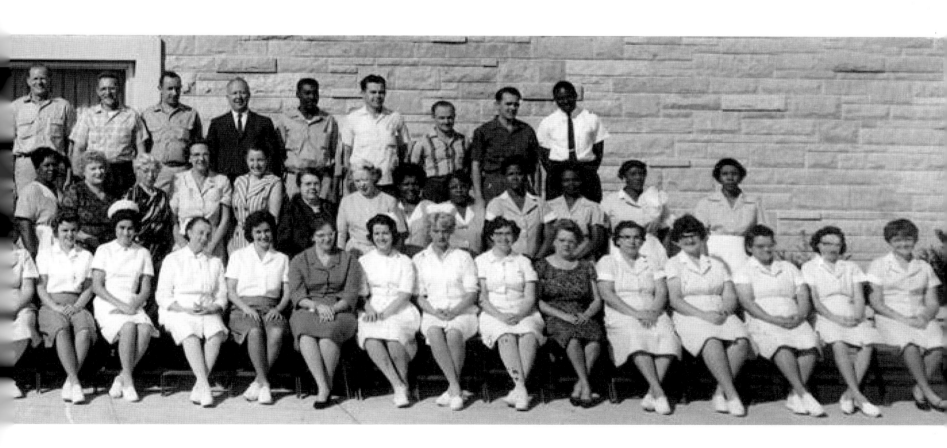

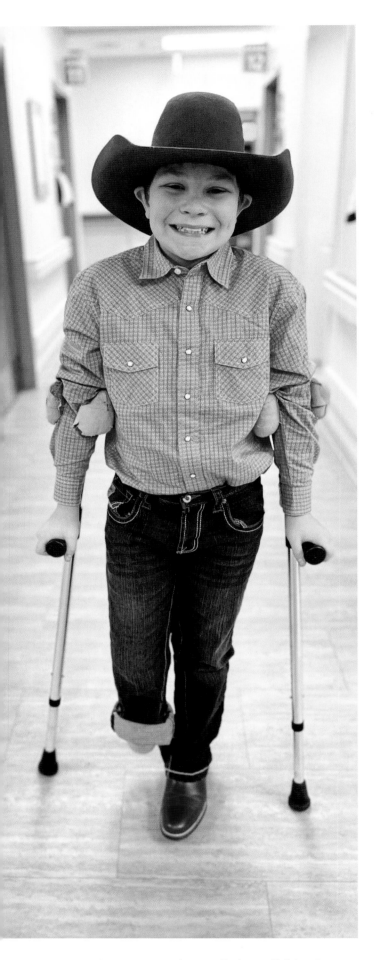

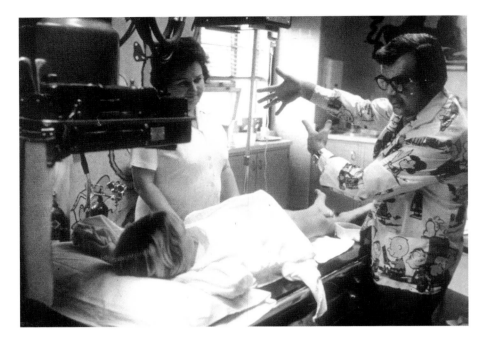

In addition to pioneering techniques in pediatric radiology,
Dr. Armand E. Brodeur was also an accomplished stage magician.
Here, he performs a trick, wearing his signature Peanuts *jacket.*

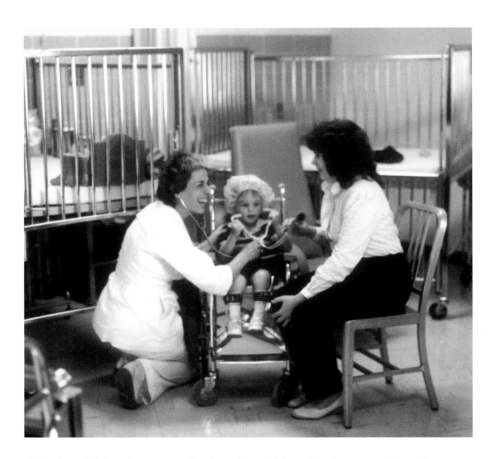

Allowing children to use medical equipment is a classic means of making
them comfortable. In this 1984 photograph, a young patient at Shriners
Children's St. Louis tries a stethoscope while being examined.

Preston, a patient at Shriners Children's
St. Louis, has a smile as big as his hat.

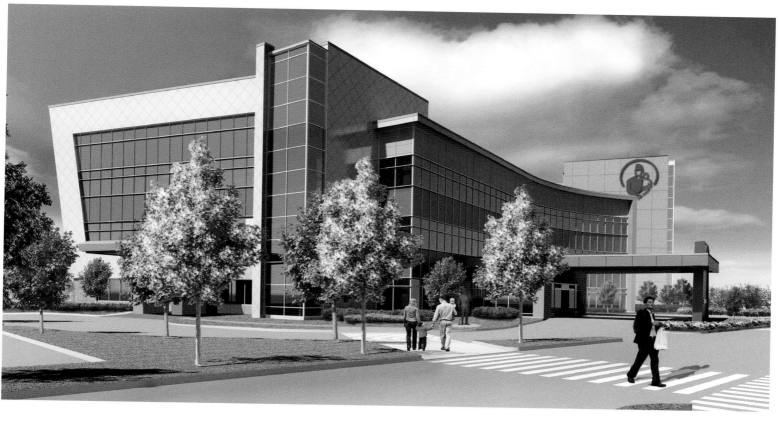

In 2015, Shriners Children's returned to St. Louis, moving into a new facility on the campus of the Washington University School of Medicine, where the long tradition of pediatric care and research continues.

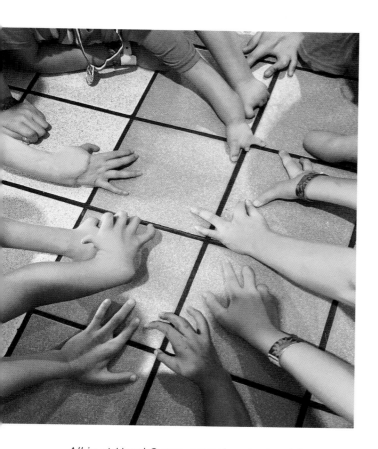

All in at Hand Camp, a weekend retreat for children with hand or upper limb deficiencies.

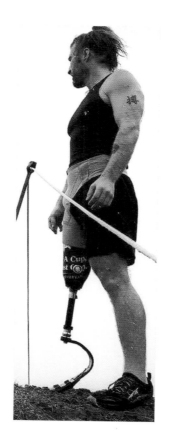

Zach was born without part of his right leg. The staff at Shriners Children's St. Louis fitted him with a futuristic prosthetic blade, and he now runs 50-kilometer ultramarathons.

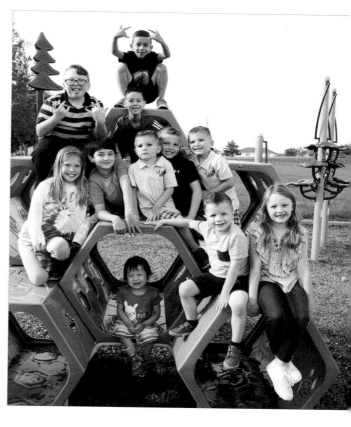

Patients at Shriners Children's St. Louis gather on the playground.

SPOKANE, WASHINGTON
NOVEMBER 15, 1924

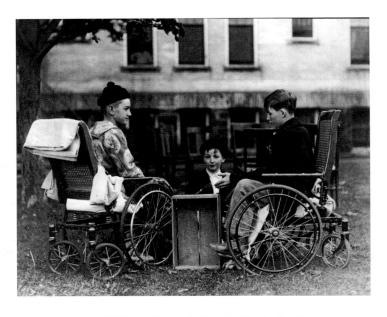

Like Shriners Children's Hawaii, the facility in Spokane was originally conceived as a mobile unit, located in a 20-bed ward of St. Luke's Memorial Hospital.

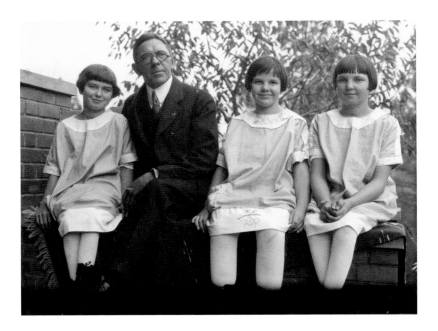

Dr. Charles F. Eikenbary, flanked here by three of his patients, served as the hospital's first medical chief of staff.

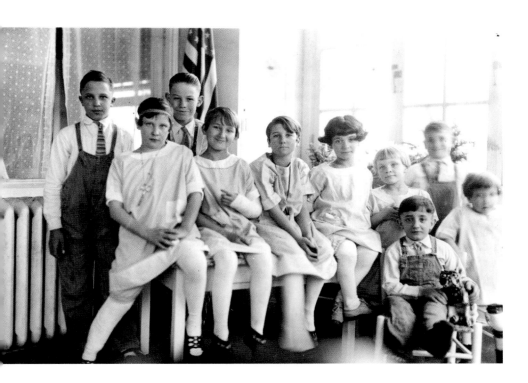

The Spokane facility was known as "the biggest little hospital" in the Shriners Children's healthcare system because it served children from such a wide area. Patients came from Montana, Northern Idaho, Washington, Alaska, British Columbia and Alberta.

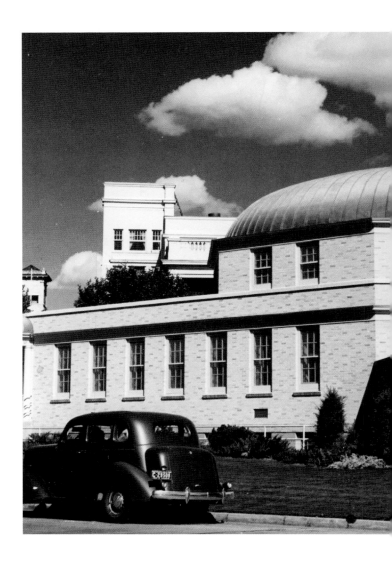

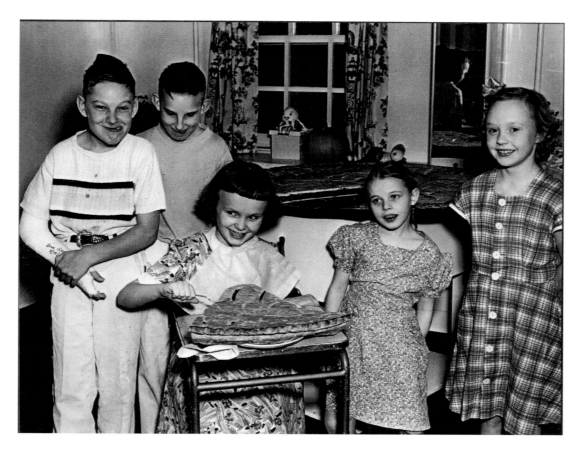

The food services staff at Shriners Children's Spokane included a baker who made extravagant cakes and pies for special occasions.

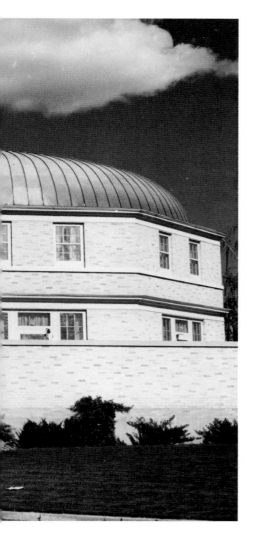

Left: The service the hospital provided for the community was so great that, in the early 1930s, local residents began a campaign to collect tin foil for sale to a metal factory to raise funds for a stand-alone facility. The publicity attracted further financial support, and in 1939, the unit moved to a new hospital built at a cost of $85,000 (almost $1.8 million in 2022 dollars).

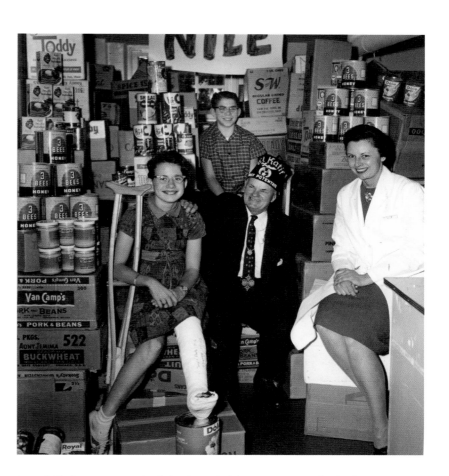

Local Shriners supported the hospital in many ways, including organizing donations of food. Here a Noble of El Katif temple surveys the bounty with a nurse and two patients from Shriners Children's.

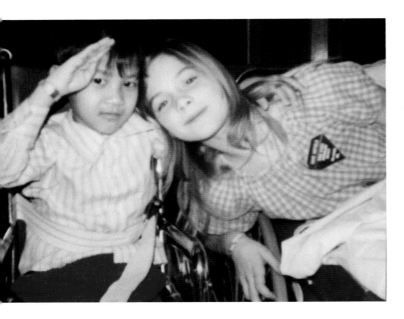

A hospital ward creates an international community. Here, Khanh, a patient from Vietnam, poses with American-born patient Arla, 1971.

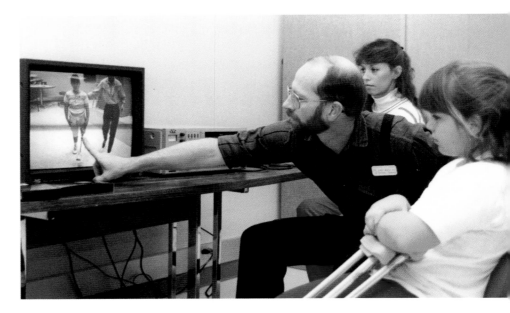

Jerry White, a researcher and physical therapist at Shriners Children's Spokane, assesses the results of a patient's trial at the hospital's motion analysis lab.

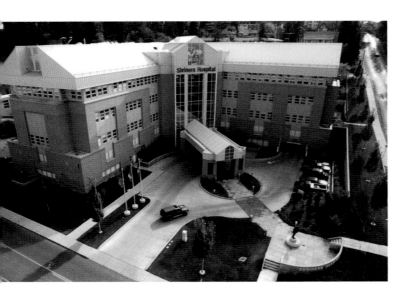

Shriners Children's Spokane continued to share resources with St. Luke's — the two facilities were connected by an underground tunnel. In 1991, the facility moved to a new, modern building that offers the latest in medical technology.

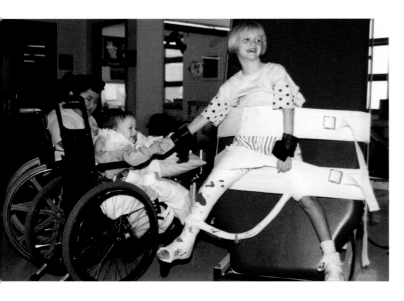

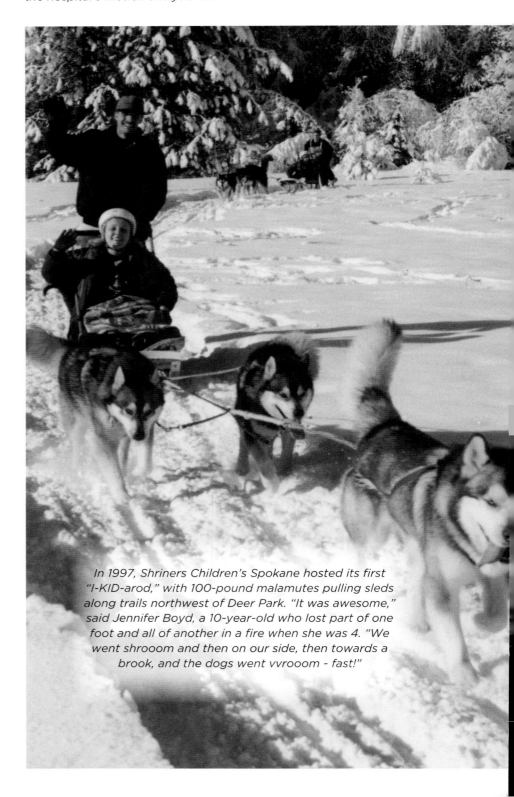

In 1997, Shriners Children's Spokane hosted its first "I-KID-arod," with 100-pound malamutes pulling sleds along trails northwest of Deer Park. "It was awesome," said Jennifer Boyd, a 10-year-old who lost part of one foot and all of another in a fire when she was 4. "We went shrooom and then on our side, then towards a brook, and the dogs went vvrooom - fast!"

A patient recovering from a hip operation connects with two friends at Shriners Children's Spokane, 1980s.

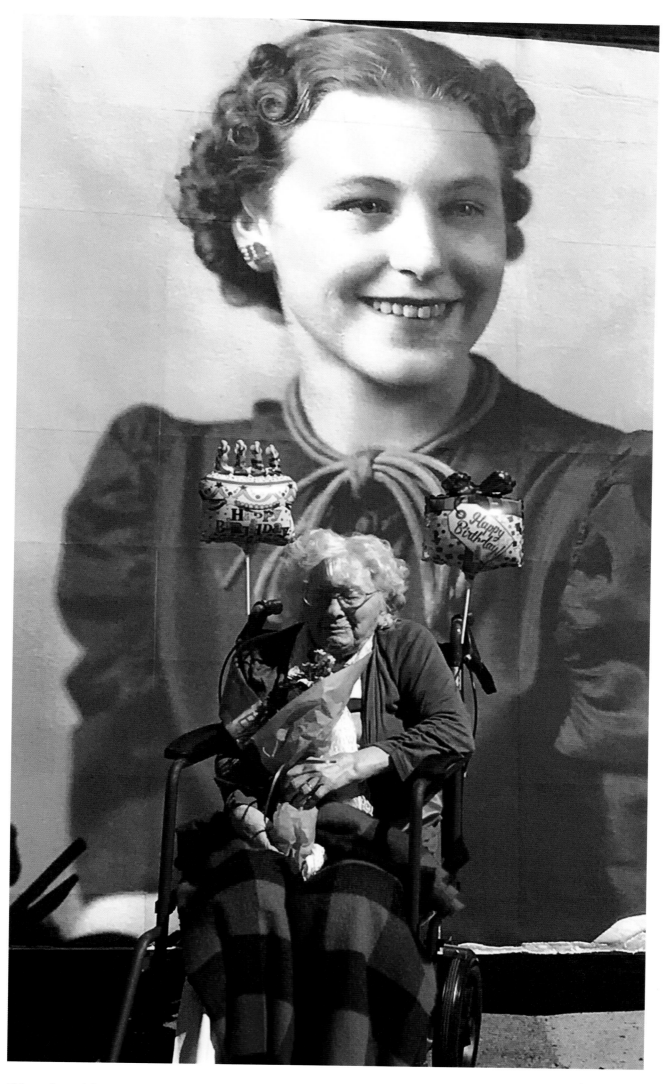

When she celebrated her 103rd birthday in 2020, Irene was Shriners Children's oldest living patient.

SALT LAKE CITY, UTAH
JANUARY 22, 1925

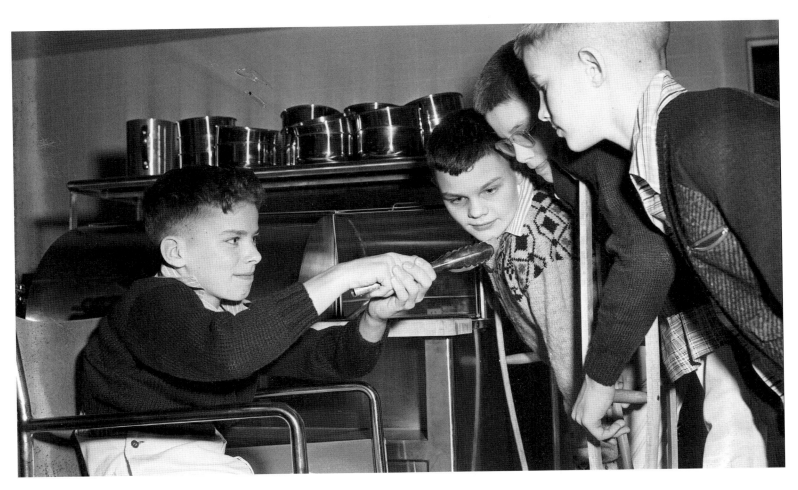

Boys learn practical skills in the kitchen at Shriners Children's Salt Lake City, 1951.

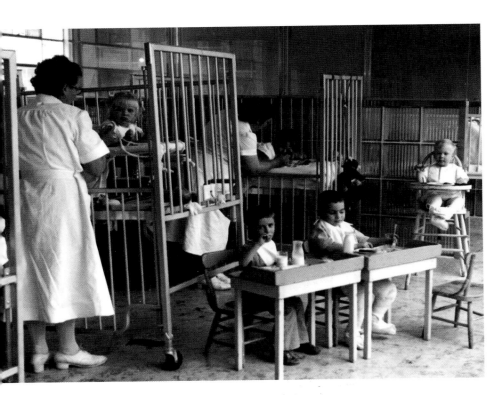

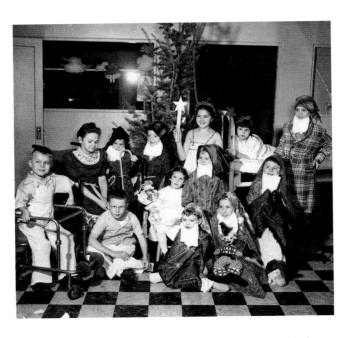

Every Christmas, patients at Shriners Children's Salt Lake City performed in a pageant. Schoolteachers wrote and directed the production. Costumes were designed by the same volunteer sewing circle that prepared gowns and linens for the hospital.

Mealtime in the boys' ward of Shriners Children's Salt Lake City. Thanks to annual food caravans from the Shriners fraternity, there was always plenty to go around.

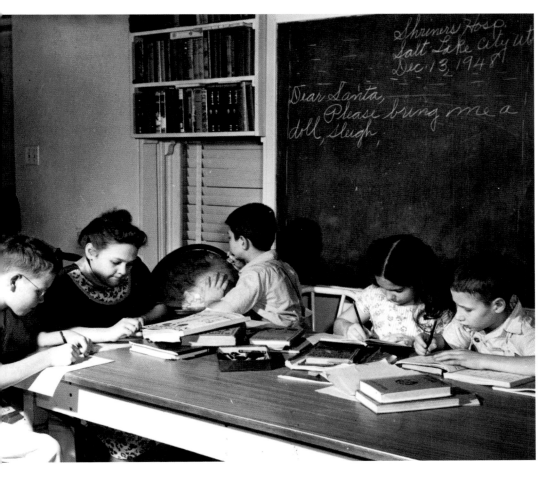

Patients at Shriners Children's Salt Lake City kept up with their studies while hospitalized, sometimes for months at a time. Utah state law required long-term care facilities for children to provide schooling. State-certified teachers were provided by the Salt Lake City school district.

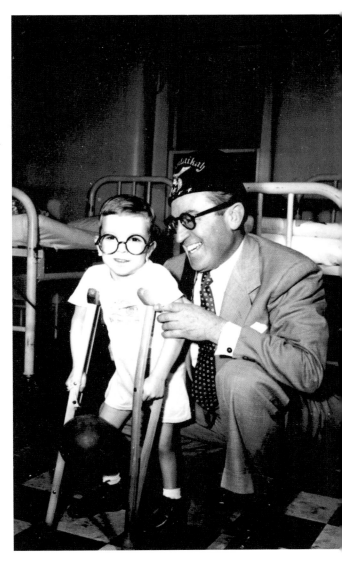

Actor, comedian and stunt performer Harold Lloyd served as the 1949–1950 Imperial Potentate of Shriners International and in 1963 would be appointed Chairman of the Board of Shriners Children's. He made frequent visits to the hospitals to cheer up the kids — and let them try on his spectacles.

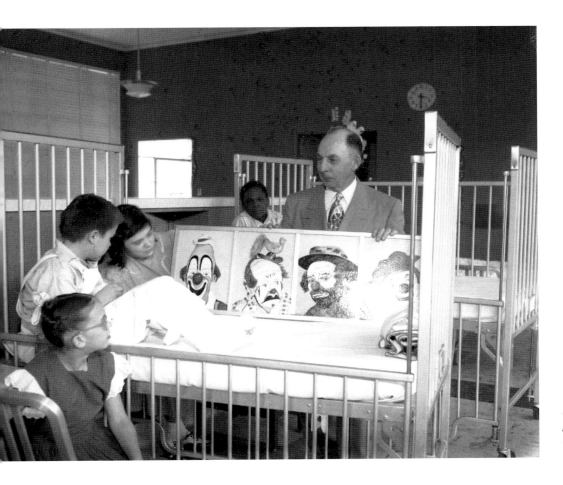

Lester L. Patten, an artist in Ogden, Utah, presents a selection from his series of paintings of 20 famous American clowns to RaNae (front), Kent, Nelda, and R.C., 1951.

65

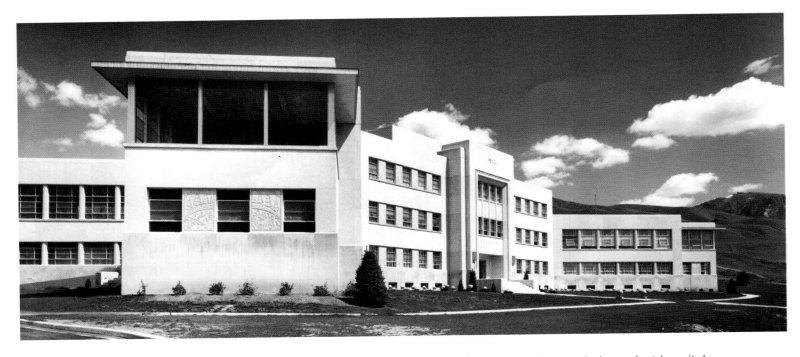

After leasing space at the old St. Mark's Hospital since 1925, Shriners Children's began work on an independent hospital high in the Greater Avenues neighborhood of Salt Lake City. It took an Act of Congress signed by President Truman, himself a Shriner, to appropriate government land for the site. The new hospital opened in 1951.

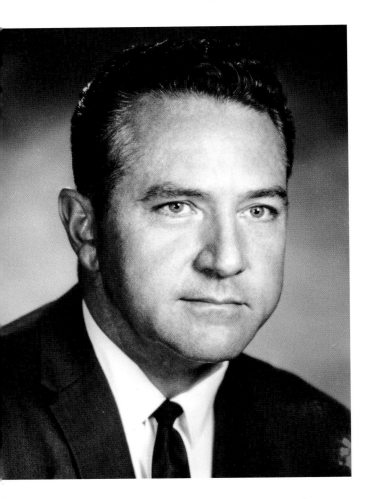

To keep the facility at the forefront of medical knowledge, Chief of Staff Sherman S. Coleman, who served the hospital for 33 years, organized a conference of orthopedic surgeons that has convened every year since 1962. Dr. Coleman also founded an outreach clinic in Juárez, Mexico.

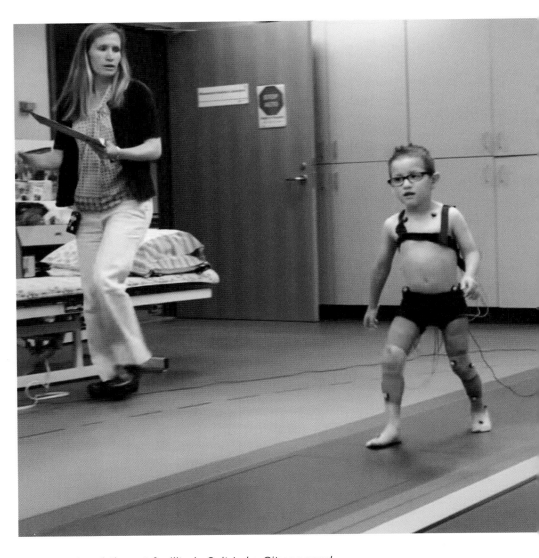

A new state-of-the-art facility in Salt Lake City opened in 1995 to offer expanded services, including a motion analysis center that was one of the first accredited gait laboratories in the United States.

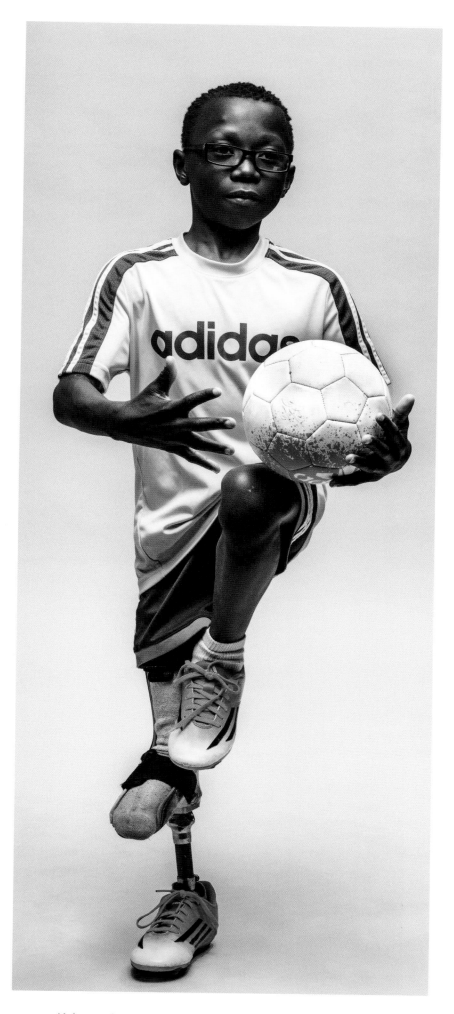

Kai, a patient at Shriners Children's Salt Lake City, bounces a soccer ball while standing on his prosthetic leg, 2017.

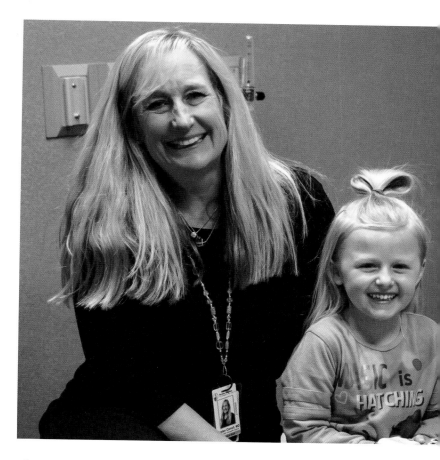

Elena with Dr. Kristen Carroll, Chief of Staff at Shriners Children's Salt Lake City.

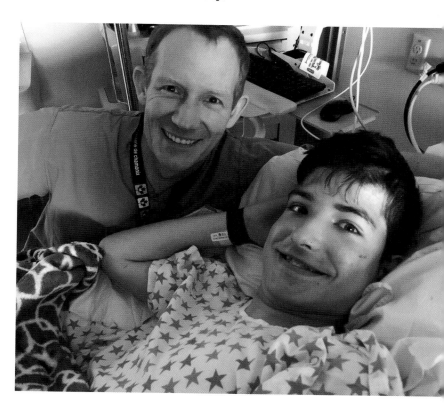

Born prematurely with cerebral palsy, microcephaly, and fetal alcohol syndrome, Miles has thrived under the care of Dr. Josh Klatt and other staff at Shriners Children's Salt Lake City.

MONTREAL, QUEBEC, CANADA
FEBRUARY 18 AND MARCH 15, 1925

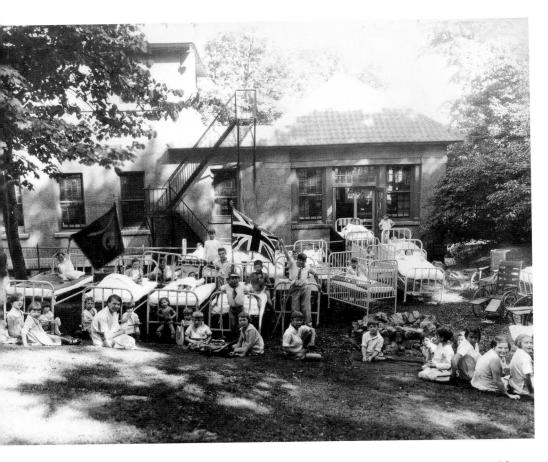

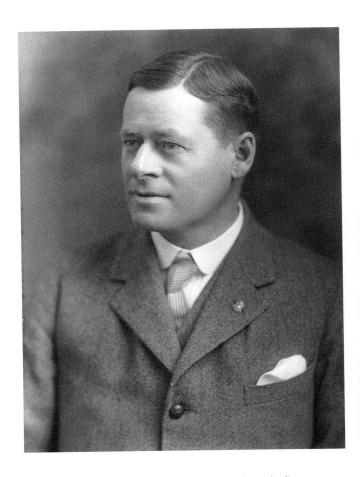

Shriners Hospitals for Children Canada, located in Montreal, has allowed for close collaboration between the pediatric hospital and McGill Medical School from the very beginning. A second location in Winnipeg, Manitoba, operated from 1925 to 1977.

Dr. Alexander MacKenzie-Forbes, the hospital's first chief of staff, was a pioneer in Canadian orthopedics, and his successors were no less distinguished. One developed the Petrie cast, widely used in the rehabilitation of hip issues. Two others invented the Fassier Duval nail, a bone connector that extends as a child grows, reducing the need for surgery.

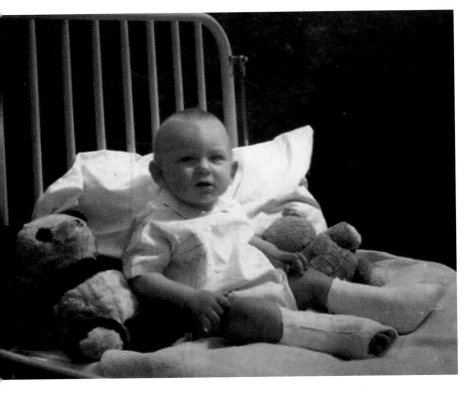

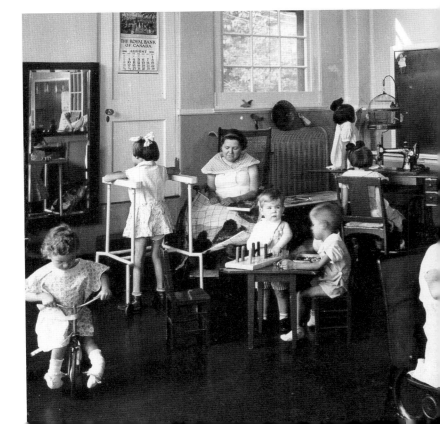

An early patient at Shriners Hospitals for Children Canada, recovering from surgery for clubfoot.

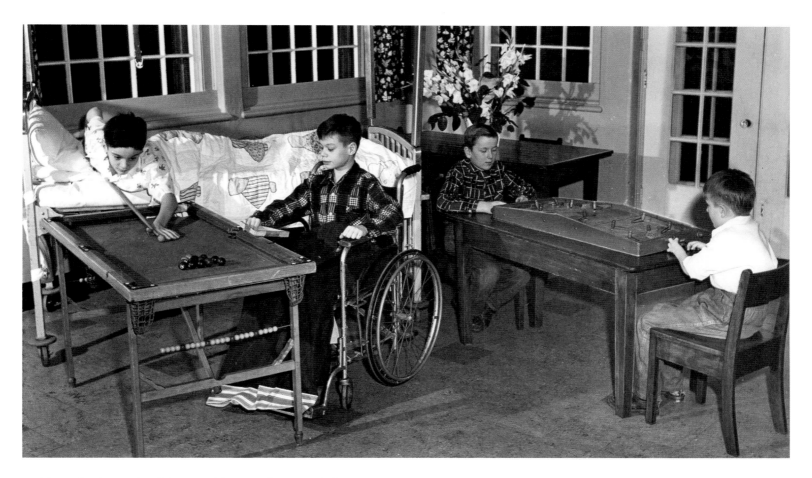

Neither a bed nor wheelchair could get in the way of these patients playing their favorite games — billiards and table hockey.

There were a wide range of possibilities for occupational therapy at Shriners Hospitals for Children Canada. In this photograph from August 1931, the options include sewing, leatherworking, and whittling.

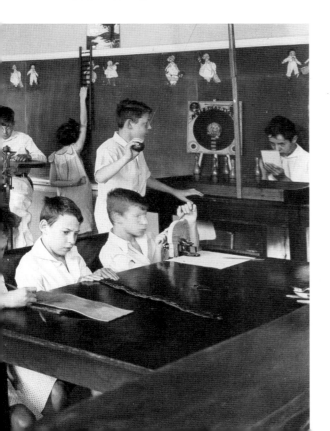

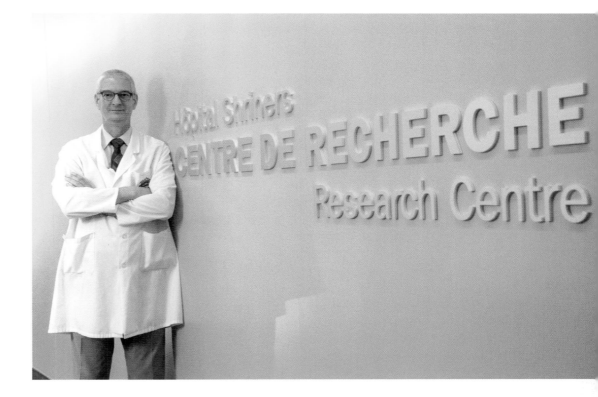

In 1973, Shriners Hospitals for Children Canada opened the first department in a Shriners Hospital dedicated solely to research, generating key innovations and discoveries in the treatment of rickets, osteogenesis imperfecta (brittle bone disease) and other conditions.

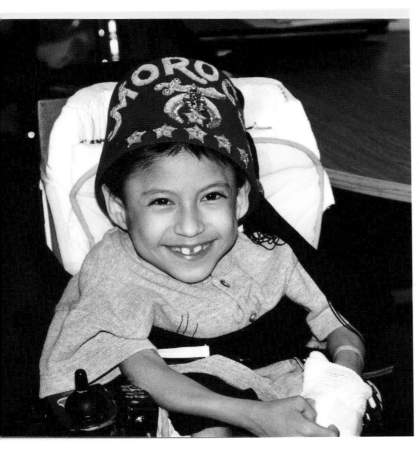

Carlo, born with osteogenesis imperfecta (brittle bone disease), proudly sports a Shriners International fez.

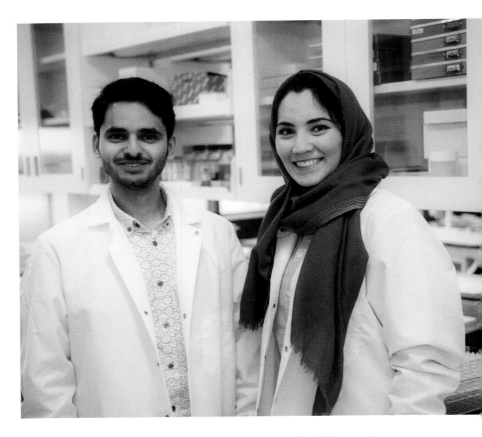

This historical cooperation between the hospital and the academy has been so fruitful that, when the McGill University Hospital Centre (MUHC) was compelled to move to a new site, Shriners Children's followed, ensuring that the treatment it offered to patients would always be state of the art.

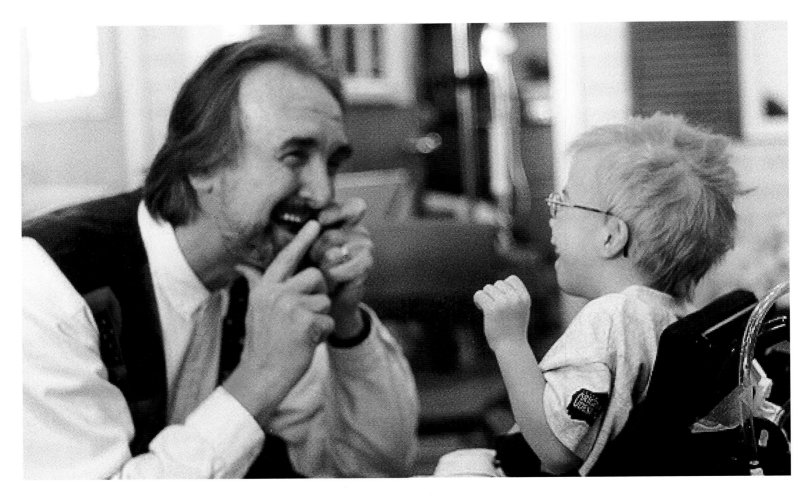

Beloved children's entertainer Fred Penner, renowned for his song "The Cat Came Back," laughs with one of his fans.

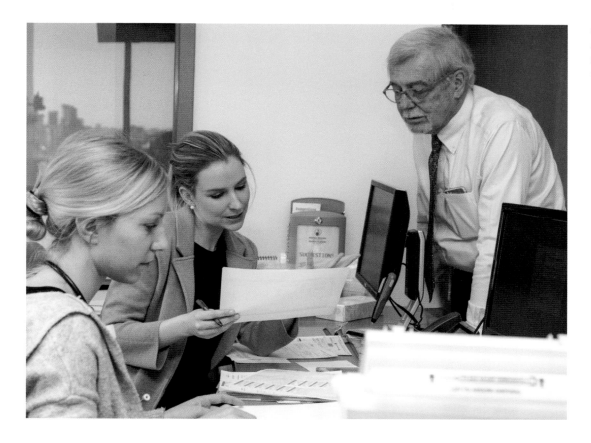

Dr. Francis Glorieux, a medical researcher at Shriners Hospitals for Children Canada since 1973, with two colleagues.

Michael, a patient from Ghana, was confined to a wheelchair until his treatments at Shriners Hospitals for Children Canada. Now, he can walk on his own.

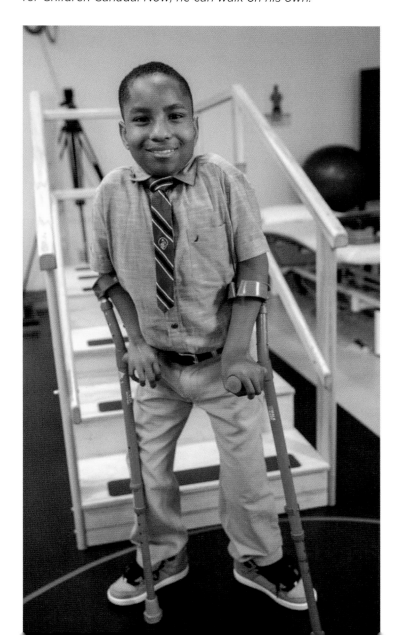

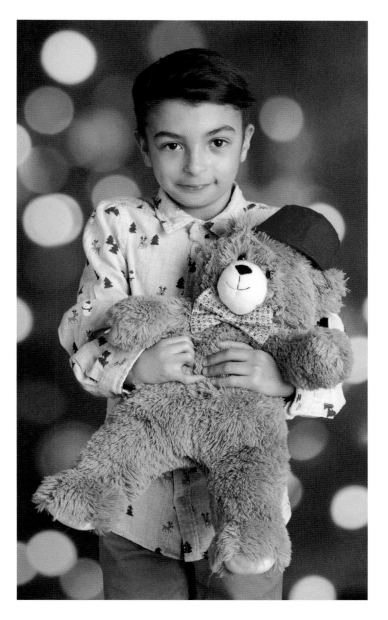

Olivier with Fezzy, the official mascot of Shriners Hospitals for Children.

SPRINGFIELD, MASSACHUSETTS
FEBRUARY 21, 1925

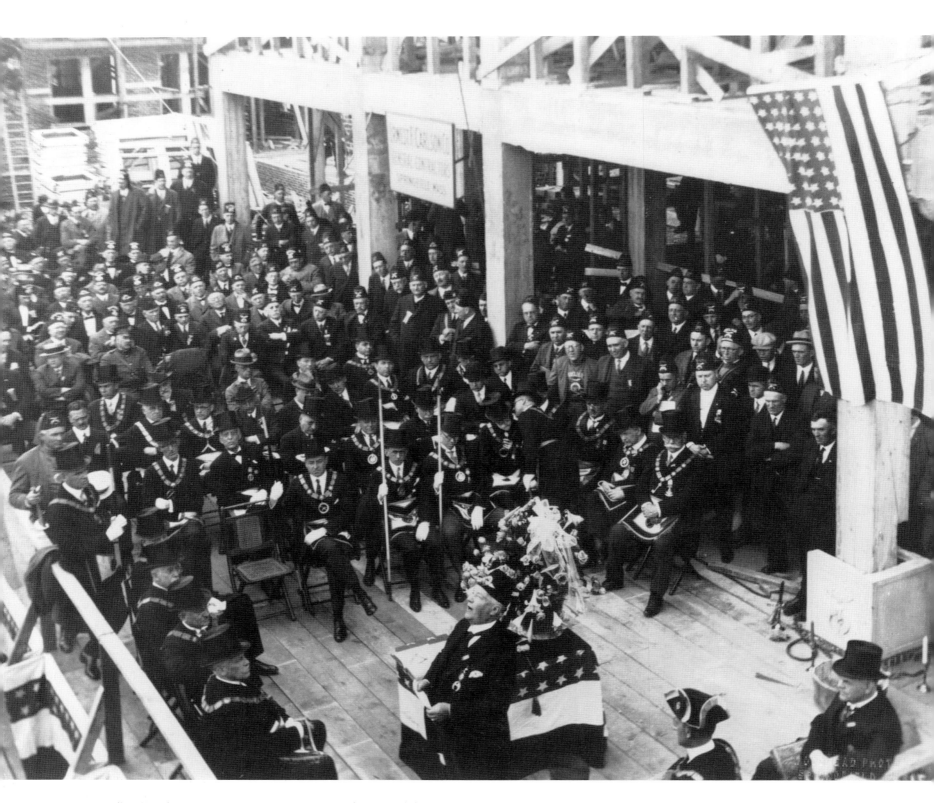

Dedicating the cornerstone, 1924. Having a Shriners Children's hospital in one's city was recognized as a great honor, so when the Board decided to build one in New England, there was a fierce competition between members of Aleppo Shriners in Boston and Melha Shriners in Springfield. Aleppo was the older, wealthier and more influential of the two temples, but Springfield had an ace up its sleeve — there was a Rolls Royce factory in town. When the Board arrived, the Melha Shriners transported them in a caravan of luxury cars during their visit. Aleppo couldn't top that!

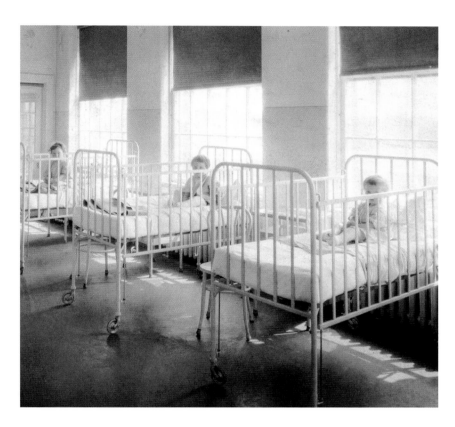

Toddlers recover from operations on their legs in this early photograph from Shriners Children's New England.

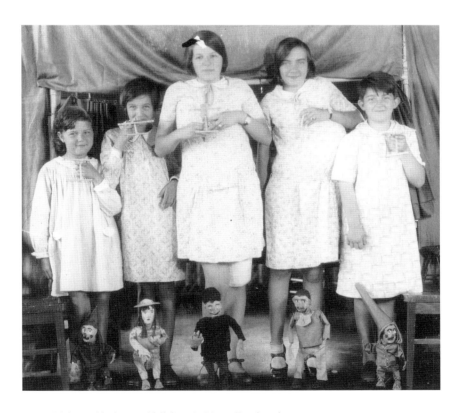

Girls at Shriners Children's New England practice the art of puppetry.

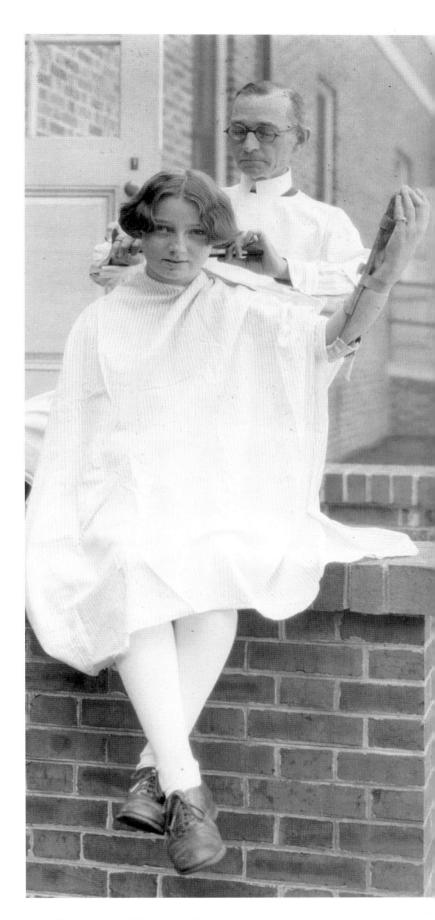

Hospital stays could last months, even years, so the range of patient care was extensive. This young woman, her arm in a splint, gets a coiffure in the latest style.

Gift Of Goat As Thanks For Shriners' Hospital Work

William E. Bissell Has Taken 68 Crippled County Children to Hospital for Operations; Grateful Family Gives Dr. Hatt a Goat

(By Roger W. Tubby)

Sixty-eight crippled children from Bennington county have undergone operations at the Shriners' hospital in Springfield, Mass., during the last ten years and many others during that time have gone to the hospital for clinical observation and treatment.

Many of these children were seriously crippled. Many had given up hope of ever living normal lives. That the great majority were restored to good health is due primarily, of course, to Dr. R. N. Hatt, the hospital's great surgeon, and his staff. However, they were all enabled to enter the hospital in the first place through the help of William E. Bissell, Bennington Shriner.

Recently the writer visited the Springfield hospital with Mr. Bissell. Perhaps what impressed him most was not so much the efficient staff, the modern operating rooms, the many splendid features of the hospital which help the children in mind as well as body. What impressed him most was a billy goat.

accomplishments that the public at large may become more deeply interested in the steady advance of this humanitarian cause.

Surprising growth has followed a small beginning. The object was to start but one hospital for the relief of crippled children. It was advanced by Noble W. Freeland Kendrick of Philadelphia, at Portland, Oregon, in 1920 and provided for a small annual contribution from each member of the Shrine. These contributions would establish and develop such an institution. In 1921 at the Imperial Council at Des Moines a resolution was adopted making the annual assessment $2.00 per year per member for the purpose of building and equipping and putting in operation such a hospital.

Thus the greatest charity ever undertaken was brought to life and developed until now there are 15 hospitals in operation; twelve in this country, two in Canada and one in Honolulu.

Much thought was given to the location of these hospitals so that the territory served might be as extended as possible. The population of the districts chosen and the determination to locate units only in cities where there was a Shrine Temple were factors considered.

The total bed capacity in all hospitals is 831 and the beds are practically filled at all times.

As with all hospitals in the network at that time, Shriners Children's New England offered its services, regardless of a family's ability to pay. In 1941, one family showed their gratitude by presenting the staff with a goat.

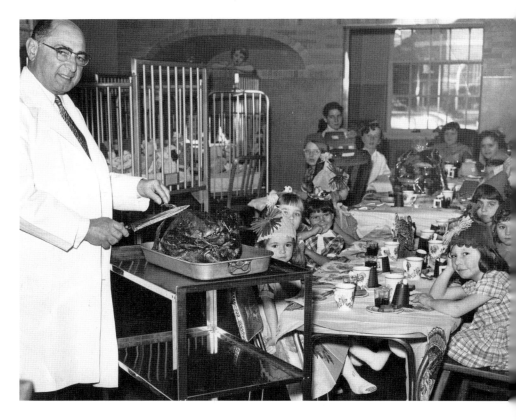

Dr. Garry deNeuville Hough, Jr., who served Shriners Children's New England from 1925 to 1963, prepares to practice his surgical skills on a Thanksgiving turkey.

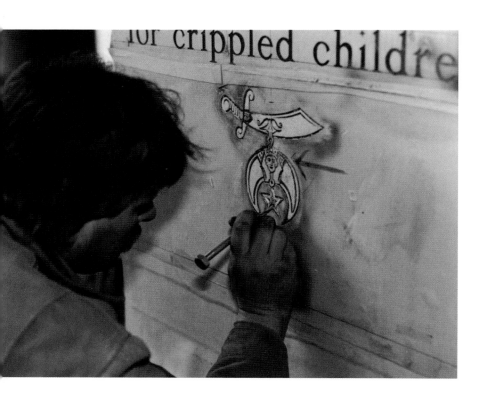

After 65 years in its original location, Shriners Children's New England moved to a new facility. Here, a stonecarver inscribes the cornerstone of the new facility, which opened in September, 1990.

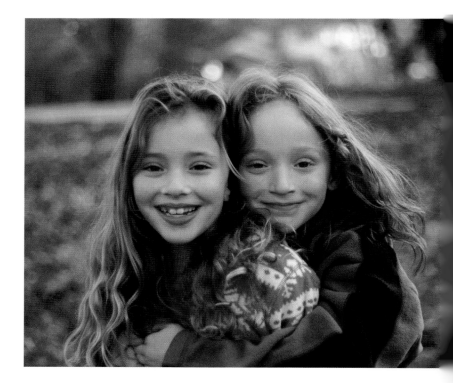

Twins Clarissa (left) and Elliot (right) were both patients at Shriners Children's New England. She was treated for scoliosis; he was fitted with an ankle-foot orthosis to stabilize his joints.

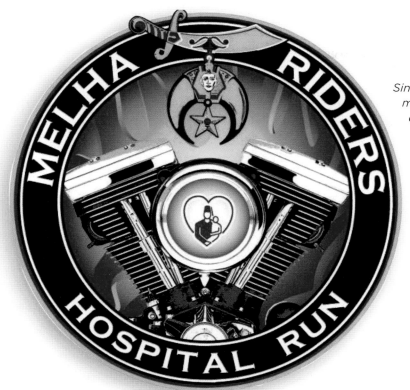

Since 1989, motorcycle enthusiasts have staged an annual Fall Run — a fundraising ride of 60 miles that has raised more than $575,000 for the hospital.

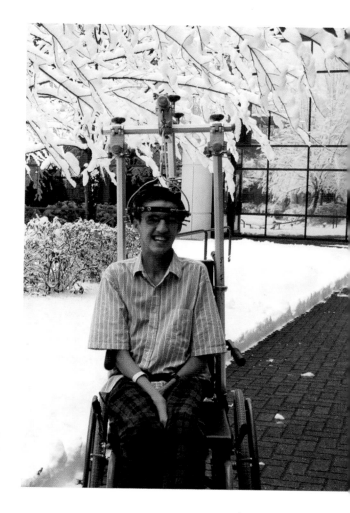

Right: The hospital's original facilities expanded over the years, and were replaced entirely in 1991. In 2022, Shriners Children's Springfield transitioned to an outpatient model to meet shifting medical needs. To more accurately reflect its coverage area, it is now called Shriners Children's New England.

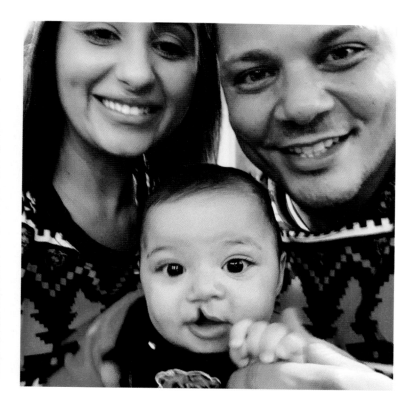

Shriners Children's New England offers full range of care, including treatment for cleft lip and cleft palate. Here is Jovani with his parents before his operation.

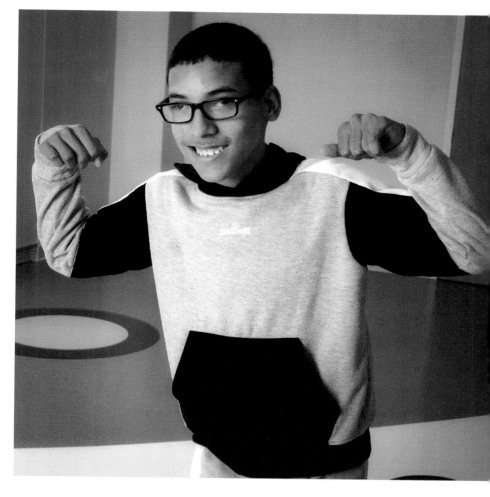

Emmanuel, a cerebral palsy patient at Shriners Children's New England, stays strong.

CHICAGO, ILLINOIS
MARCH 20, 1926

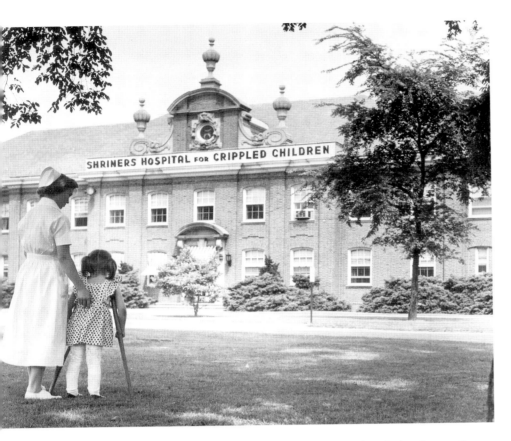

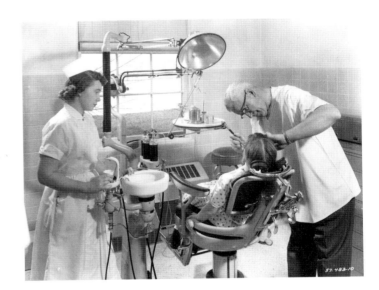

The Great Depression of the 1930s hit Chicago hard, and the war posed a new set of challenges: most doctors worked without pay, including this dentist.

Funded by one of the Shriners' wealthiest temples during boom times, Shriners Children's Chicago was built at a cost of nearly $600,000 — $9.8 million in today's dollars.

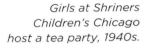

Girls at Shriners Children's Chicago host a tea party, 1940s.

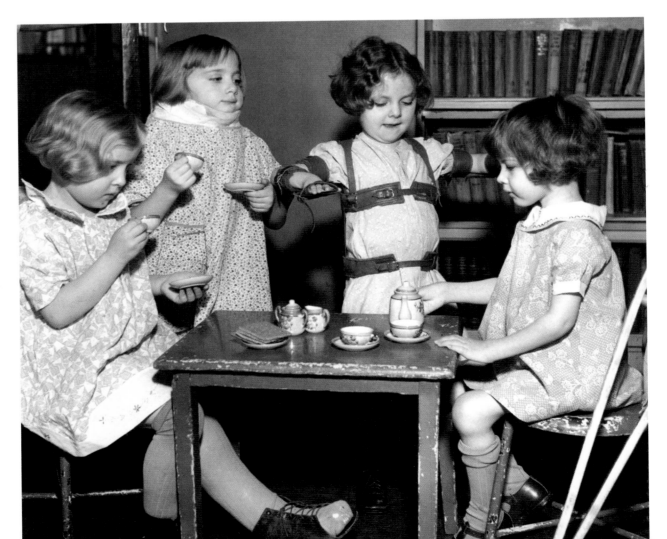

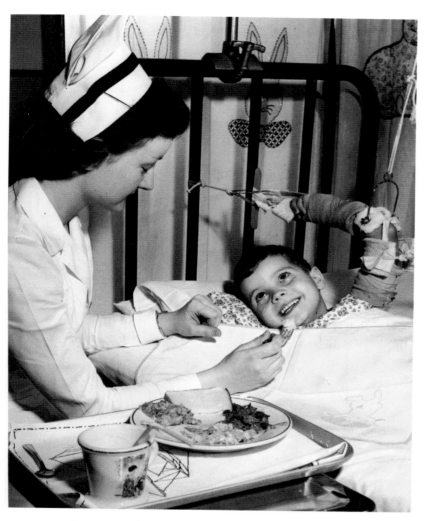

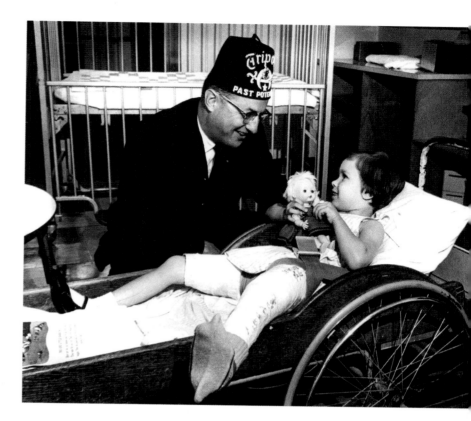

Shriners take supporting both the hospital and its patients as a joyous duty. Here, a Noble of Tripoli Temple of Milwaukee, Wisconsin, gives a doll to a girl recovering from an operation.

A nurse at Shriners Children's Chicago feeds a grateful patient.

Chicago is famed for its music scene, and Shriners Children's was no exception. Here, young patients wearing Shrine Circus fezzes attend an outdoor piano concert.

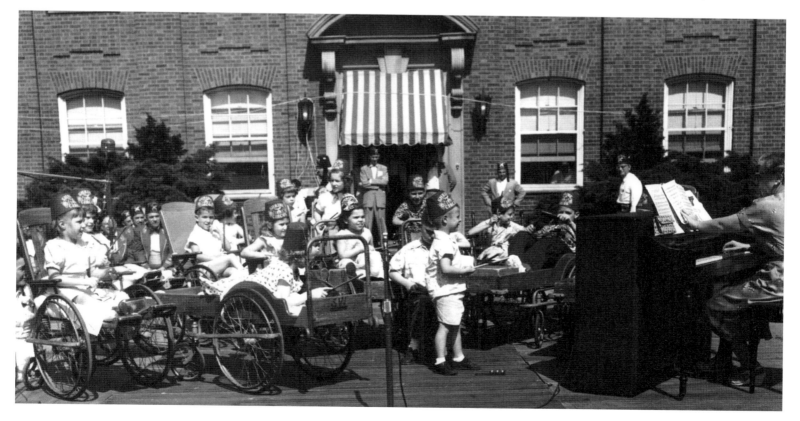

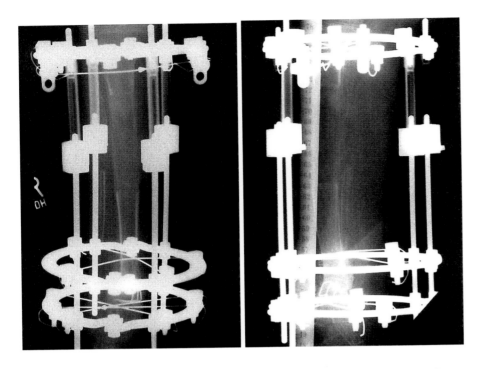

In the post-war era, the hospital became a center of medical invention. One doctor developed one of the first surgical interventions for osteogenesis imperfecta (brittle bone disease). The halo skeletal fixator was still in its beta stage when it was first used at the hospital in 1966.

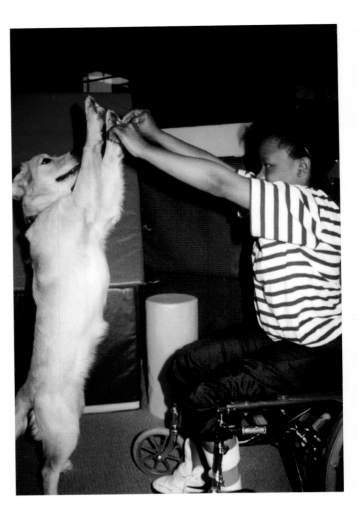

Above: Linda with Doozer, a registered pet therapy dog. Specially trained pets work in supportive roles to help meet treatment goals. For example, dogs may be used in physical therapy to encourage a child to walk a few more steps.

After a complete hospital overhaul in 1981, Shriners Children's Chicago started programs in cleft lip and palate and craniofacial surgery that have since been expanded to other Shriners Children's hospitals. Here are Evan and his mother after surgery.

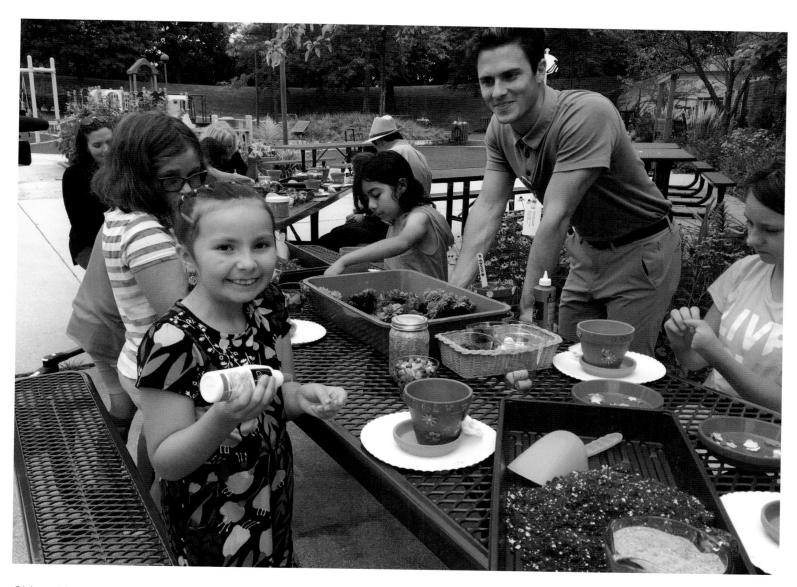

Girls at Shriners Children's Chicago design their own flowerpots at the Chicago Botanic Garden, 2018.

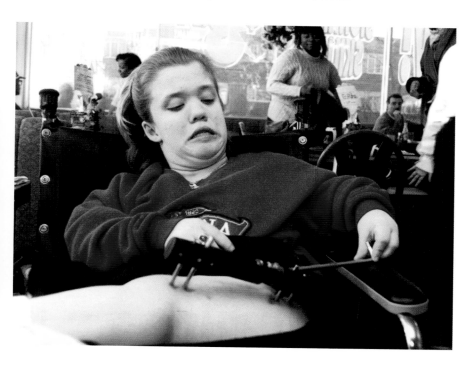

A renovation completed in 2009 added a new clinic wing and updated the pediatric intensive care unit and inpatient facilities. Here, Melissa, born with achondroplasia, a form of dwarfism, turns the pins that help her legs grow in a process that potentially could extend her height by up to 10 to 12 inches.

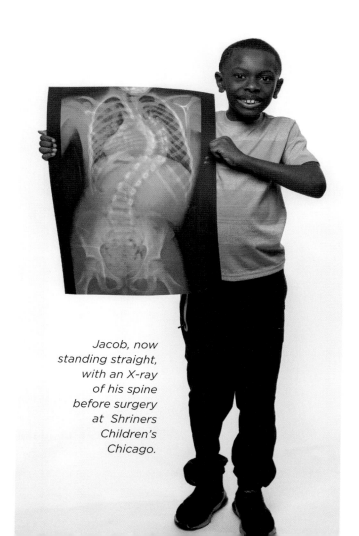

Jacob, now standing straight, with an X-ray of his spine before surgery at Shriners Children's Chicago.

PHILADELPHIA, PENNSYLVANIA
JUNE 24, 1926

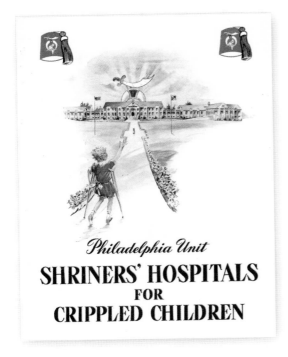

W. Freeland Kendrick was a Philadelphian, so this facility of the Shriners Children's system naturally was dearest to his heart. He served as chairman of the hospital until his death in 1953.

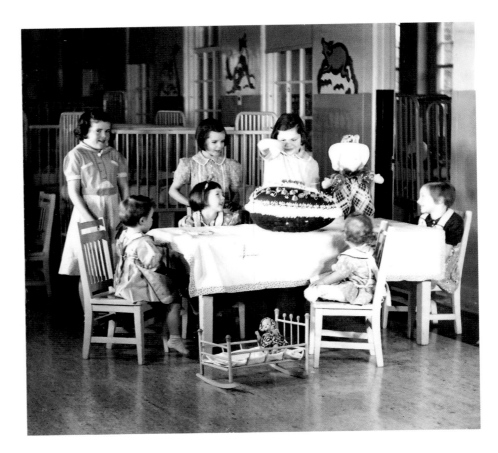

Girls at Shriners Children's Philadelphia prepare to open an Easter surprise, 1929.

Sporting their new baseball caps, boys at Shriners Children's discuss the Phillies.

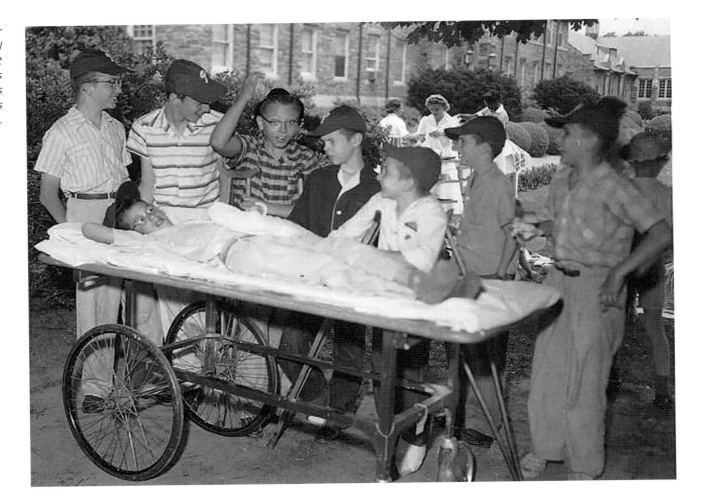

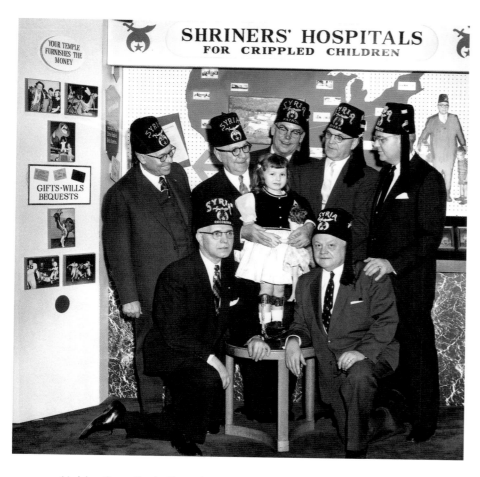

Nobles from Syria Temple, Pittsburgh, visit Shriners Children's Philadelphia.

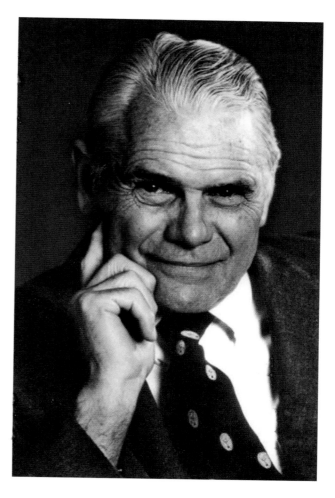

In 1966, Chief of Staff Dr. Howard H. Steel founded an outreach clinic that sees more than 1,000 children in Puerto Rico each year.

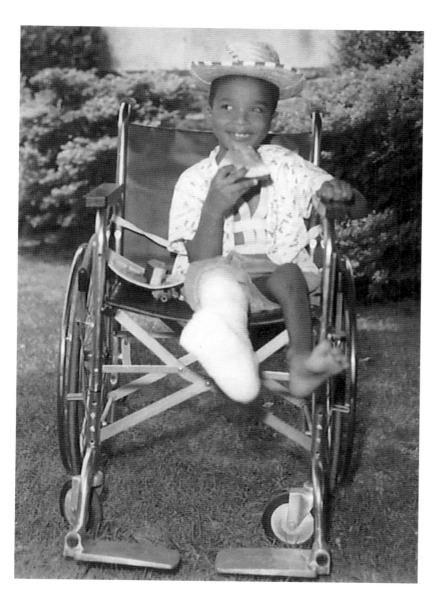

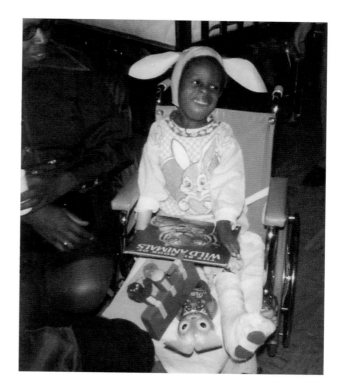

A joyous patient at Shriners Children's Philadelphia celebrates Easter in style, 1971.

Being in a wheelchair did not stop this patient at Shriners Children's Philadelphia from enjoying his summer.

81

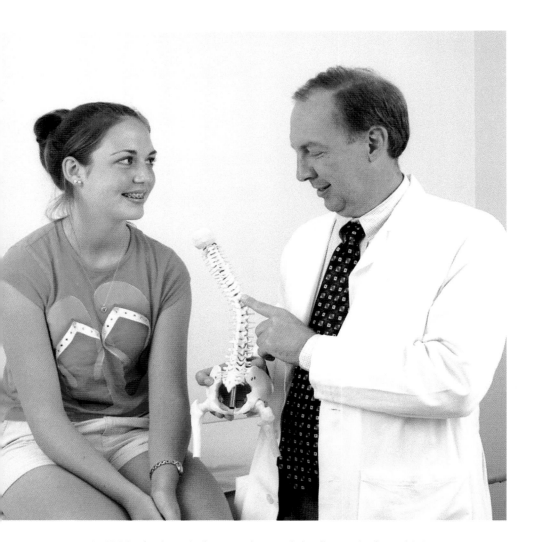

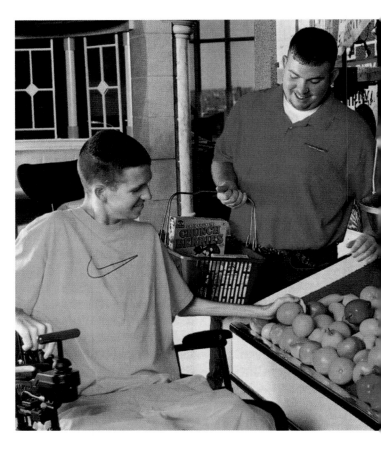

Above: Reese practices grocery shopping in Independence Square, an area of the Philadelphia hospital that replicates a town square and allows patients to practice skills they will need when they return to their homes and communities.

In 1980, the hospital opened one of the first spinal cord injury rehabilitation units in the country and, in 1991, helped to pioneer titanium rib surgery as an approach to scoliosis. More recently, the medical team in Philadelphia helped pioneer Vertebral Body Tethering, an alternative to spinal fusion surgery for certain patients with scoliosis. Here, Dr. Randal R. Betz discusses treatment with Katie.

Below: In 1998, the hospital moved to a modern facility in north Philadelphia to work in close collaboration with Temple University Children's Hospital. This partnership with an academic research institution has facilitated the development of a number of new treatments and techniques in pediatric medicine.

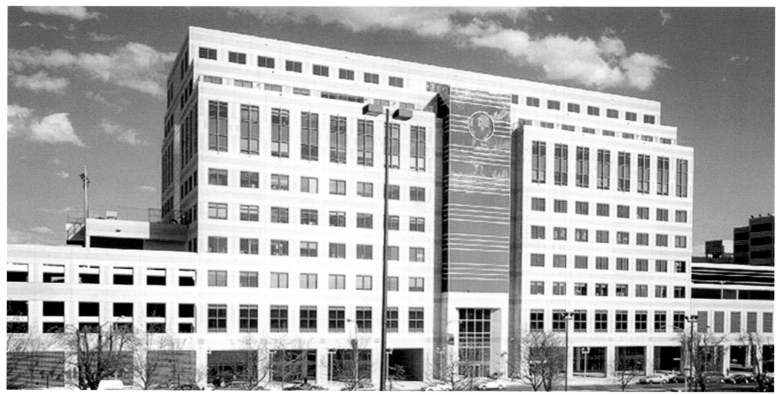

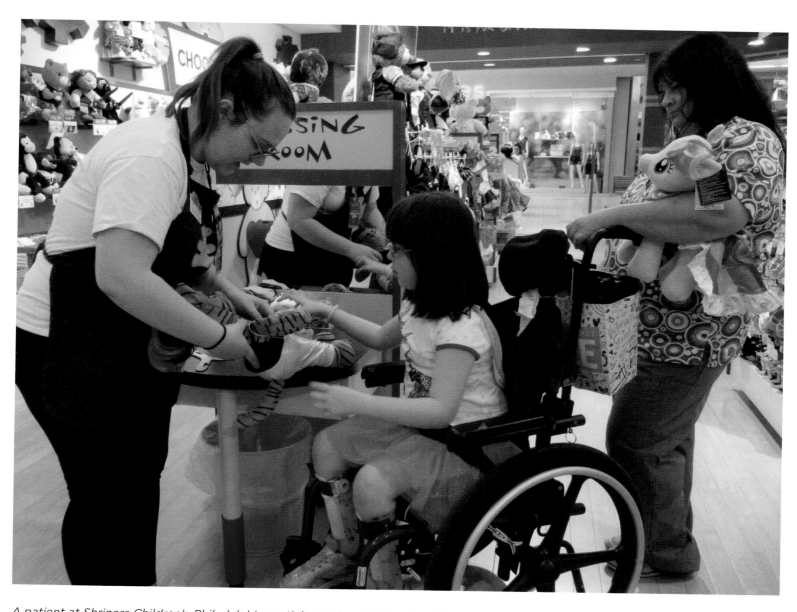

A patient at Shriners Children's Philadelphia participates in a Build-A-Bear® workshop, 2019. The Build-A-Bear Foundation supports Shriners Children's with financial contributions and donations of over 5,000 furry friends annually.

Even getting a new cast can be fun, as Kristin, howling with glee, learns at Shriners Children's Philadelphia.

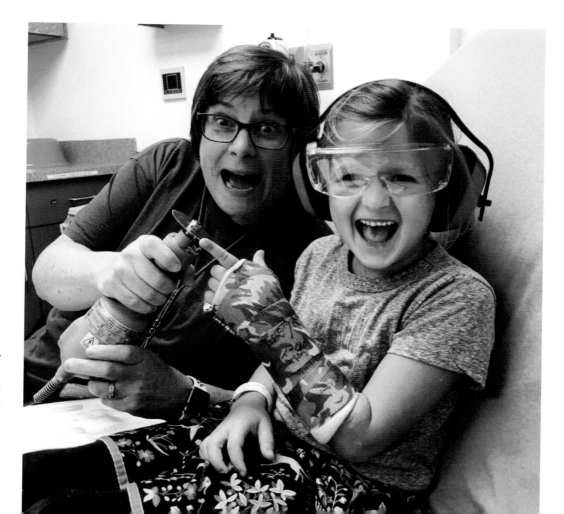

LEXINGTON, KENTUCKY
NOVEMBER 1, 1926

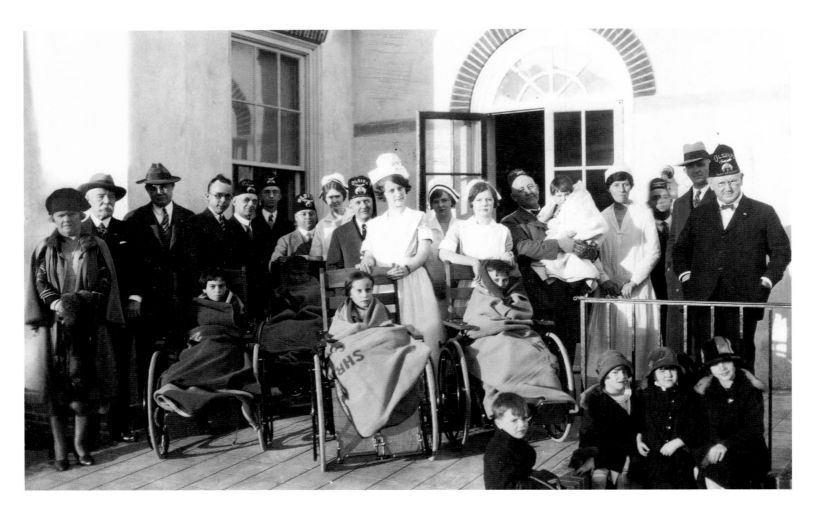

Shriners Children's Lexington started as a mobile unit, occupying a 20-bed ward in the Good Samaritan Hospital. It was clear early on that the demand for pediatric orthopedic services far outpaced capacity, but the Great Depression and World War II delayed hopes of expansion. Here, Florence Potts and Sam Cochran (far left) pose with staff and patients of the unit.

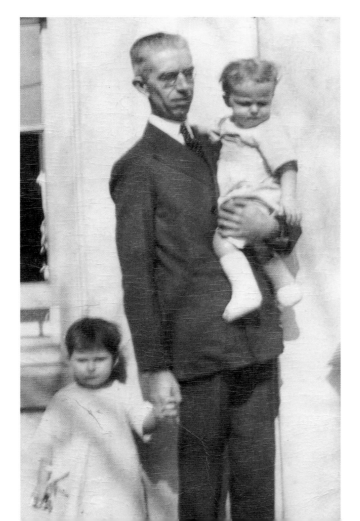

Theo L. Jones, Recorder of Oleika Temple, with Theodore Roosevelt Tweed and Ulah Floyd, the first patients to be admitted to Shriners Children's Lexington, 1926.

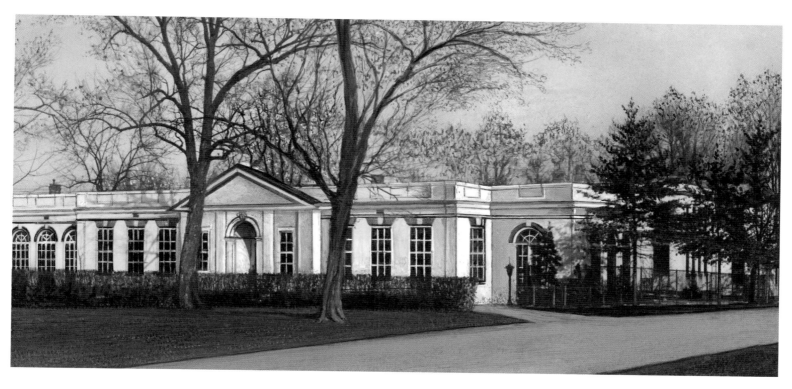

*In 1951, the process began to build a free-standing hospital on a 27.8-acre tract.
The new facility, which opened in 1955, included housing for the nursing staff.*

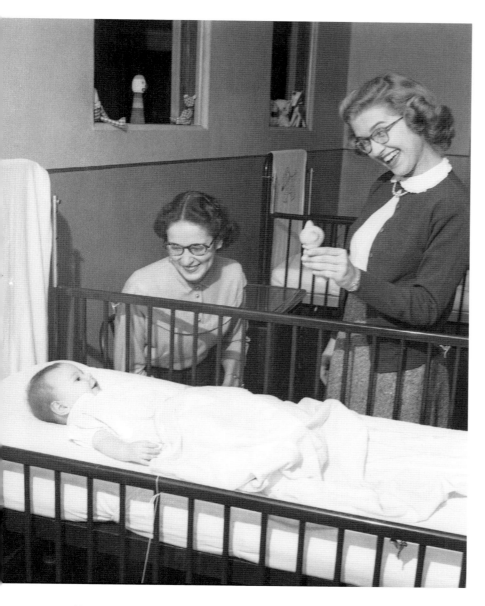

*Nurses at Shriners Children's Lexington
entertain a child with a kewpie doll.*

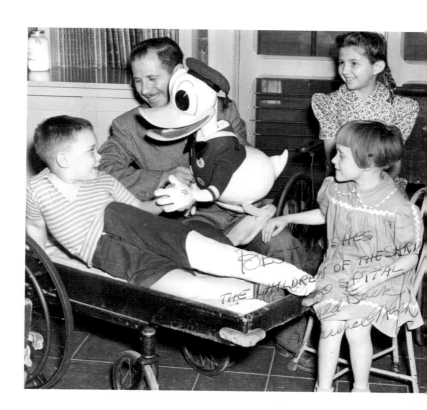

*Clarence Nash, the original voice of Donald Duck,
visits Shriners Children's Lexington.*

A patient peals with laughter as clowns work their wonder at Shriners Children's Lexington, mid-1950s.

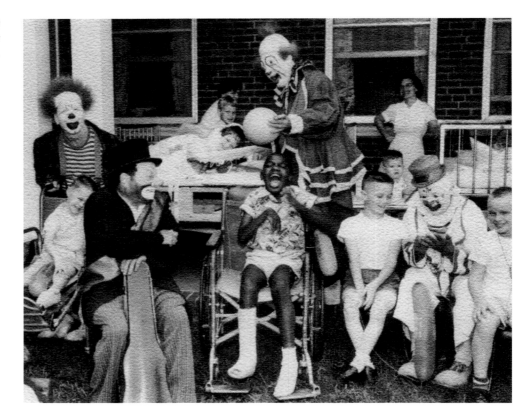

Below: Two patients at Shriners Children's Lexington mold figures with plaster and bandages, 1980s.

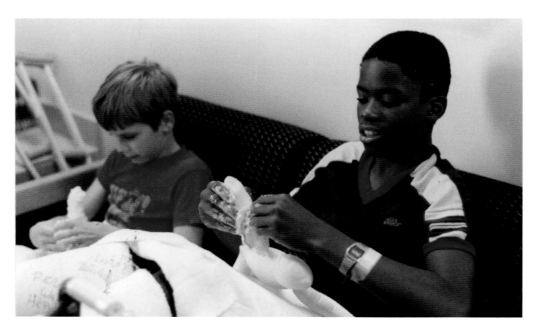

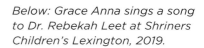

Below: Grace Anna sings a song to Dr. Rebekah Leet at Shriners Children's Lexington, 2019.

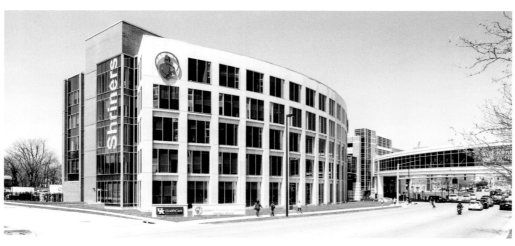
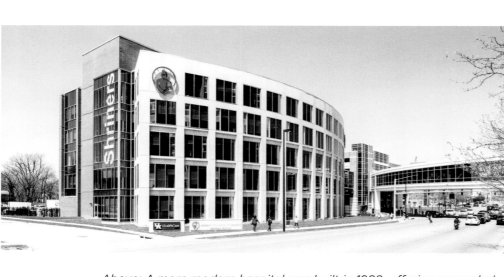

Above: A more modern hospital was built in 1988, offering expanded medical services and an increased focus on outpatient care. In 2017, Shriners Children's Lexington relocated to the University of Kentucky's HealthCare Campus to better coordinate its cooperative program with Kentucky Children's Hospital.

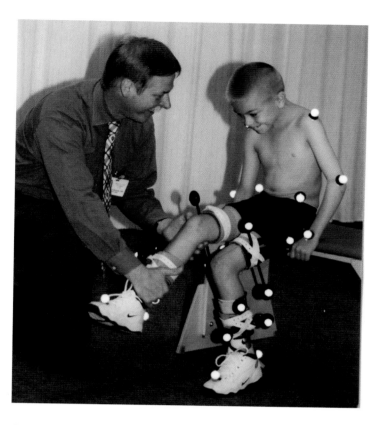

Dr. Chester M. Tylkowski ensures that all of Casey's reflective markers are in place before the youngster begins his gait analysis at Shriners Children's Lexington.

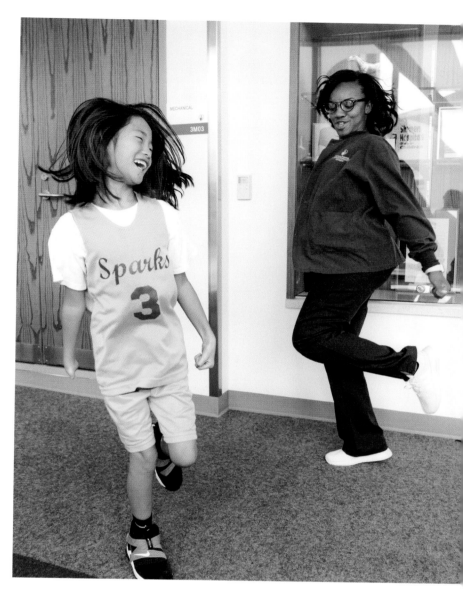

Organized into three units covering specialty care, rehabilitation and ambulatory surgery, Shriners Children's Lexington now treats more than 16,000 active patients, including Addlee, dancing in the foreground.

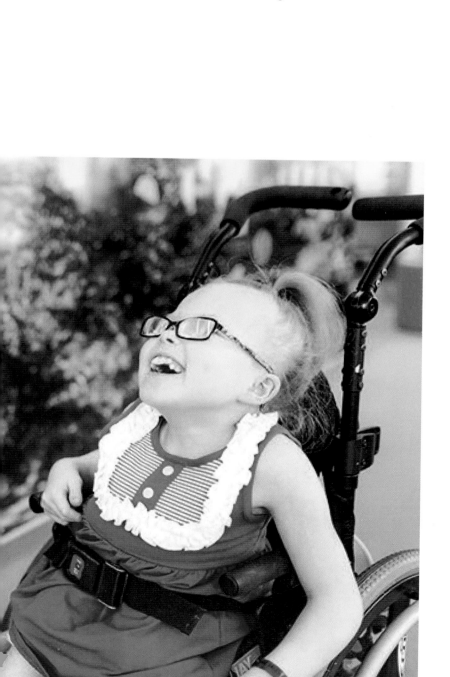

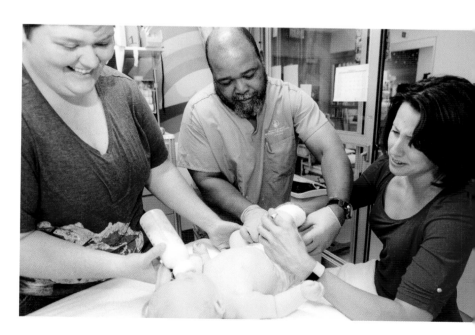

Kristy soothes her son Brantley with a bottle as staff at Shriners Children's Lexington fit him with a new cast.

GREENVILLE, SOUTH CAROLINA
SEPTEMBER 1, 1927

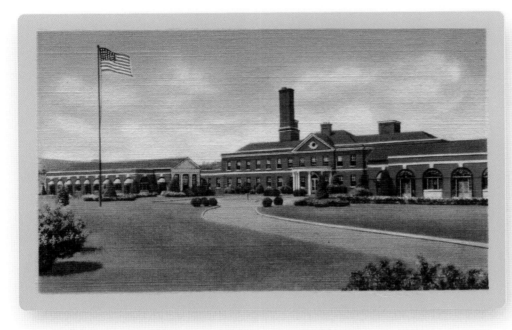

Shriners Children's would not have been founded without the generosity of thousands of individual donors, but the Greenville unit stands out in owing its existence to one benefactor, W. W. Burgiss, a local businessman who wrote a check for $350,000 (about $5.9 million in today's dollars) to buy the land and build the facility.

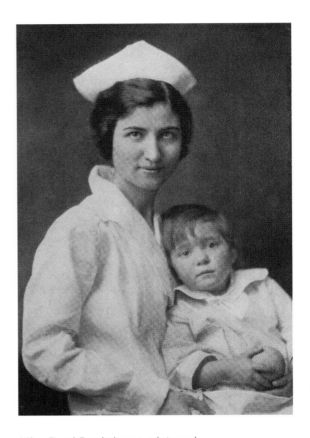

Miss Byrd Boehringer, pictured here with a patient, was the first superintendent of Shriners Children's Greenville.

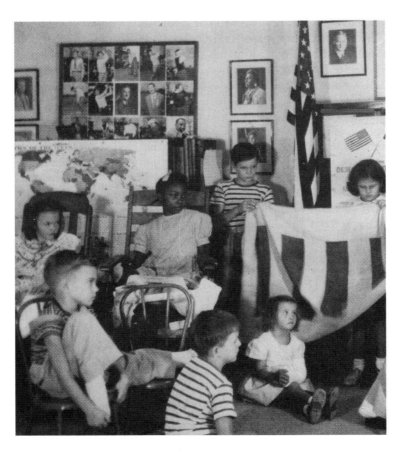

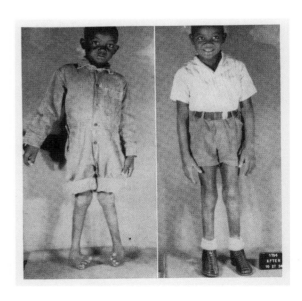

In 1932, 5-year-old Hilton was admitted to Shriners Children's Greenville for a series of operations on his feet. In 1947, he joined the staff.

All Shriners Children's hospitals admitted children, regardless of race. This was controversial in the South during the Jim Crow era. Bravely, the staff resisted local pressure and upheld the hospital's standards of inclusivity.

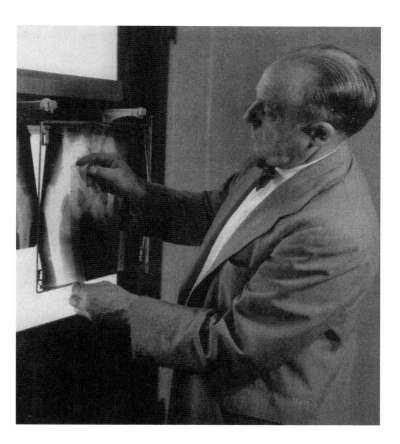

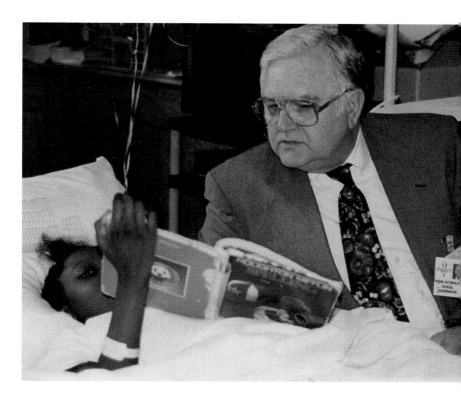

After retiring as principal of a local elementary school, Frank Sutherland continued to volunteer at Shriners Children's Greenville.

Dr. J. Warren White served at Shriners Children's Hawaii before accepting a position as Chief Surgeon at the Greenville hospital.

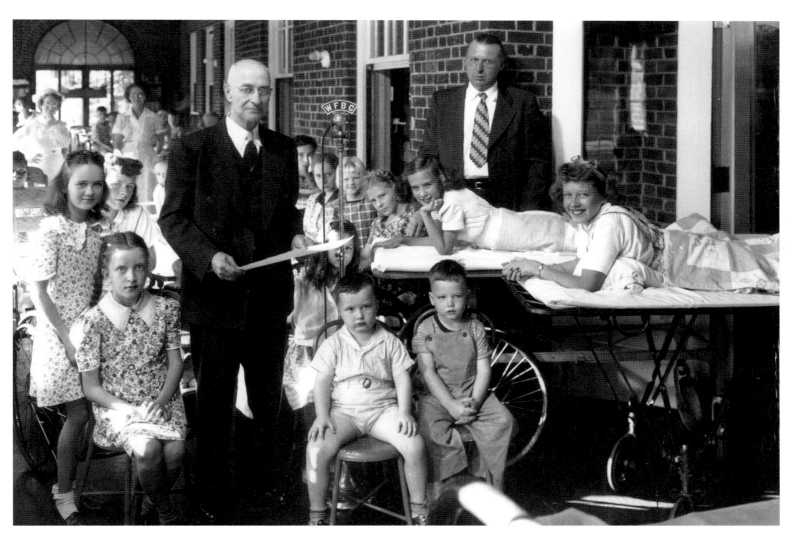

In 1946, Jacob T. Solomons, Jr., a member of the board of Shriners Children's Greenville, standing at the center, was honored for his service to children on the "Big Little American" feature of "The Coke Club," a nationwide radio program hosted by Morton Downey.

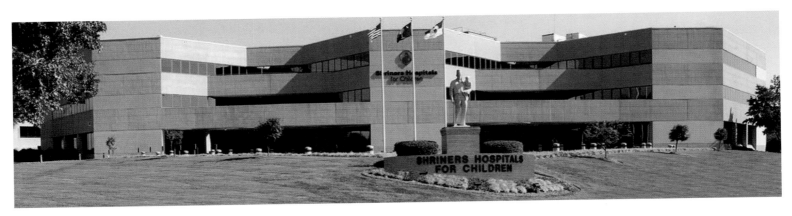

Shriners Children's Greenville was expanded several times in the 1950s and 1960s, and was finally replaced with a new $25 million facility in 1989.

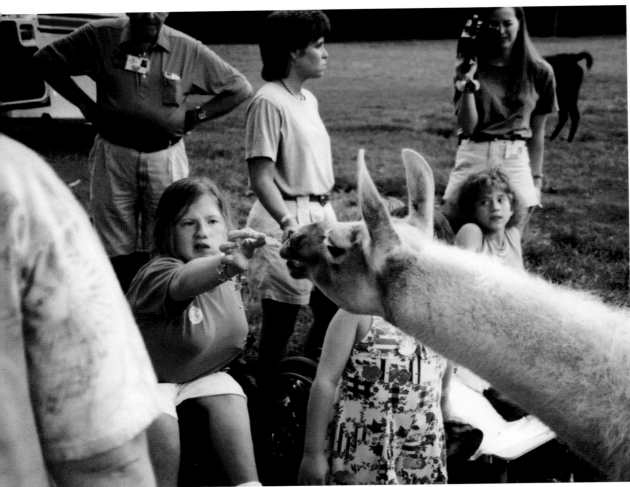

Patients at Camp Eagle's Wing, a 12-day in-house rehabilitation program at Shriners Children's Greenville for children with spina bifida, 1993.

9-year-old Sheera has the world in hand after rehabilitation at Shriners Children's Greenville, 1993.

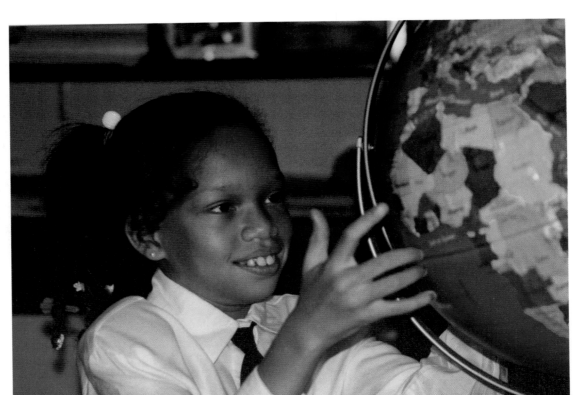

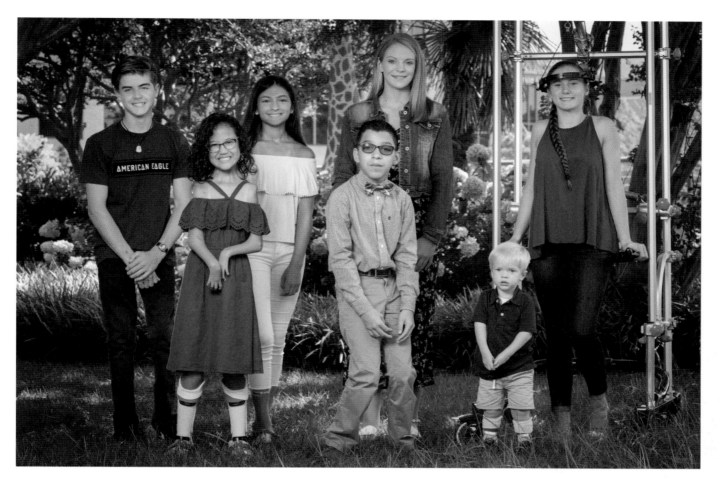

Today, patients at Shriners Children's Greenville are treated for a wide variety of medical conditions.

Members of the medical team at Shriners Children's Greenville strike a heroic pose, 2021.

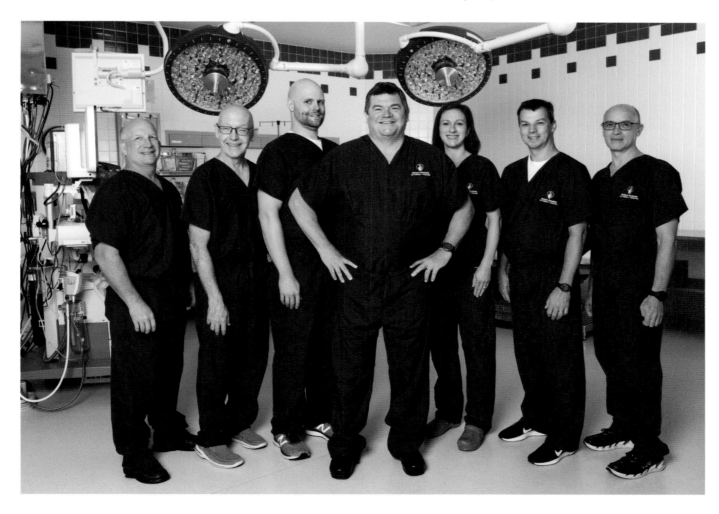

MEXICO CITY, MEXICO
MARCH 10, 1945

The leadership of Shriners International had long determined not to build more hospitals than their membership dues could sustain; so in 1928, they decided to stop establishing new facilities — a prescient choice given the financial impact of the Great Depression. But in 1944, they voted to make an exception. A new public hospital for children had recently opened in Mexico City, and the leaders of the local Shriners saw an opportunity. Anezeh Temple would commit $10,000 a year (over $166,000 in today's money) to sponsor a Shriners Children's facility within the Hospital Infantíl de Mexico if the Imperial Council would provide matching funds. It was an easy decision.

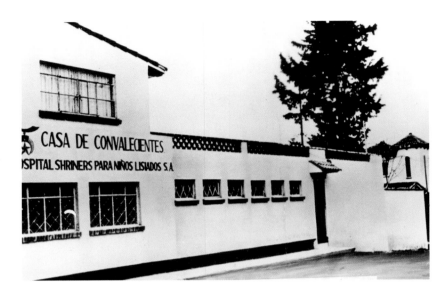

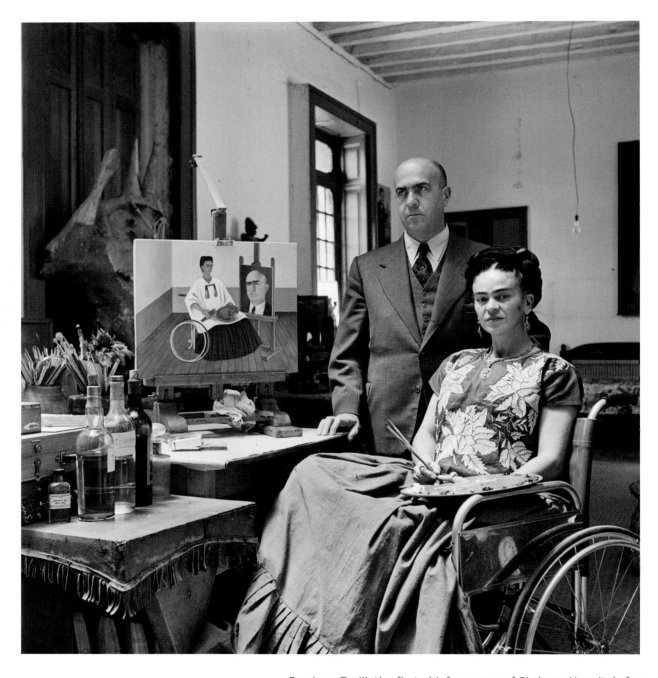

Dr. Juan Farill, the first chief surgeon of Shriners Hospitals for Children Mexico, with his most famous patient, Frida Kahlo, 1948.

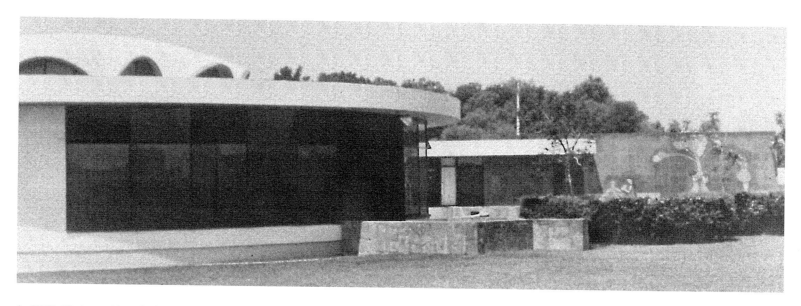

In 1961, Shriners Hospitals for Children Mexico moved to a new facility in Xotepingo, a suburb of Mexico City, which ultimately served thousands of children from Latin America over the course of 45 years.

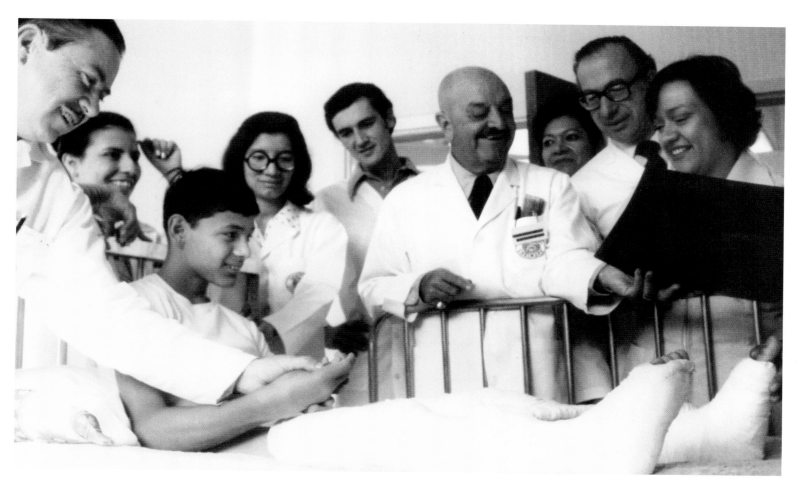

Above: The medical staff at Shriners Hospitals for Children Mexico examine the results of a successful treatment.

Right: A young patient examines the credentials of Dr. Nelson Cassis, Chief of Staff at Shriners Hospitals for Children Mexico, during an outreach clinic in Ciudad Juarez, 1992.

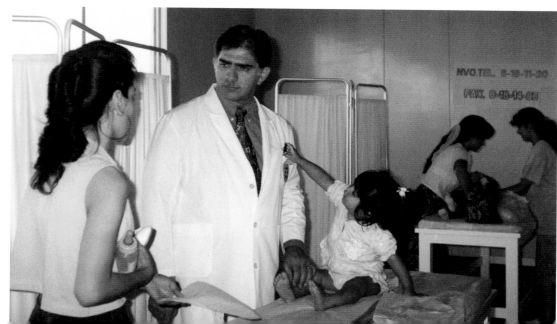

93

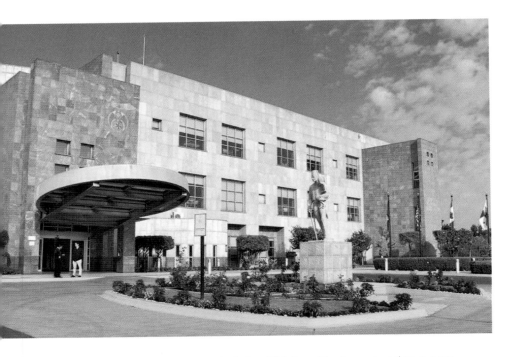

In 2006, Shriners Hospitals for Children Mexico moved to a new modern building in Pedregal de Santa Úrsula, with expanded facilities for both treatment and medical research.

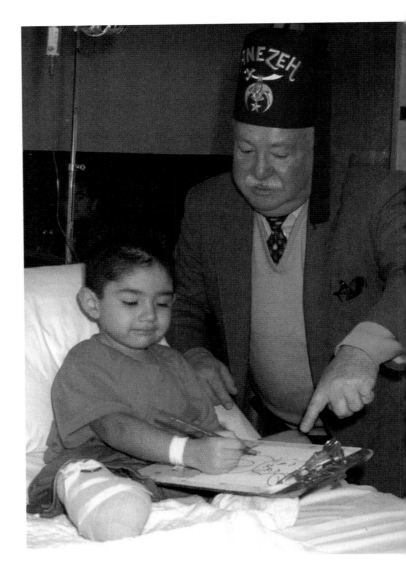

Right: Anezeh Past Potentate Victor Montalvo visits with Bruno, recuperating from leg surgery, 2001.

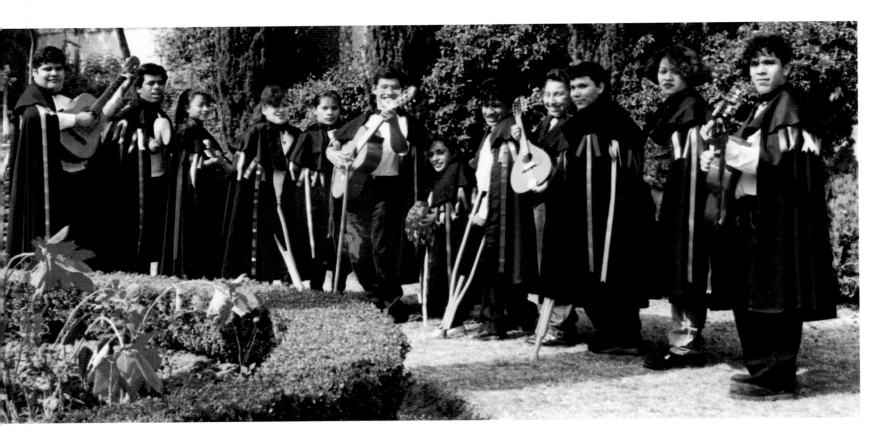

An Estudiantina comprised of former patients performs in the gardens at Shriners Hospitals for Children Mexico.

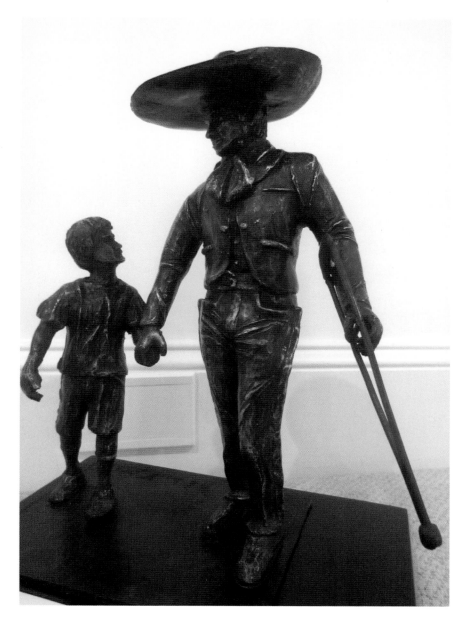

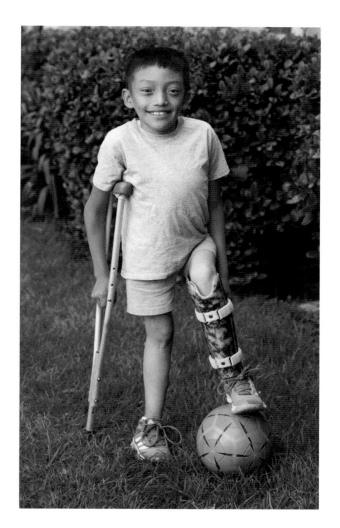

Above: Nothing can keep Abdiel away from his soccer ball.

Left: A uniquely Mexican variant of the Editorial Without Words at the hospital trades the fez for a sombrero.

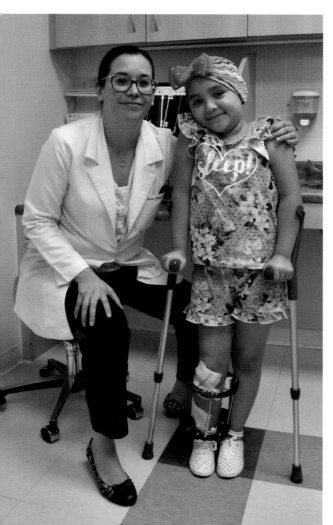

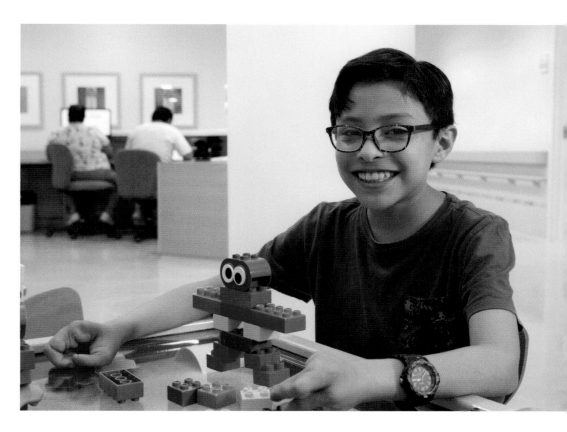

Above: Saul uses construction blocks to improve his dexterity.

Left: Dr. Daniela Velázquez and one of her grateful patients at Shriners Hospitals for Children Mexico, 2021.

95

GALVESTON, TEXAS
FEBRUARY 1, 1952 AND MARCH 20, 1966

The present Shriners Children's facility in Texas combines two units that were established separately. In 1919, Arabia Shriners in Houston founded a small pediatric clinic. In 1946, Houston Shriners initiated a fund drive to expand the clinic into a 40-bed hospital. In only 10 days, they raised over $541,000 — over $8.2 million in today's dollars. The Arabia Shriners' new clinic opened in 1952. In 1966, it was formally adopted into the Shriners Children's healthcare system.

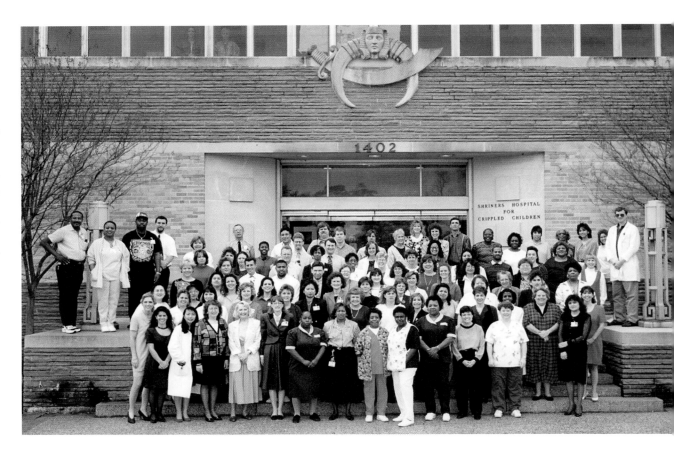

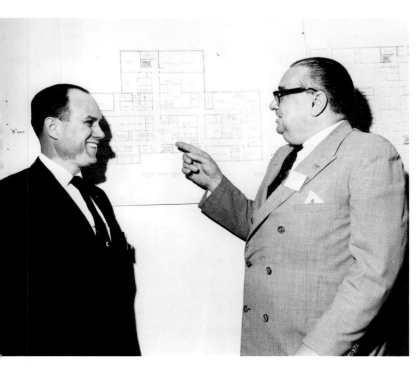

That same year, Shriners Children's embarked on a bold new venture, building its first pediatric hospital dedicated to treating burn injuries in Galveston, Texas. Here, Harvey A. Beffa (right), founder of the Shriners Burns Institutes, reviews plans with Dr. Jack B. Lee of Alzafar Temple, San Antonio.

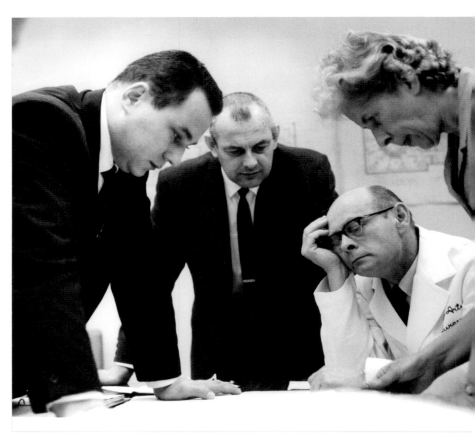

Dr. Curtis Price Artz, seated, was the first Chief Surgeon of the Galveston unit and the first burns specialist in the Shriners Children's hospital system.

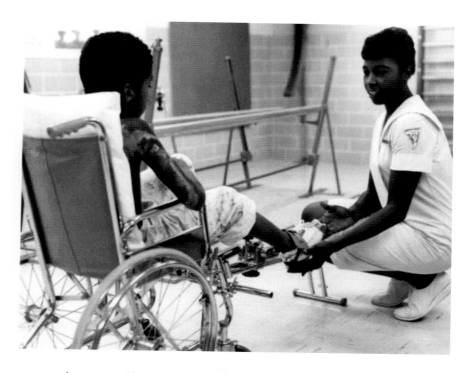

A nurse at Shriners Children's Texas prepares a patient for physical therapy on the parallel bars.

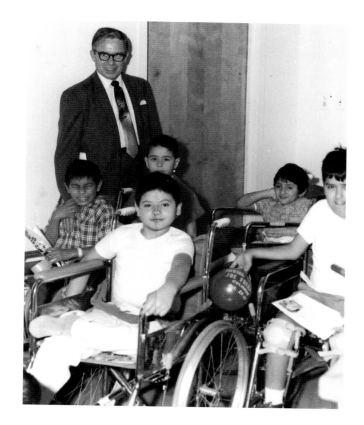

James F. Hull, administrator of Shriners Children's Texas in Houston, with some of his charges, 1970s.

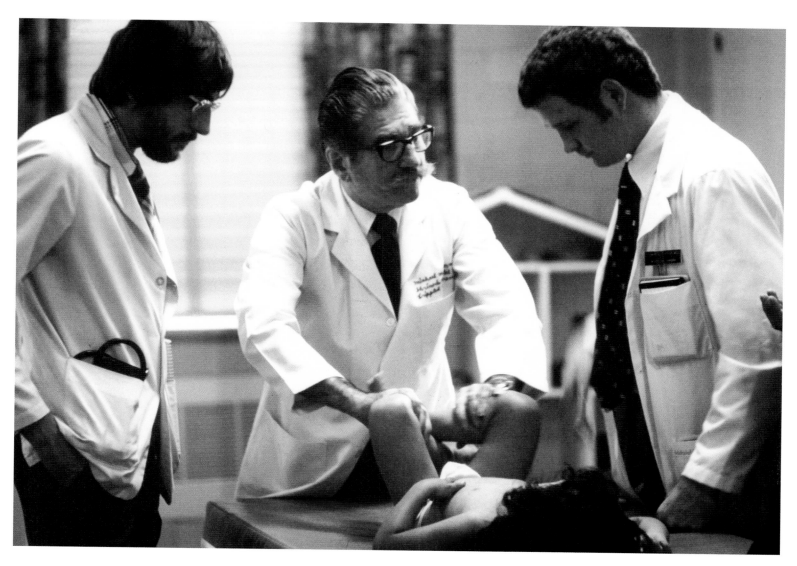

Dr. Michael M. Donovan, Chief Surgeon of the Houston unit from 1969 to 1980, models patient care for medical residents.

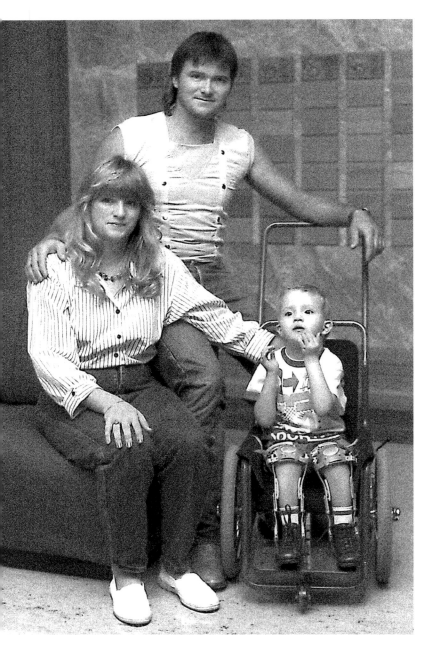

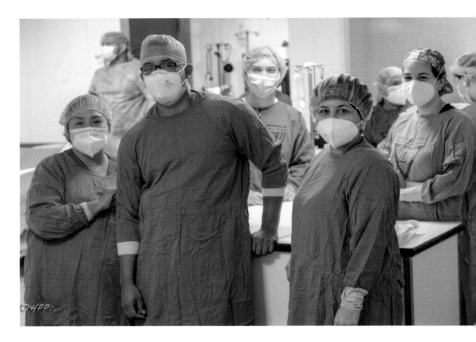

The Houston unit focused on microvascular orthopedics and established one of the system's first gait labs. In association with the University of Texas Medical Branch, the Galveston hospital worked on developing new techniques for healing wounds and grafting skin. In 2021, the two hospitals merged, with the staff and programs of the Houston hospital moving to the facility in Galveston.

Bullard, Texas, residents Michele and Shannon did not know what to do to help their son Jesse, born with cerebral palsy and other congenital conditions, until they met a Shriner from Sharon Temple. "It's not just the medical care," Michele said in 1990, praising the staff at Shriners Children's Texas. "Everyone here is always available for moral support."

When a volcano erupted in Guatemala in 2018, the U.S. Air Force transported six badly injured burn victims 1500 miles aboard a C-17 Globemaster III aircraft to Shriners Children's Texas for emergency treatment.

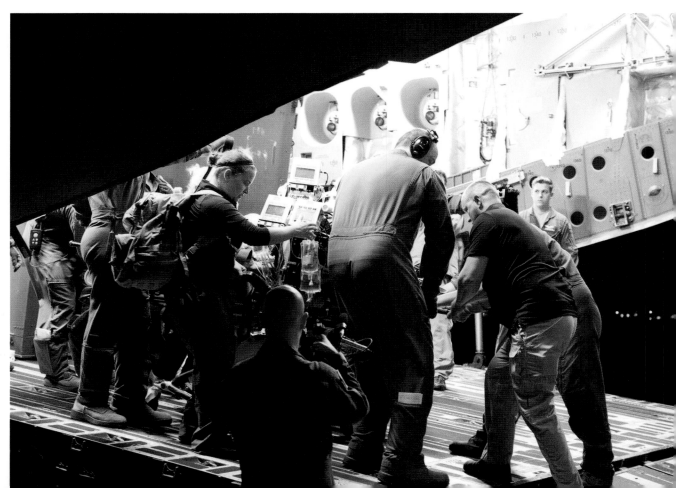

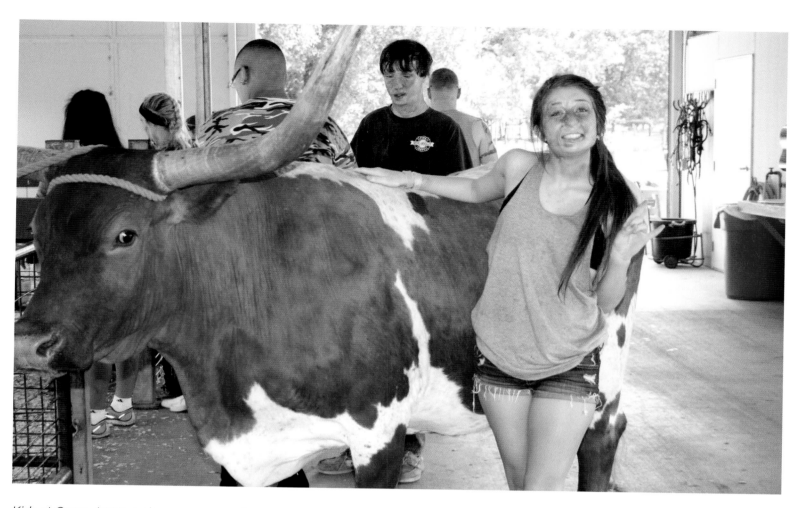

Kids at Camp Janus, a sleepaway camp for young burn patients in Burton, Texas, 2018.

Nancy Chapman of Shriners Children's Texas displays her 2020 DAISY Award® for extraordinary nursing.

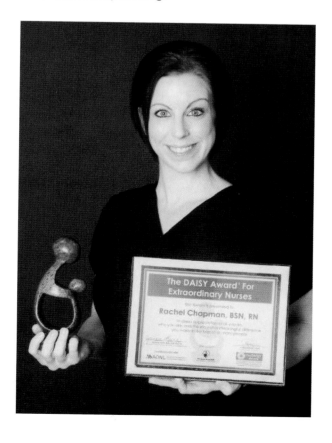

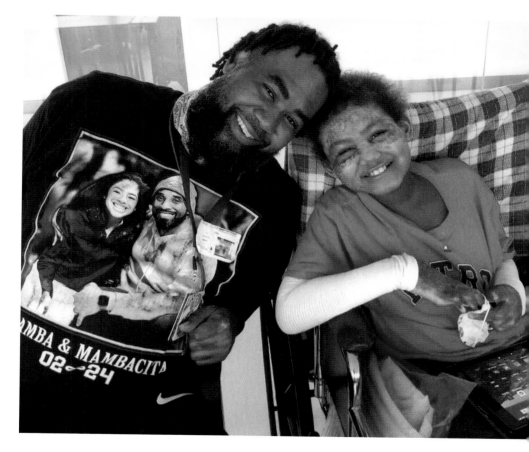

John was badly injured when his house burned down in 2020, but it was worse for his son TJ. After almost 30 surgeries at Shriners Children's Texas, TJ is on the road to recovery. "From the Chief of Staff, all the way down to the techs — everyone's been great. I just can't speak enough about them, how they made us feel as parents and patient," said John. "This is an amazing place."

PASADENA, CALIFORNIA
FEBRUARY 25, 1952

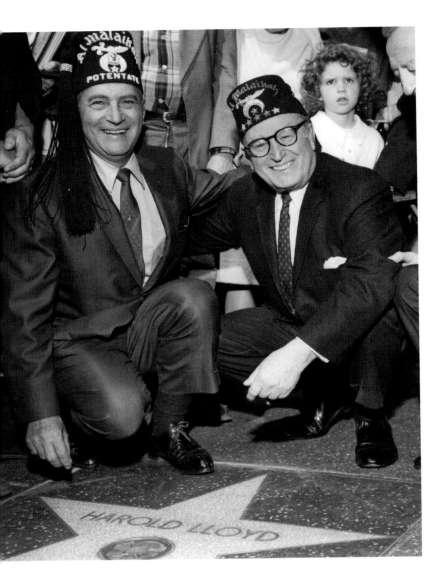

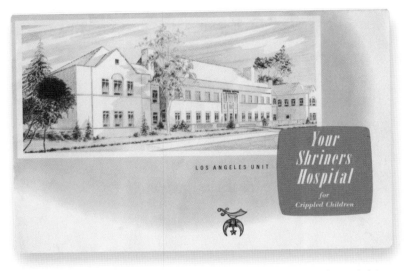

In 1944, Al Malaikah Potentate Francis Stearns initiated an eight-year project to build a new hospital. In 1952, Shriners Children's Southern California opened to the community. The construction cost $1.5 million — almost $17 million in today's dollars. The facility was completely retrofitted between 1983 and 1985.

In 1928, one member of Al Malaikah personally funded the production of a feature film to showcase the work of the hospitals at a cost of $50,000 — over $845,000 in today's dollars. The film, now lost, featured child star Philippe de Lacy and was screened nationwide.

Located next to Hollywood, Al Malaikah, in Los Angeles, California, has supplied the fraternity with more than its share of celebrities, including John Wayne, Mel Blanc, and Buzz Aldrin. Here Harold Lloyd (in spectacles), one of the greatest film comedians of the silent era and a proud member of the Shrine, squats near his star on the Hollywood Walk of Fame. A past Imperial Potentate, Lloyd served as Chairman of the Board of Trustees of Shriners Children's from 1963 until his death in 1971.

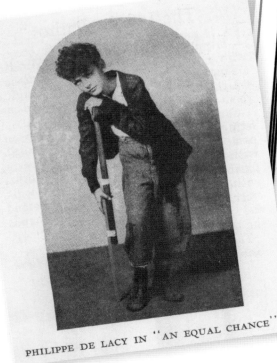

PHILIPPE DE LACY IN "AN EQUAL CHANCE"

Special Announcement
AN EQUAL CHANCE

"An Equal Chance" is the title of a three-reel film produced by the Metro-Goldwyn-Mayer Company, telling the story of the Shriners' Hospital for Crippled Children. The picture has been indorsed by the Imperial Council and is being shown by the temples of the Shrine throughout the country.

The cost of the film is being defrayed by Noble Allen H. Ratterlee of Al Malaikah Temple, Los Angeles, as his contribution to the Shriners' Hospital for Crippled Children.

It is a wonderfully well acted film story, starring Philip De-Lacy, Metro star, showing the greatest piece of welfare work ever undertaken by any organization in the world.

In addition to this film, another one will be shown, the actual work done at the Greenville, S. C., Hospital for Crippled Children. This is an actual picture taken of actual cases in the hospital.

DON'T MISS SEEING THESE PICTURES AT THE
LYRIC THEATER
BILLINGS
THURSDAY, JUNE 7th

Performances at 5:30 p. m., 6:30 p. m., 7:30 p. m. and 8:30 p. m.

Admission Free to all Masons and Their Friends
Children Only Accompanied By Adults

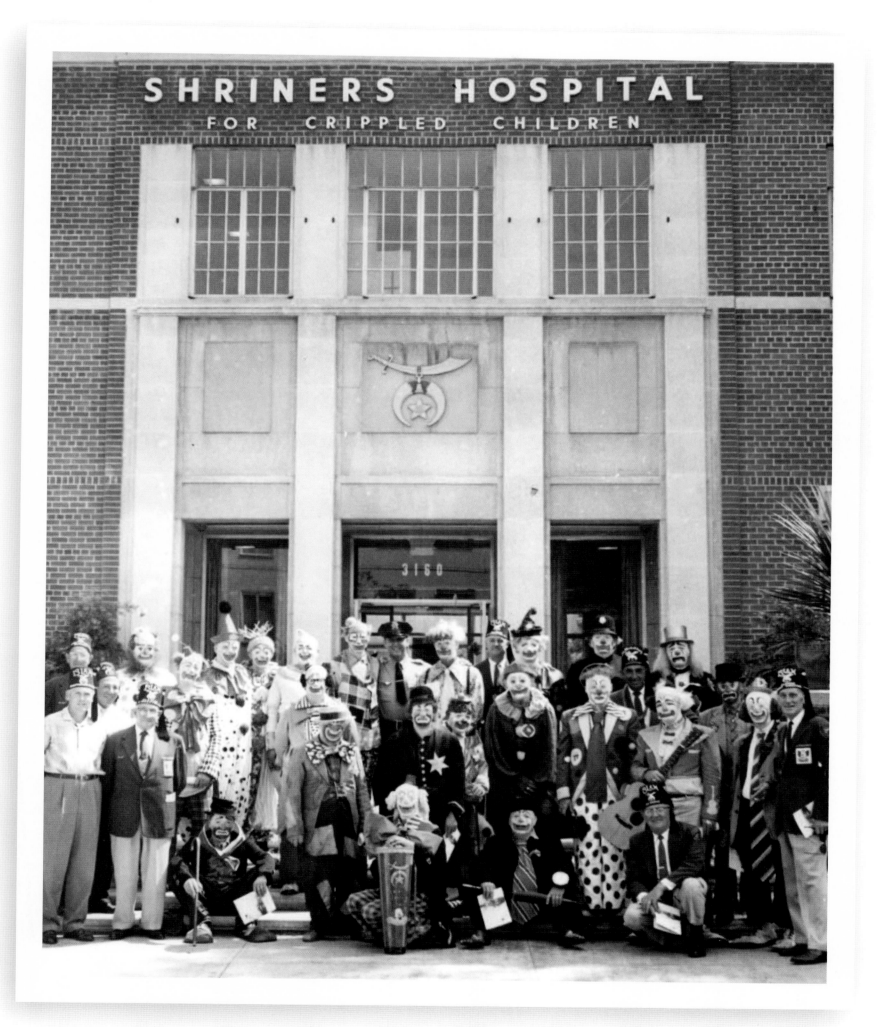

Clowns and other Shriners assembled at Shriners Children's Los Angeles, early 1960s.

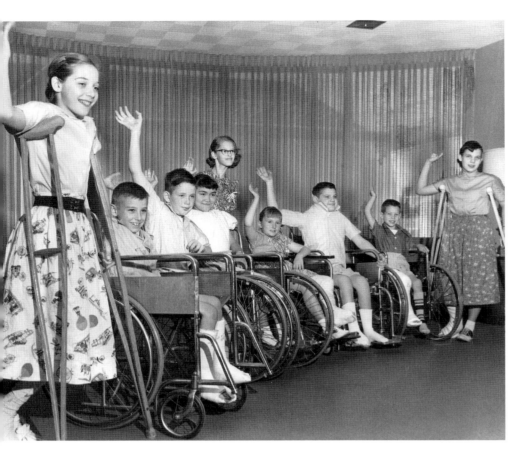

Patients at Shriners Children's Southern California afflicted with polio cheer the news of that a vaccine has been invented to curb the disease, 1955.

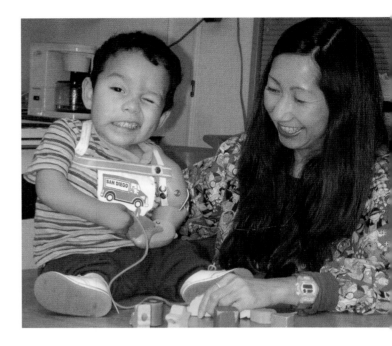

Kevin, age 2, practices stringing beads with his new prosthetic left arm as Joanne Shida, a registered occupational therapist, looks on, 2001.

Shriners Children's Southern California patient Gianna performs a sun salutation on the beach of Los Angeles, 2013.

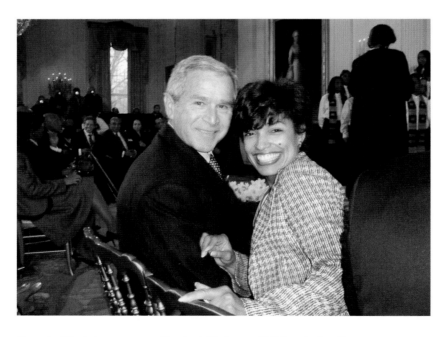

Bonnie St. John was a patient at Shriners Children's Southern California from kindergarten through high school. She went on to graduate with honors from Harvard and win a Rhodes Scholarship. She made sports history by being the first African American to medal in any winter Olympic event, competing at the 1984 Winter Paralympic Games in Innsbruck, Austria. Bonnie served as a director of the National Economic Council in the Clinton White House and as an Olympic emissary for President Barack Obama. She was honored by President George W. Bush as "the kind of person that shows that individual courage matters in life."

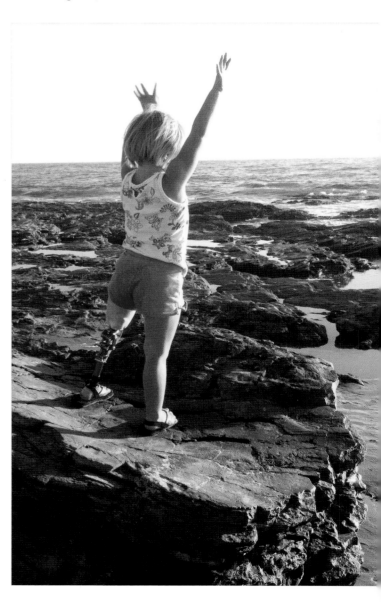

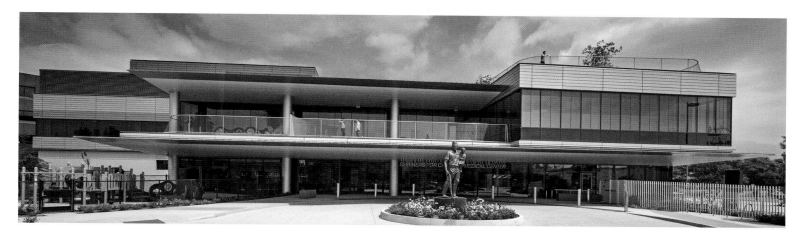

In 2017, to comply with new seismic regulations, the entire unit moved from Los Angeles to a new state-of-the-art facility in Pasadena.

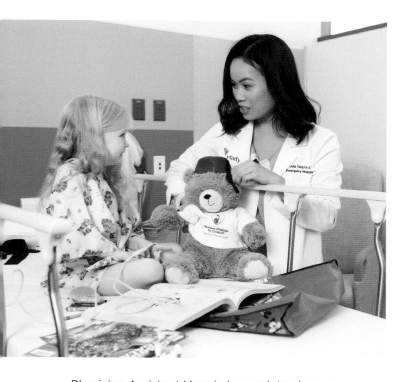

Physician Assistant Vangie Luong introduces a young patient to Fezzy, the official mascot of Shriners Hospitals for Children.

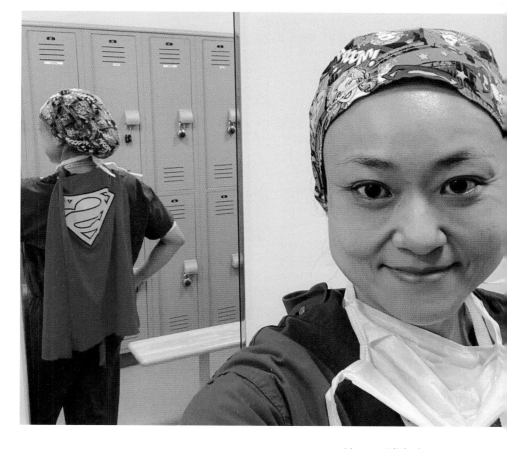

Team members at Shriners Children's Southern California celebrate May the Fourth, 2022.

Above: Blithely unaware of the mirror behind her, Dr. Selina Poon, an orthopedic surgeon at Shriners Children's Southern California, inadvertently reveals her secret identity, 2020.

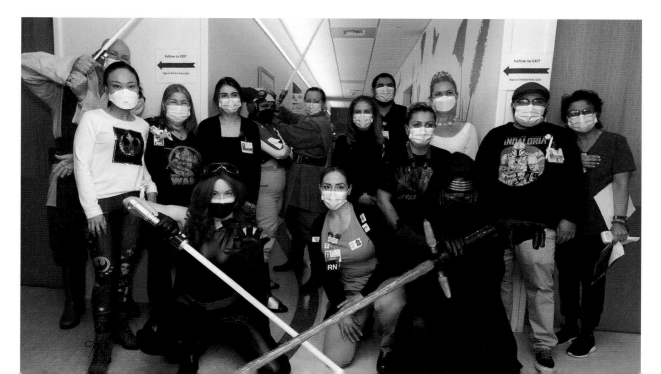

ERIE, PENNSYLVANIA
APRIL 1, 1967

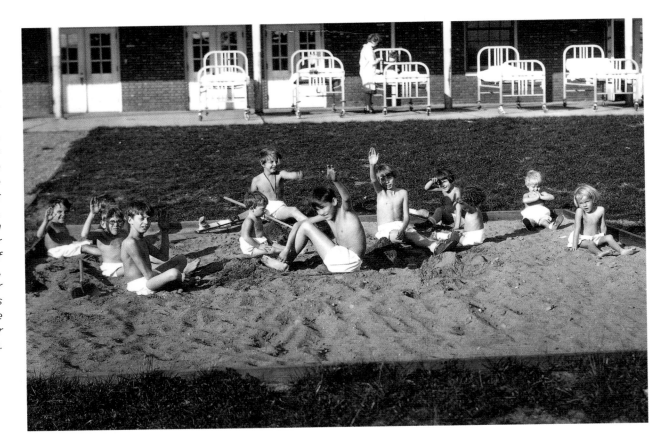

Shriners Children's Erie started in 1924, with a summer camp sponsored by Zem Zem Shriners for pediatric patients at the Hamot Hospital. This venture was so successful that, in the fall, the board of the temple determined to establish a permanent institution. In 1927, the Zem Zem Hospital opened for the rehabilitation of children with polio, tuberculosis and other conditions. Patients were referred to the Hamot Hospital for major surgeries.

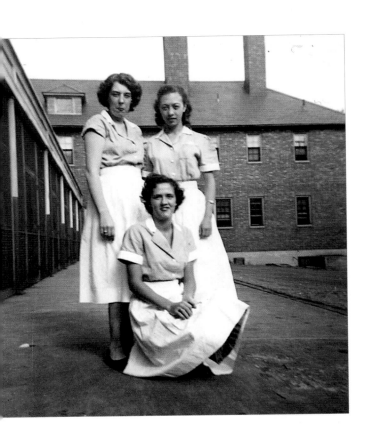

Nurses at the original Zem Zem Hospital, 1930s.

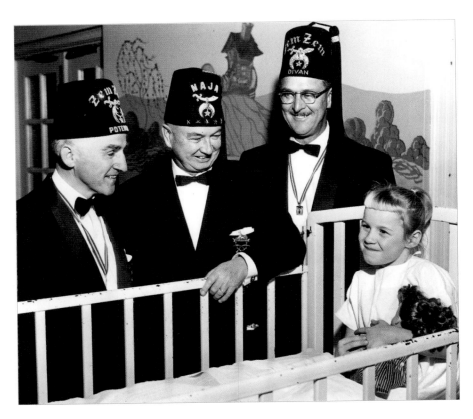

A contingent of Nobles visit the hospital, 1956.

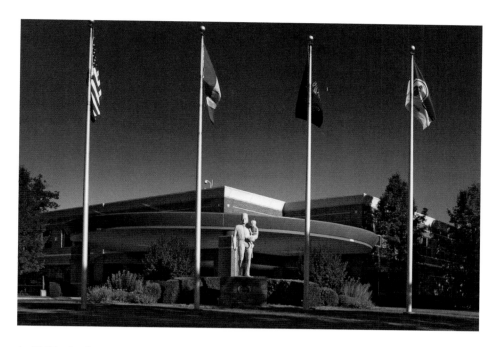

In 1967, the hospital was welcomed into the Shriners Children's healthcare system, which expanded the Erie facility to make it fully operational as a center for pediatric surgery. A continuing series of improvements culminated in a $2 million expansion in 1994.

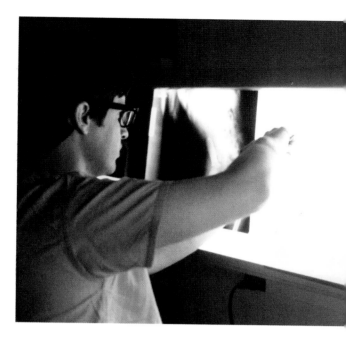

Dr. Joao Tavares, orthopedic surgeon at Shriners Children's Erie, examines an X-ray, 1978.

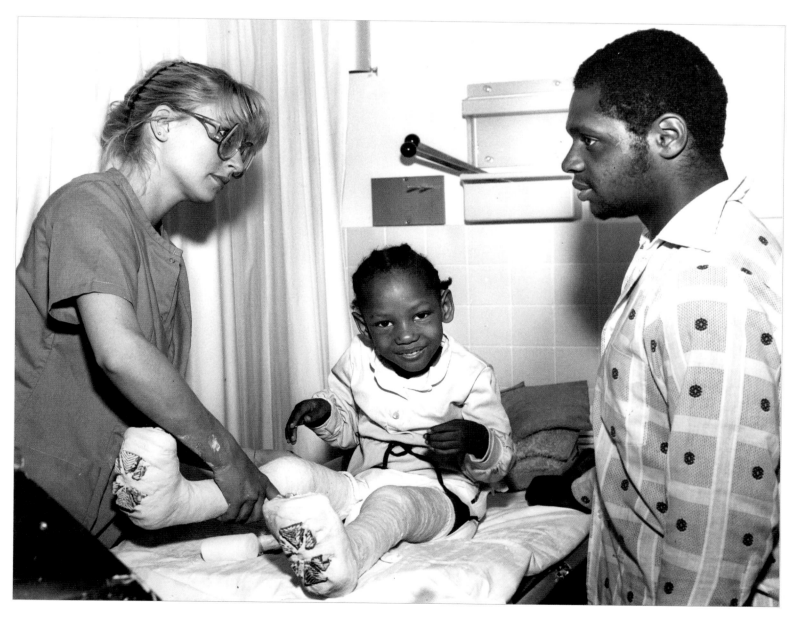

Nurse Sue Margraf checks Tonia's dressings, as her father looks on, 1970s.

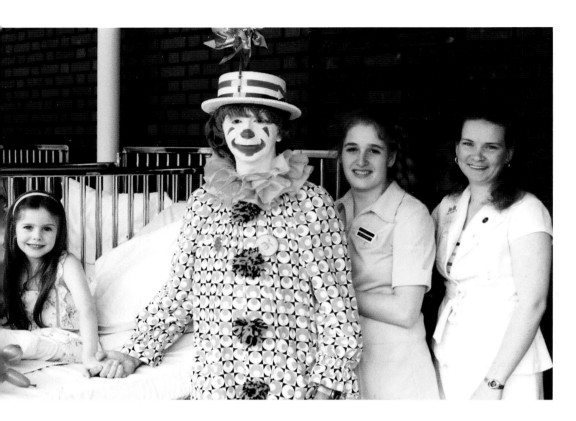

A clown brings joy to patients and staff alike at Shriners Children's Erie, early 1980s.

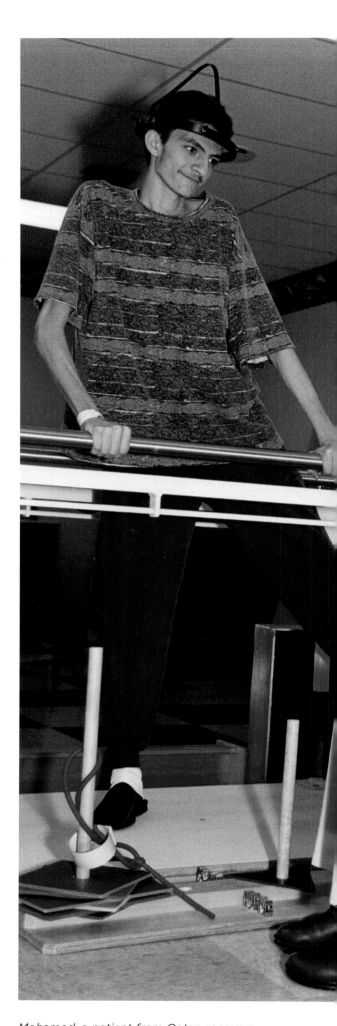

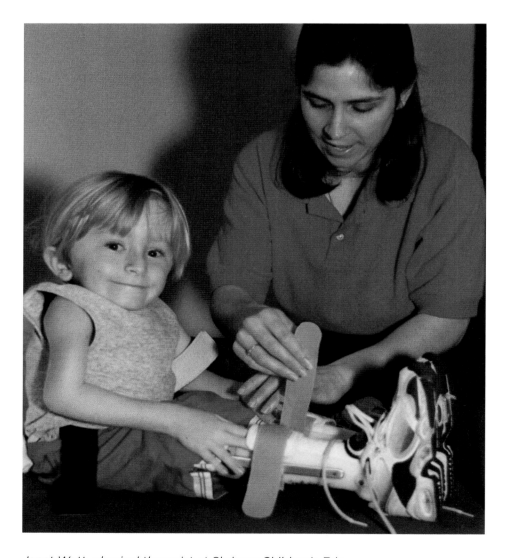

Janet Watt, physical therapist at Shriners Children's Erie, straps leg braces on Colton, who has ostogenesis imperfecta.

Mohamed, a patient from Qatar, recovers after surgery for severe scoliosis with the help of physical therapist Alicia Malinowski, 2000.

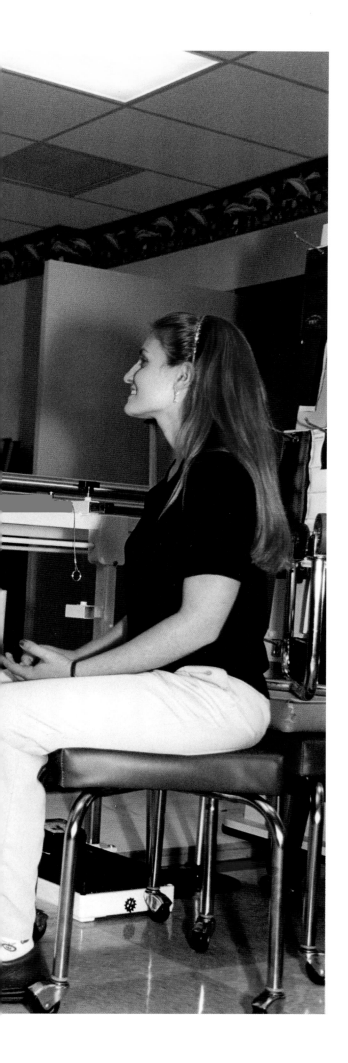

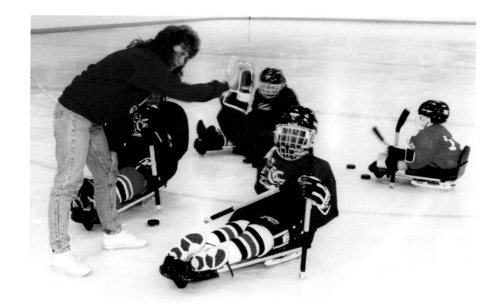

Sue Berkmire, RN, coach of the Mighty Otters — the sled hockey team at Shriners Children's Erie — gives Melissa a high five, 1997.

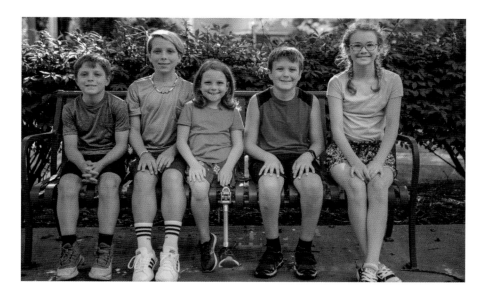

In 2012, Shriners Children's Erie met changing healthcare needs by transitioning from an inpatient model to an ambulatory medical model focusing on scoliosis, cerebral palsy, torticollis and orthopedic conditions.

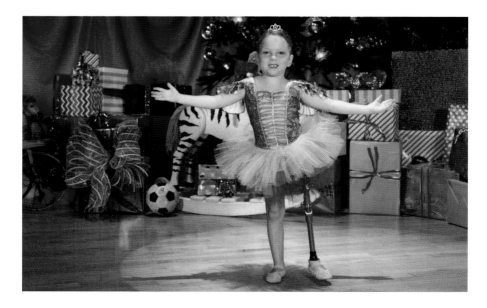

Sarah, ballerina, 2020.

DAYTON, OHIO
FEBRUARY 19, 1968

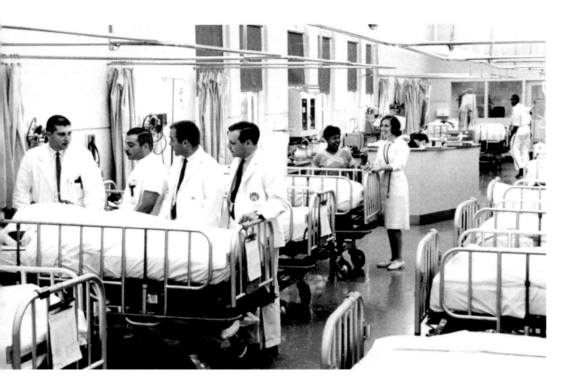

Shriners Children's Ohio was founded as part of the system's expanded mission for burn care, operating for four years before officially opening in Cincinnati in 1968. Together with the Shriners Children's burn hospitals in Galveston and Boston, the Ohio facility focused not only on treating patients, but also on developing protocols and procedures for fire safety and on promoting awareness through such campaigns as Burn Awareness Week.

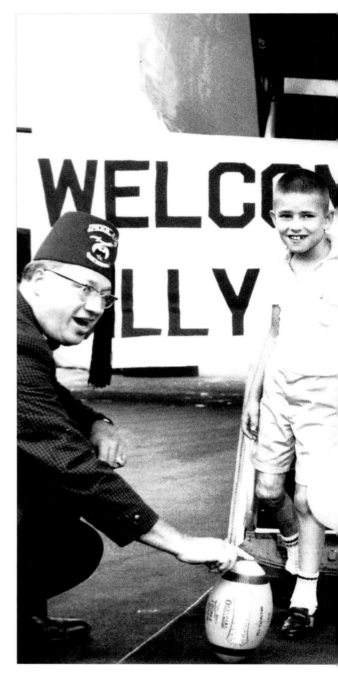

Harvey A. Beffa, Sr., the Potentate who organized the Shriners burns program, with Billy, the first patient admitted to Shriners Children's Ohio, February 1, 1964.

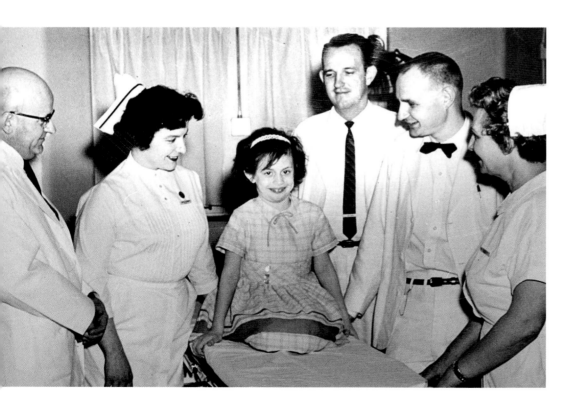

Seven-year-old Juanita, a resident of Chicago, was the first patient to be air evacuated to Shriners Children's Ohio, February 8, 1964.

Right: Imperial Barney W. Collins parades in a Shriners Children's Ohio car, flanked by young men from DeMolay International, a fraternal order for young men aged 12 to 21, 1965.

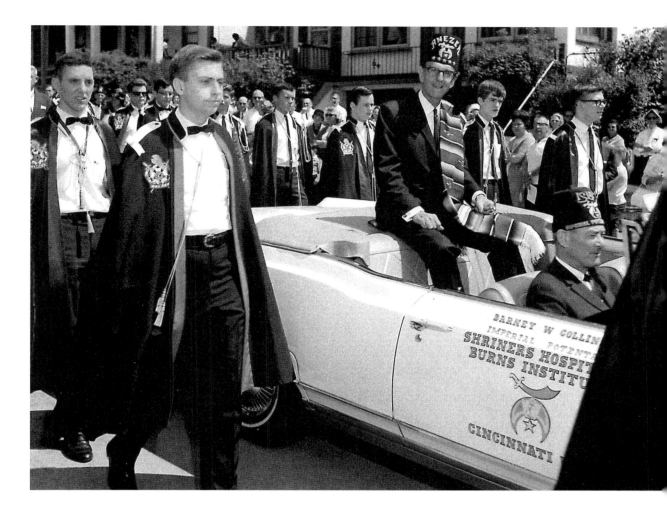

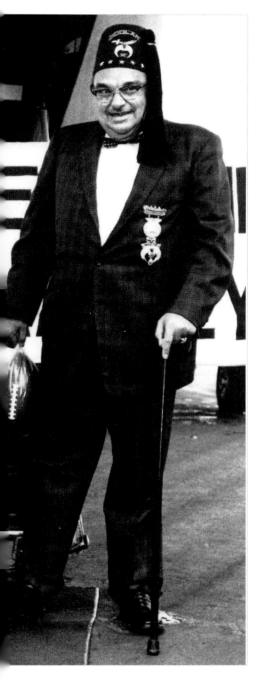

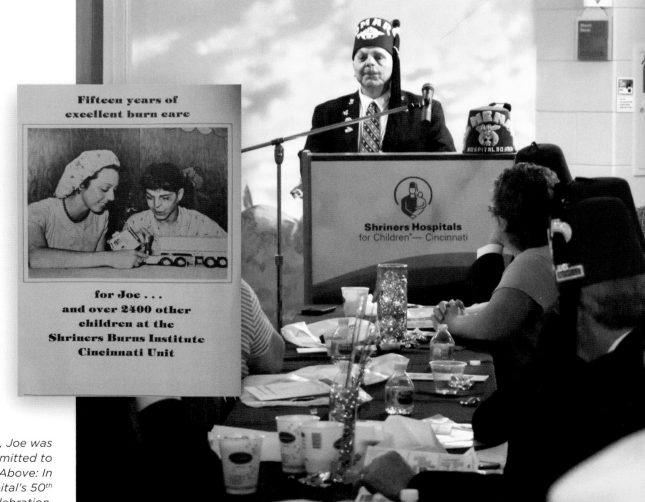

Fifteen years of excellent burn care

for Joe . . . and over 2400 other children at the Shriners Burns Institute Cincinnati Unit

Severely burned in 1965, Joe was one of the first patients admitted to Shriners Children's Ohio. Above: In 2018, he spoke at the hospital's 50th anniversary celebration.

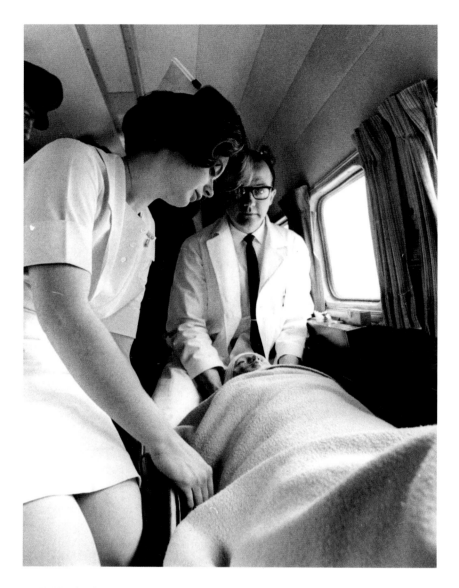

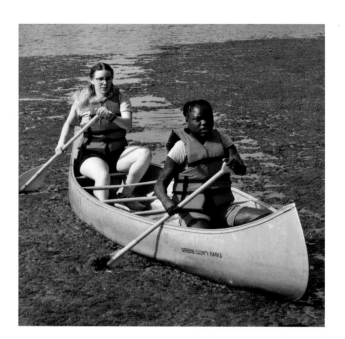

Since 1989, Camp Ytiliba ("Ability" spelled backward), sponsored by Shriners Children's Ohio, has helped recovering children to reintegrate into social life.

In 1968, the hospital organized its first air transport team to bring burn victims and other critically injured children to the hospital.

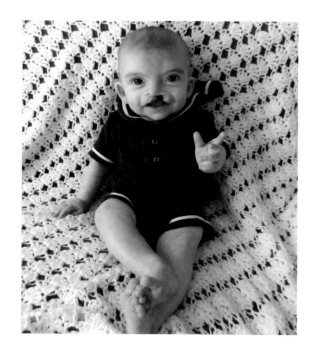

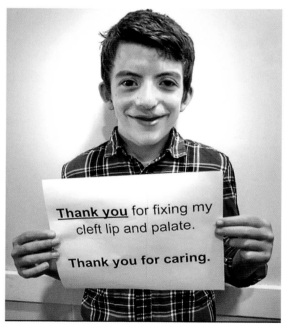

In the 1990s, Shriners Children's Ohio moved to a new facility and began to expand its burn program to address other complex wound and skin conditions, such as port wine stains, congenital ear deformities, cleft lip and palate, and other craniofacial conditions. Liam, now 10 years old (above right), was treated when he was a baby (above left).

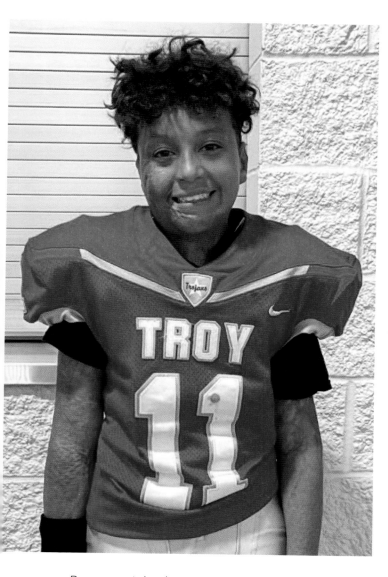

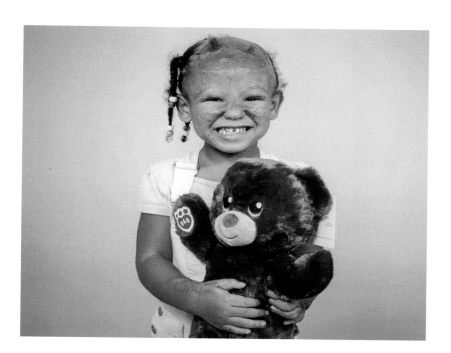

Shriners Children's Ohio has a long tradition of medical research. Here, a medical technician monitors brain activity during a study of sleep and burn recovery in 1994.

Bryson sustained second- and third-degree burns over 87% of his body when he was 8 years old and went through more 40 surgeries. Today, he competes in four sports: football, baseball, basketball, and track.

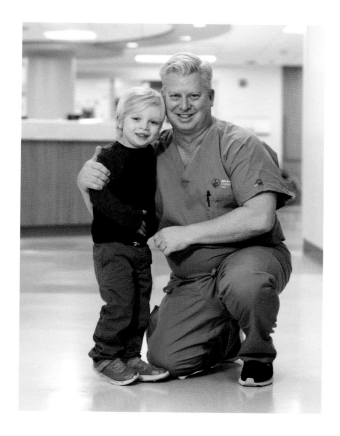

Nyla received life-saving care at Shriners Children's Ohio following a house fire when she was four weeks old. Today, she charms the world with her smile.

In 2021, Shriners Children's Ohio moved to Dayton to further expand access to services. Dr. Christopher B. Gordon, division chief of plastic surgery, poses with one of his patients.

BOSTON, MASSACHUSETTS
NOVEMBER 2, 1968

Right: Like the facilities in Galveston and Cincinnati, Shriners Children's Boston was founded as part of the burn care program. Here, Captain Lewis Goldstein of Aleppo Temple raises the flag at the new hospital as Colonel Malcolm G. Stevens, Jr. salutes.

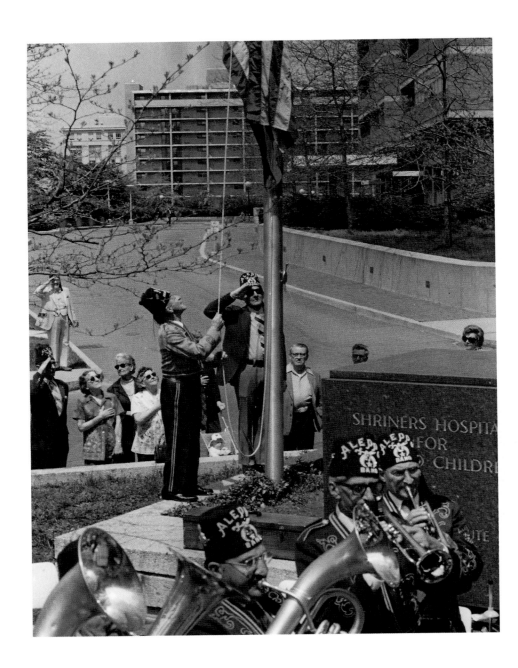

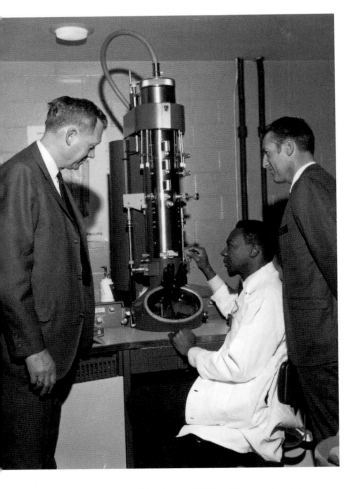

Located in the middle of a worldwide hub for medical research, the Boston facility has pioneered a number of crucial approaches to treatment. These range from developing a program to reintegrate children with burn injuries back to school and social life to instituting the world's first bank of human skin tissue. In this 1971 photograph, a researcher describes his work to visitors.

In the early days, some specialized medical equipment was made by volunteers. When doctors said they needed a toddler-sized hay-rake splint, used to straighten burned fingers, one Shriner called upon two friends, an industrial designer and a metalworker at Harvard Medical School. The two men designed and built this apparatus over 21 lunch hours.

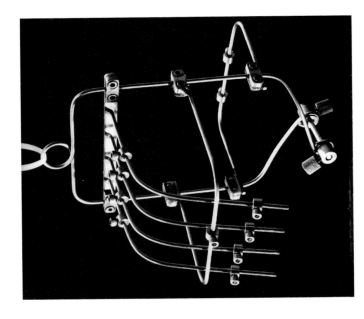

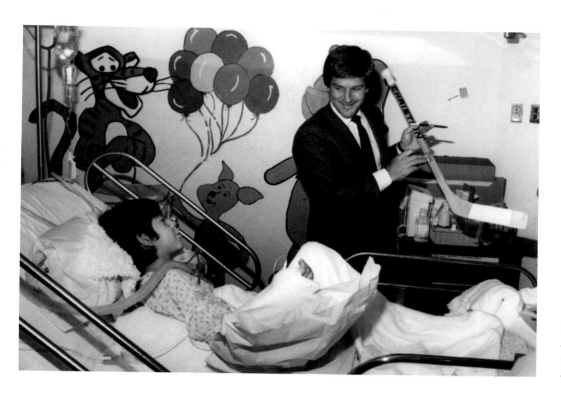

Recovering from surgery, José discusses hockey puck dynamics with Boston Bruins legend Bobby Orr, early 1970s.

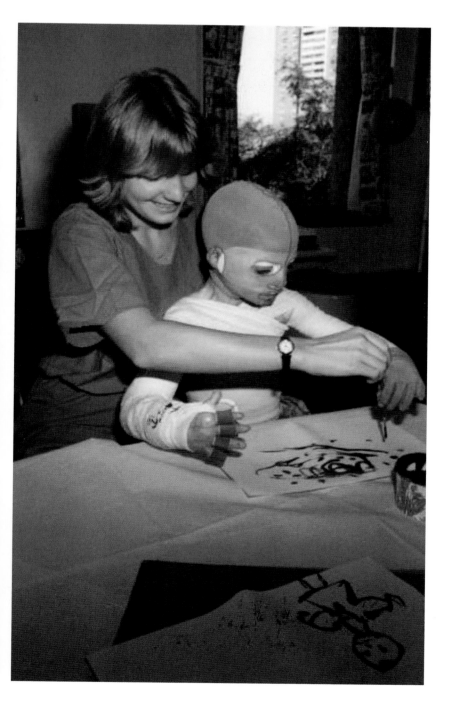

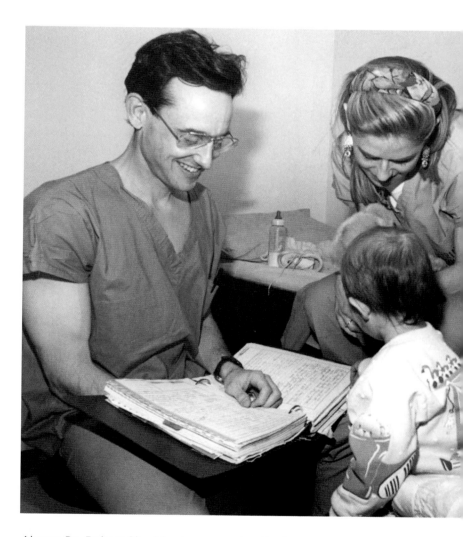

Above: Dr. Robert Sheridan has served patients at Shriners Children's Boston for over 30 years.

Left: A patient at Shriners Children's Boston wearing pressure garments – used to help prevent swelling and minimize scarring in burn patients — gets a helping hand, 1982.

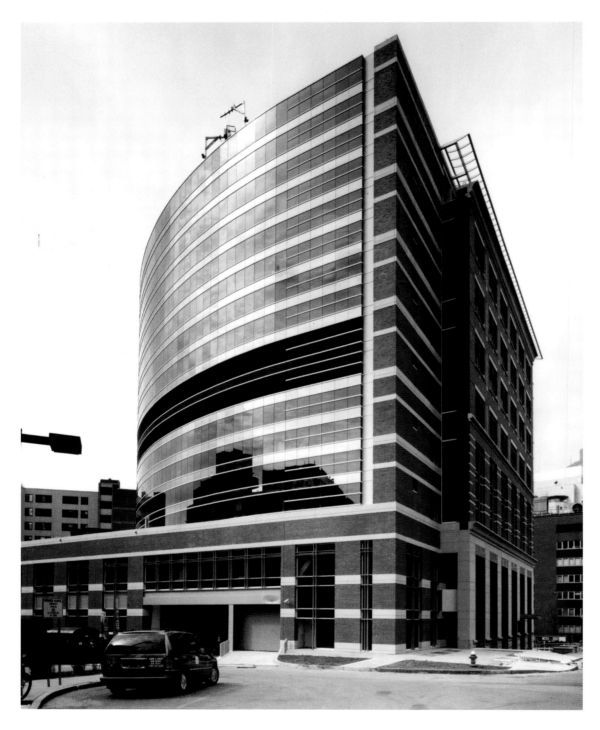

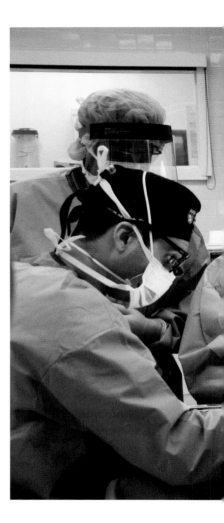

Shriners Children's Boston moved to a new building in 1999, expanding its services to cleft lip and palate, as well as reconstructive and plastic surgery.

Recovering from severe injuries is easier with support from a range of specialists. Kenia (center, in pink), a 21-year-old who was burned as a child in El Salvador, stands with her treatment team at Shriners Children's Boston

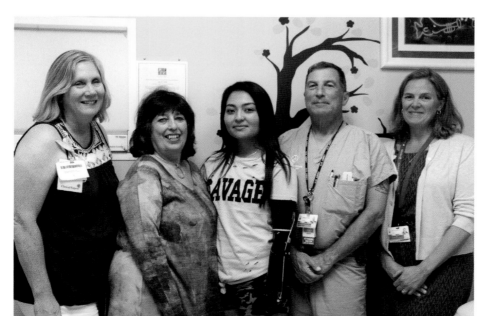

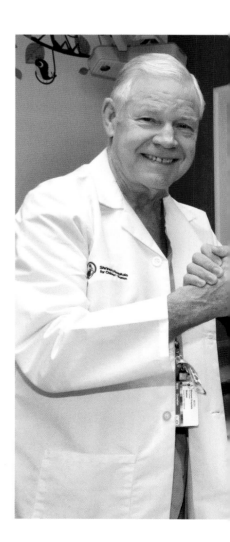

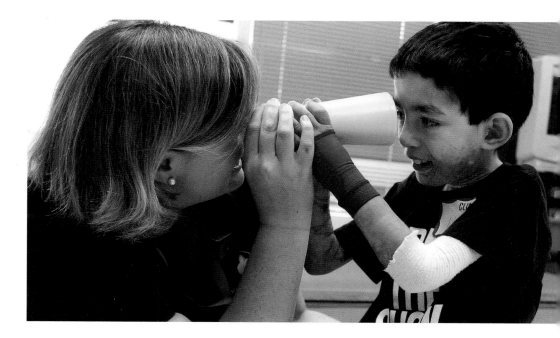

Ihor, an 11-year-old orphan from Ukraine, came to Shriners Hospital for Children in Boston severely malnourished and with life-threatening injuries. Thanks to his team, including occupational therapist Katherine Hartigan, he is able to walk again. "He'll be unstoppable," she predicted.

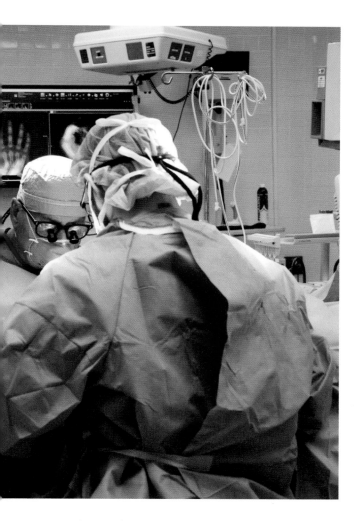

Above: Through its partnerships around the United States and across the globe, the facility has treated patients from over 70 countries, effecting cures in cases that other hospitals feared were hopeless.

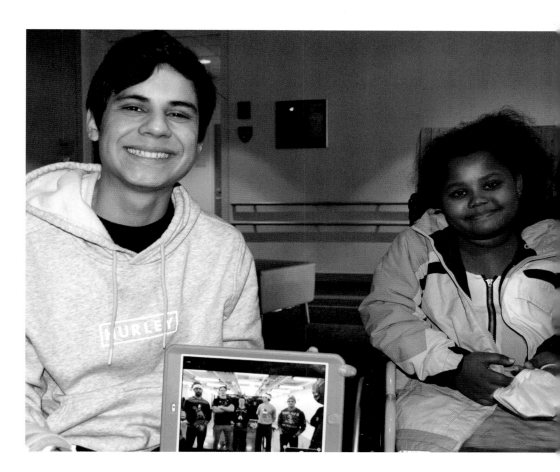

The COVID-19 pandemic restricted guests at the Shriners Children's hospitals, but that didn't stop the Boston Bruins from visiting Juan Diego and Iris virtually in 2021.

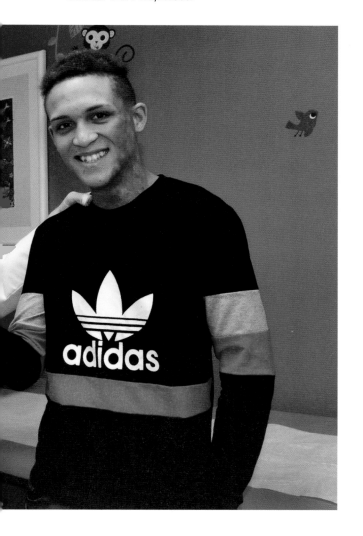

Left: Leufry, a teenager from the Dominican Republic, suffered burns on over 30% of his body at the age of 6, when a live high-tension wire fell on him. He thrives today thanks to novel laser treatments from Dr. Matthias Donelan, Chief of Staff at Shriner's Childrens Boston.

115

TAMPA, FLORIDA
OCTOBER 16, 1985

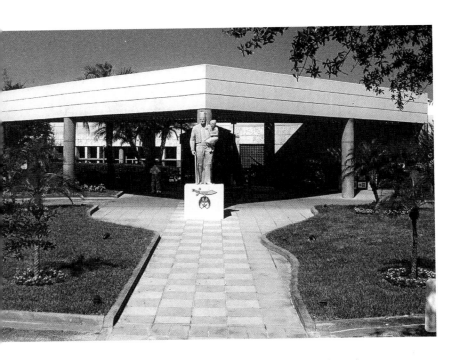

In 1985, Shriners Children's Florida opened its doors on the campus of the University of South Florida in Tampa to provide specialty care to children with orthopedic conditions. In the years since, nearly 70,000 patients received life-changing care at the hospital thanks to the unique contributions of the staff and their supporters, including members of Shriners International and other volunteers and donors.

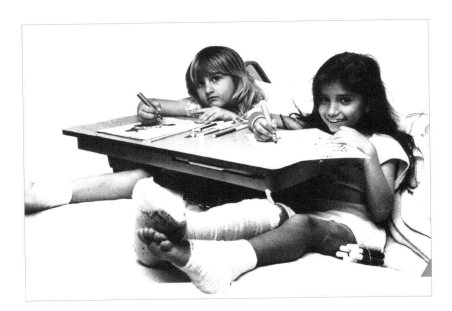

In October 1986, Luz (right) made headlines when she was attacked by a shark off the West Coast of Florida. Here, she relaxes with a friend at Shriners Children's after follow-up surgery on her leg.

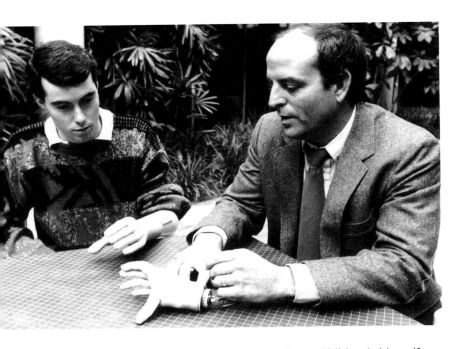

Ron Gingras, once a patient at Shriners Children's himself, served as director of Pediatric Orthotic and Prosthetic Services (POPS) at Shriners Children's Florida for 43 years. In this photo from the 1980s, he fits a patient with a new set of hands.

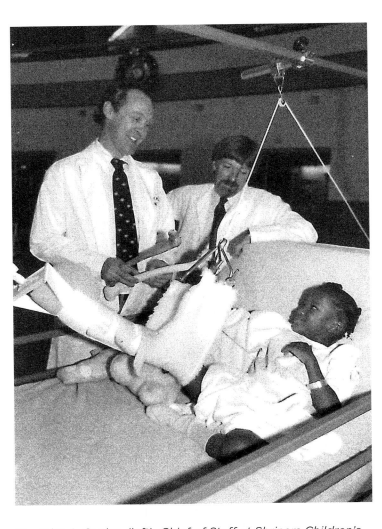

Dr. John A. Ogden (left), Chief of Staff at Shriners Children's Florida, checks on a grateful patient as a resident looks on.

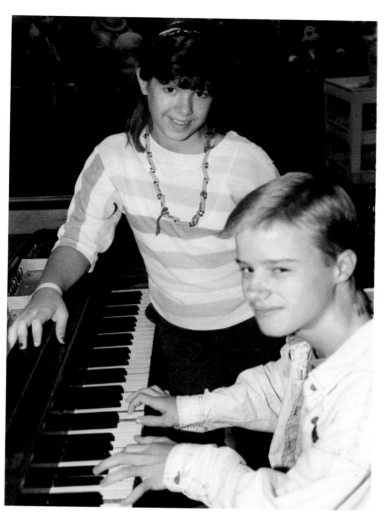

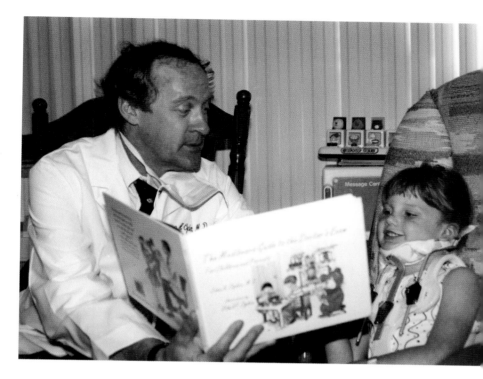

In 1991, Dr. Ogden published a children's book to help children prepare for medical visits, The Medibears Guide to the Doctor's Exam. *Here, he reads a copy to one of his patients.*

Steven plays the piano as another patient at Shriners Children's Florida looks on, 1991.

Orthopedic surgeon Dr. Maureen Maciel with Carleigh.

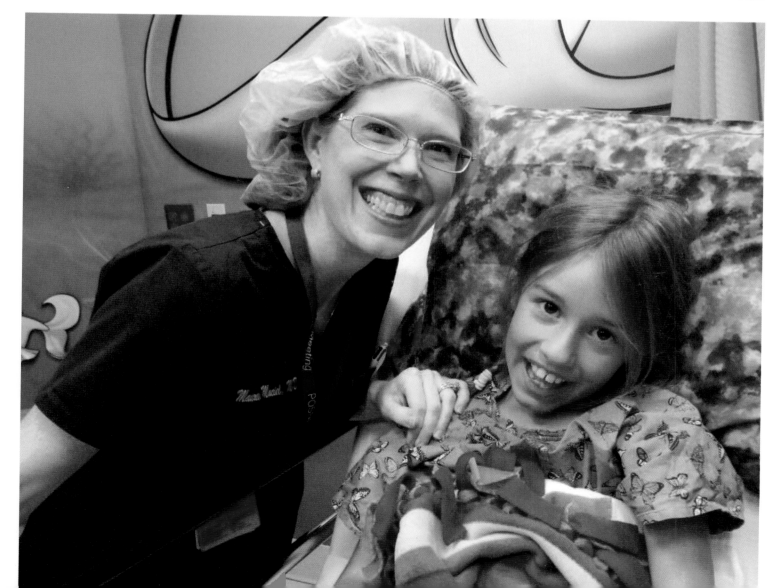

117

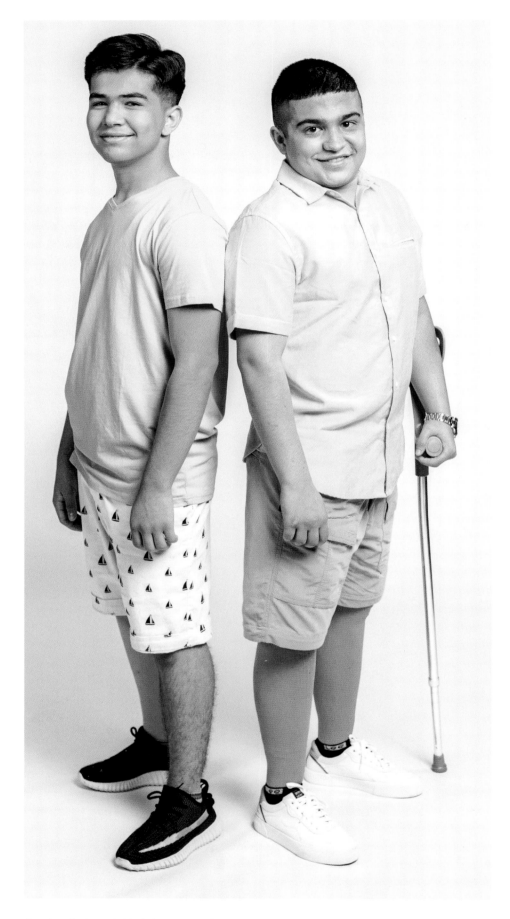

Doniyorbek and Abdulaziz, two friends at Shriners Children's Florida, show off their new legs.

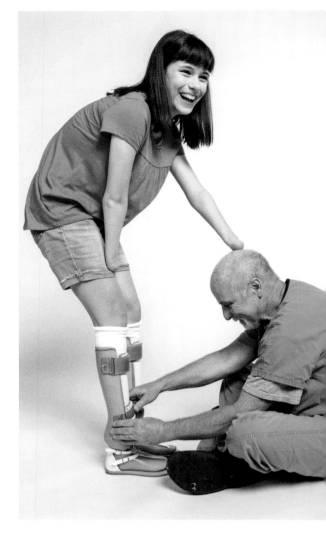

Grace steadies herself on the closest available surface as prosthetist Bryan Sinnott makes final adjustments on her leg.

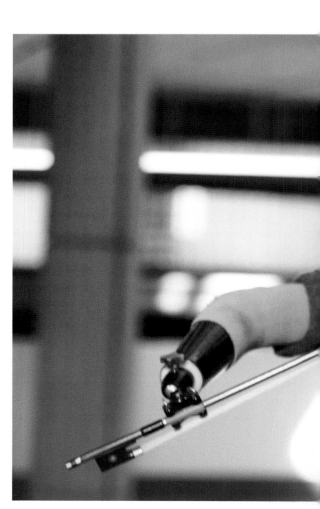

13-year-old Momo, treated at Shriners Children's Florida, plays a violin with a specially designed prosthetic attachment, 2021.

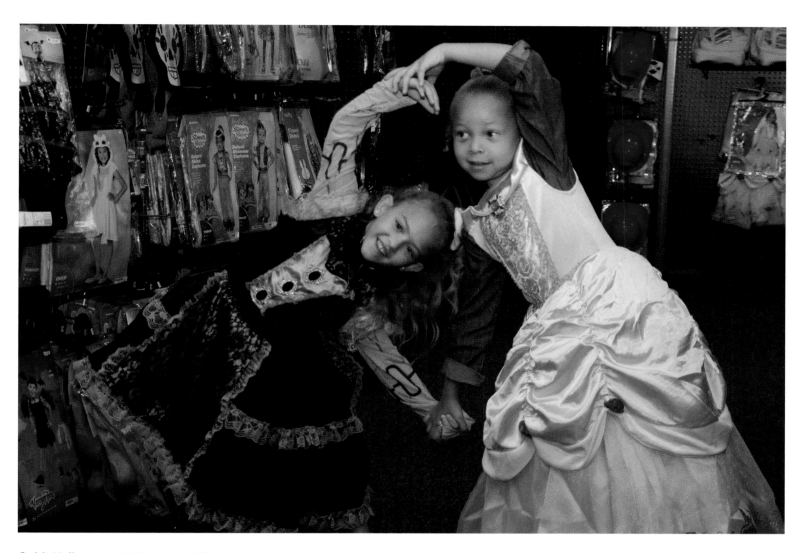

Spirit Halloween, LLC, is one of the largest seasonal retailers in the United States. Since 2007, the company's Spirit of Children fundraising campaigns have raised over $10 million for Shriners Children's child life program. Spirit Halloween also hosts parties and provides costumes for patients such as these two princesses at Shriners Children's Florida.

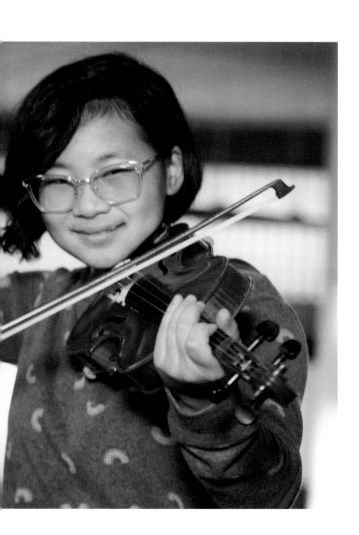

Innovation and change are deeply rooted in the history of Shriners Children's. In 2022, the Florida facility resolved to serve more children in more places by shifting to a new decentralized model. Identifying pediatric orthopedic providers throughout the state as affiliates, Shriners Children's Florida now offers pediatric orthotic and prosthetic services at multiple access points, including Tampa, Gainesville, and Miami.

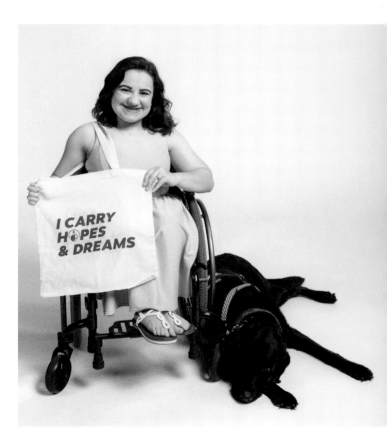

119

EXPANDING ACCESS

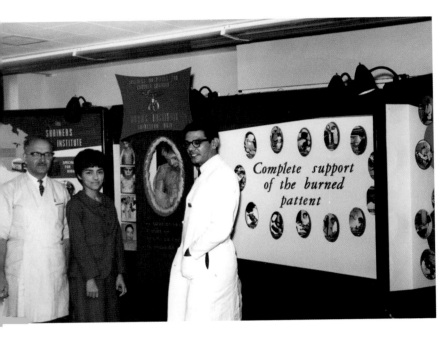

Education and outreach to raise awareness and promote safety has been central to the Shriners Children's burns program from the very beginning.

ENSURING ACCESS TO SPECIALIZED CARE HAS always been one of the greatest challenges in medicine. Answering that challenge is central to the mission of Shriners Children's. Over the years, Shriners Children's has worked to help patients receive the expert medical attention they need, wherever they may live. Medical advances have increasingly changed the model of care from inpatient to outpatient, and this has created both new challenges and new opportunities. Today, Shriners Children's offers advanced medical care not only through its major hospitals and medical centers, but also through smaller-scale and pop-up clinics, affiliated medical facilities, genomics labs and telehealth services.

In furtherance of its goal of reaching more children in more places, Shriners Children's has developed a network that is truly global. Every year, the hospitals receive patients from Asia, South America, Africa and Europe who come to receive the specialized care that only Shriners Children's can offer. In recent years, Shriners Children's has doubled down on its commitment to global health by instituting an international outreach program. Physicians and clinicians travel across the world to provide medical care to new and current patients. Specially trained rapid response teams address local, national and international emergencies. Thanks to cutting-edge research and new technologies, Shriners Children's unique approach to compassionate, innovative care reaches more patients today than ever before.

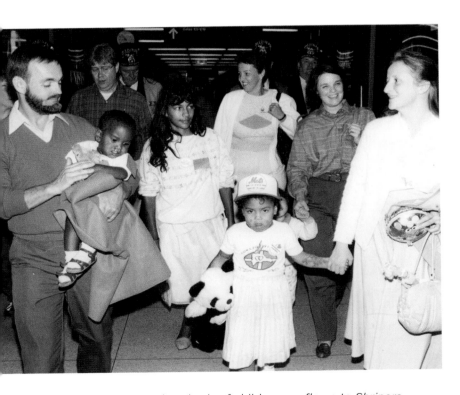

Every year, hundreds of children are flown to Shriners Children's for specialized treatment. In 1988, the hospitals saw 110 international patients, including Luis, Rosana and Maria from the Dominican Republic.

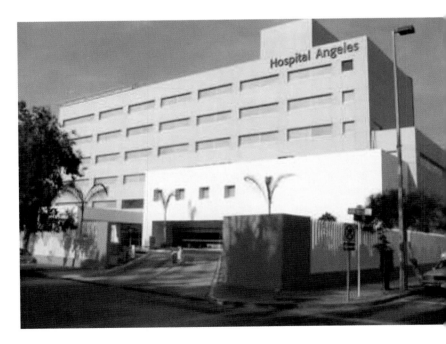

Shriners Children's Tijuana Ambulatory Clinic is an extension of Shriners Children's Southern California, conveniently located for families in Baja California, Mexico. The clinic provides comprehensive medical and surgical care to children up to the age of 18 with orthopedic conditions, burn scars, and cleft lip and palate.

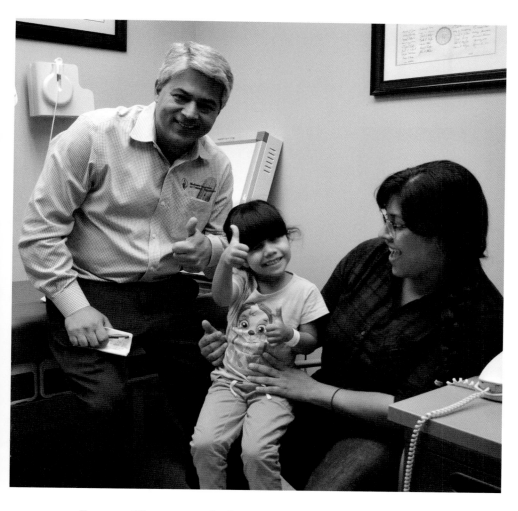

For over 50 years, medical staff at Shriners Children's Philadelphia have traveled to San Juan, Puerto Rico to provide specialized orthopedic care. Here, Dr. Amer F. Samdani gets the thumbs up from Uma, sitting on her mother's lap.

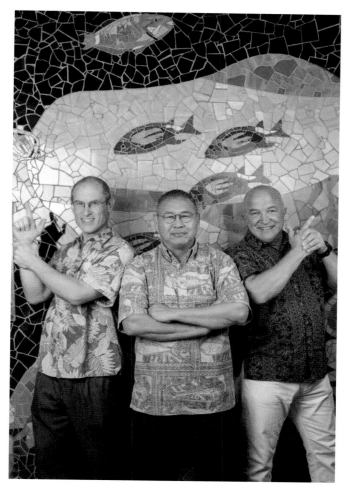

The medical staff at Shriners Children's Hawaii cover the entire Pacific basin. In 2022, Dr. Craig Ono, (center), flanked here by Dr. Jonathan Pellett (left) and Dr. Paul Moroz (right), led an outreach team to treat keiki of the Mariana Islands in Guam and Saipan.

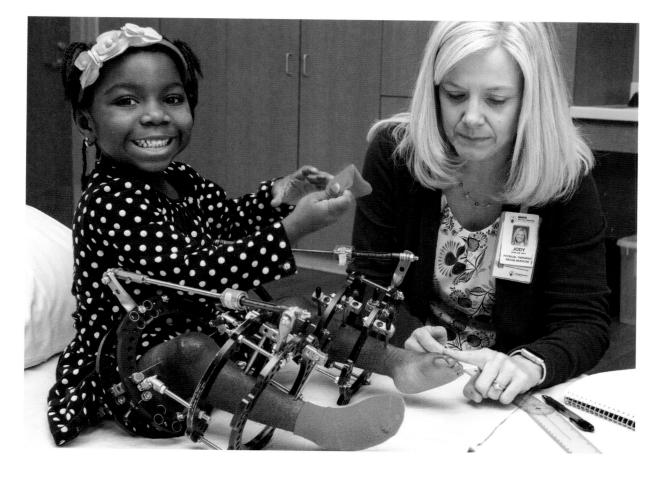

Maria Eva, a patient from the Ivory Coast, smiles as Jody Barlow, a physical therapist at Shriners Children's St. Louis, checks her progress.

GLOBALIZING EXPERTISE

AFTER 100 YEARS OF SPECIALIZED CARE, medical staff at Shriners Children's are uniquely situated to share their expertise with medical students and professionals around the globe. Today, Shriners Children's is recognized as a leader in training physicians and medical professionals throughout their residencies and fellowships. Since the initiation of the burns program in the 1960s, Shriners Children's has conducted educational outreach, hosting conferences, symposia, seminars, continuing education programs, hands-on skills labs and webinars. Doctors and nurses from Shriners Children's also travel internationally to offer training clinics for their counterparts in underserved areas, all in the service of the healthcare system's mission of helping more kids in more places.

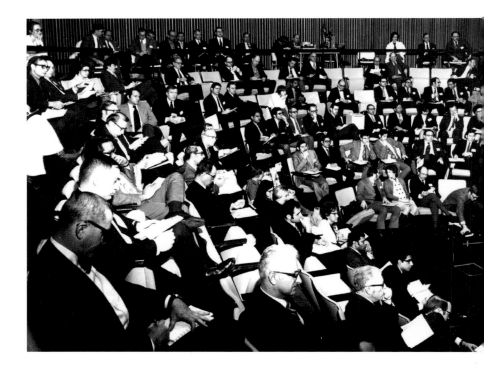

Opening session of the three-day seminar of the American Academy of Orthopedic Surgeons Committee on Injuries, Shriners Children's Boston, 1971.

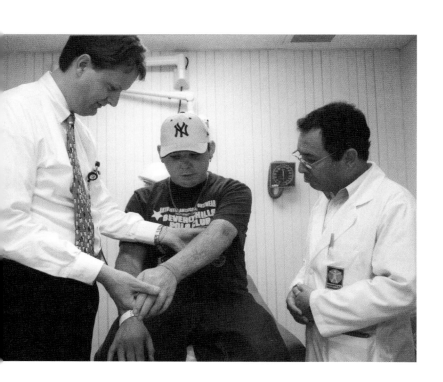

Dr. Augusto Valdivia (right), a plastic surgeon from the children's hospital in La Paz, Bolivia, spent a month at Shriners Children's Ohio in 2006 to learn from Dr. Kevin Bailey (left) and other burn specialists.

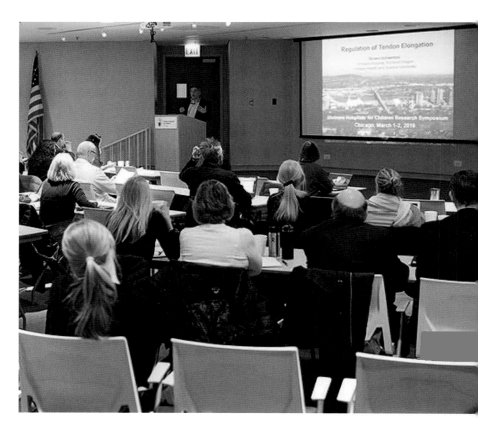

Ronen Schweitzer, Ph.D., a scientist at Shriners Children's Portland and Oregon Health and Science University, presents his findings on tendon elongation at the 2019 Shriners Children's Research Symposium in Chicago, Illinois.

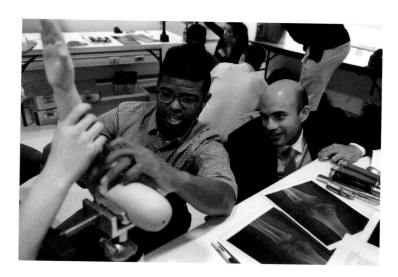

Residencies and fellowships at several Shriners Children's hospitals offer medical students the opportunity to work closely with such mentors as Dr. Vedant Kulkarni, an orthopedic surgeon at Shriners Children's Northern California.

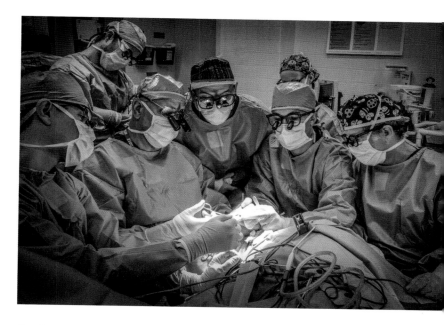

Dr. Scott Levin demonstrates surgical technique to students and colleagues at Shriners Children's Philadelphia, 2021.

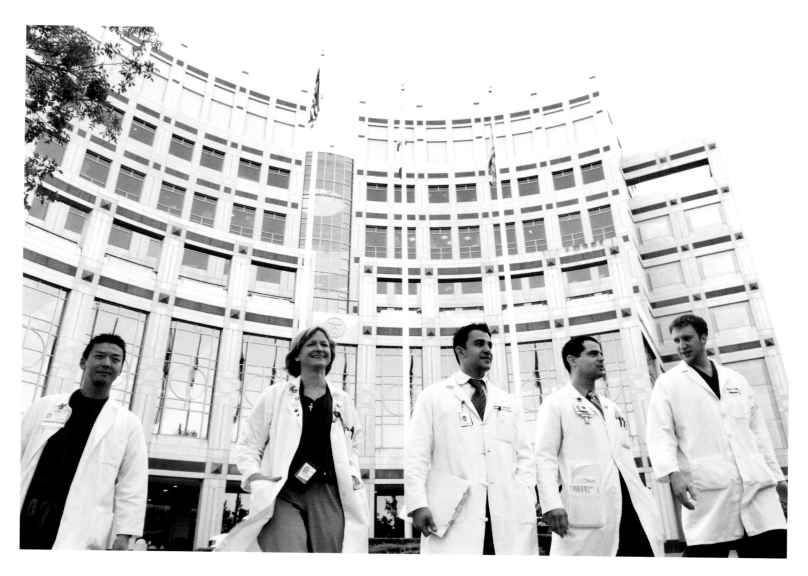

Dr. Michelle A. James of Shriners Children's Northern California heads to a medical conference to share her insights with her colleagues, 2008.

EAST-WEST SHRINE BOWL

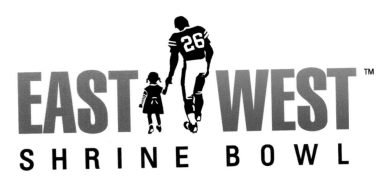

LONG HERALDED AS "Football's finest hour," the East-West Shrine Bowl is almost as old as the Shriners Children's hospitals themselves. The Bowl was born out of a friendly baseball rivalry in San Francisco between the members of the local Shriners chapter and another fraternal group. One noble suggested they play football instead, but other Shriners reasoned that "the human wreckage that might result when older men started committing mayhem on the gridiron was hardly to be countenanced." Instead, they founded an All-Star game, with William H. Coffman as director. He would continue to organize the game every year for 40 years. After the bombing of Pearl Harbor, the Army banned public gatherings on the West Coast, so Coffman moved the game temporarily from San Francisco to New Orleans.

From early on, the East-West Shrine Bowl became a key venue for showcasing the talents of college athletes and a major site of NFL recruitment. Among the many football greats who competed are Dick Stanfel, Johnny Lujack, "Mean" Joe Green, Troy Vincent, Pat Tillman, Gale Sayers, Alan Page, Dick Butkus, Brett Favre, Gino Marchetti, Walter Payton and John Elway. U.S. President Gerald Ford played center in the 1935 game. The quarterback for the 2000 East Team was a senior from the University of Michigan named Tom Brady.

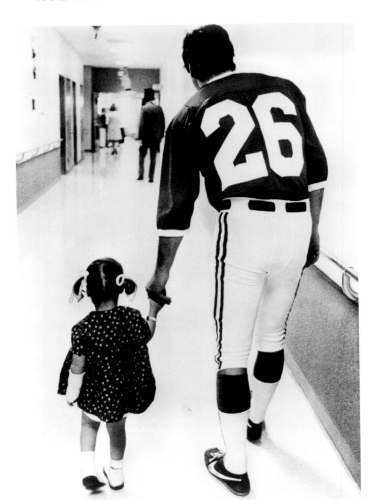

Center: Visiting Shriners Children's Northern California before the 1974 East-West Shrine Bowl, running back Mike Esposito saw 2-year-old Nicole crying. He took her hand to comfort her, and they walked down the hall together. A local photographer spotted them and took the picture that would be adapted as the official logo for the game.

Below: Wiley Smith, cartoonist for the San Francisco Examiner, was renowned for his strips Life with Homer and Football Follies. His art adorned the program for the 1948 East-West Shrine Bowl.

Islam Temple Potentate Louis Sutter and players from the 1943 Shrine Bowl sing carols with patients at Shriners Children's Northern California, December, 1942. Two of the athletes, Jim Jurkovich (left) and Tony Compagno (third from left) went on to pro careers.

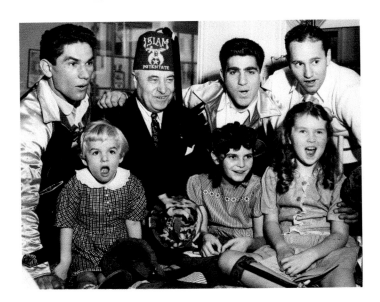

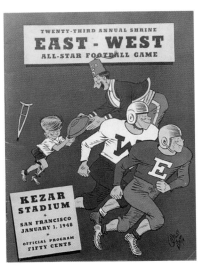

Historical pennants for the
East-West Shrine Bowl.

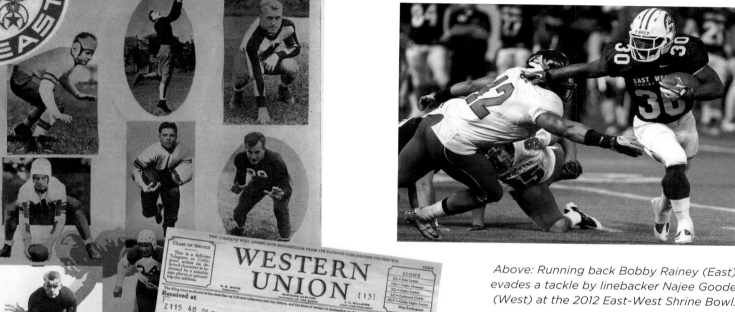

Above: Running back Bobby Rainey (East)
evades a tackle by linebacker Najee Goode
(West) at the 2012 East-West Shrine Bowl.

U.S. President Gerald Ford, perhaps the finest athlete to occupy
the White House, played center in the 1935 East-West Shrine
Game. He would later join the nobility of Shriners International.

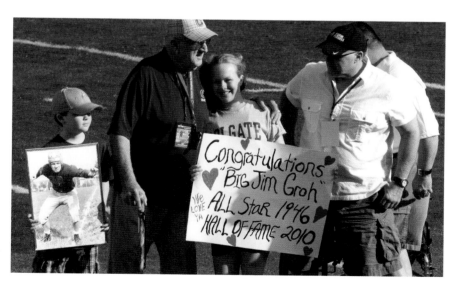

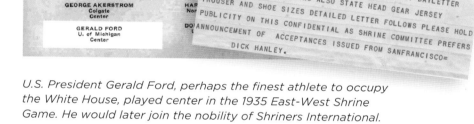

Dr. James Groh was a football star at Colgate University whose
performance as an offensive guard in the 1946 East West Shrine Bowl
was so impressive that it earned him a spot in the hall of fame. Forgoing
a professional career in sports, Dr. Groh attended medical school and
became an orthopedic surgeon, serving the population of Milwaukee,
Wisconsin, for more than 30 years.

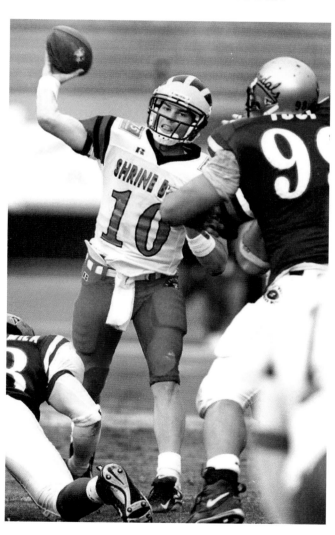

The 2000 East-West Shrine Bowl represented
a homecoming for Tom Brady, then a college
senior. He attended high school in San Mateo,
California, a few miles away from the arena.

125

COMPETITIONS FOR A CAUSE

THE EXTRAORDINARY SUCCESS OF THE EAST-WEST Shrine Bowl gave rise over the years to other sporting events to benefit Shriners Children's. The Shriners Children's Open, a PGA Tour event, is played annually in Las Vegas and draws many of the sport's greatest players. Like the East-West Shrine Bowl, the tournament event serves as a showcase for emerging talent. It was at the 1996 Shriners Children's Open that Tiger Woods, then only 20 years old, recorded his first PGA Tour victory.

Located in Houston, Texas, Minute Maid Park is the home of the Houston Astros. Since 2001, it has also been home to the Shriners Children's College Classic, one of the top collegiate baseball tournaments in the nation. The three-day, six-team, nine-game event draws fans, top-ranked programs and scouts from every Major League organization each year.

The Shriners Children's Charleston Classic is a premier college basketball tournament held each year in Charleston, South Carolina. Held early in the season, the event features eight Division 1 teams playing 12 games over three days.

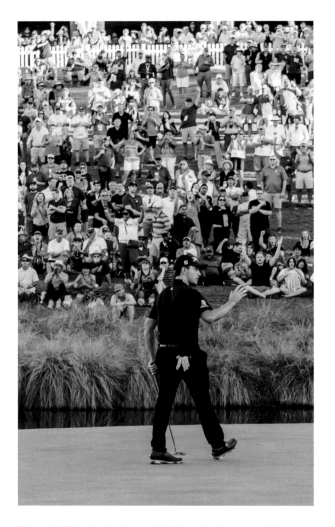

Since 1983, the Shriners Children's Open, a PGA Tour event, has drawn thousands of dedicated professional and amateur golfers in a trophy competition that supports the healthcare system.

A record crowd of more than 53,000 people attended the 2022 Shriners Children's College Classic in Houston's Minute Maid Park.

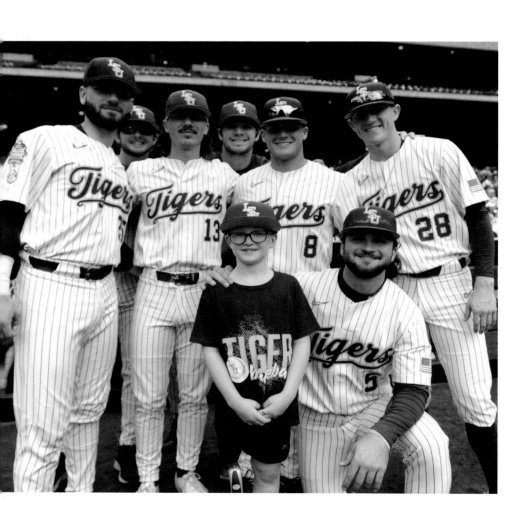

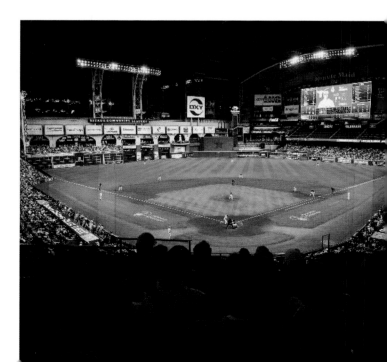

Above: The Louisiana State University Tigers welcomed Hayes, a patient at Shriners Children's Shreveport, as Team Captain during the 2022 Shriners Children's College Classic.

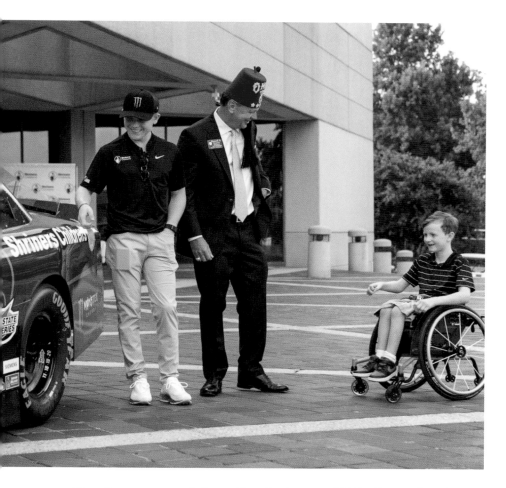

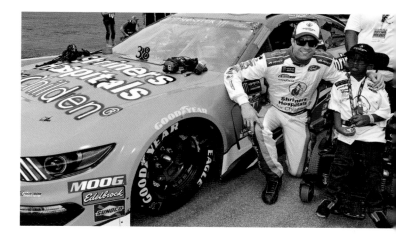

David Ragan posing with a patient at the Talladega Race in 2019.

Race Day was especially exciting for 9-year-old Wyatt, a patient from Shriners Children's Greenville. His mother said he is a lifelong NASCAR fan, 2022.

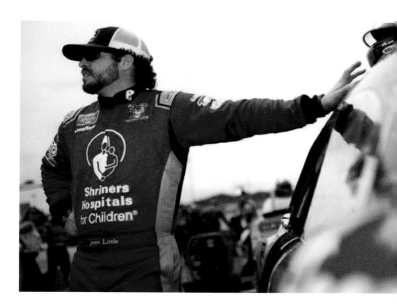

Nascar driver Jesse Little, 2021.

THE LONGSTANDING RELATIONSHIP BETWEEN Shriners Children's and NASCAR combines a great cause with a great sport, raising awareness and garnering support for the care of children with unique conditions around the world. NASCAR driver David Ragan is both a long-time supporter of Shriners Children's and a member of Shriners International. He named Shriners Children's his official charity of choice in 2008 and has taken time to visit with patients at various locations and participate in public service announcements.

NASCAR driver Jesse Little first became aware of Shriners Children's when his cousin, April, was a patient. During his rookie season in 2020, he forged a formal partnership with Shriners Children's, promoting the work of the hospitals by decorating his cars with pictures of the children they serve. In 2021, Jesse doubled down on his philanthropic commitment by becoming a Freemason and a Shriner, supporting the hospitals even when off the track.

In 2022, Shriners Children's presented the traditional Labor Day Race Weekend at Darlington Raceway, NASCAR's original superspeedway, nicknamed "The Lady in Black" and "The Track Too Tough to Tame." During the Shriners Children's centennial celebration, Ty Gibbs became the latest NASCAR driver to pledge his support, unveiling a special edition of his race car painted with the Shriners Children's logo.

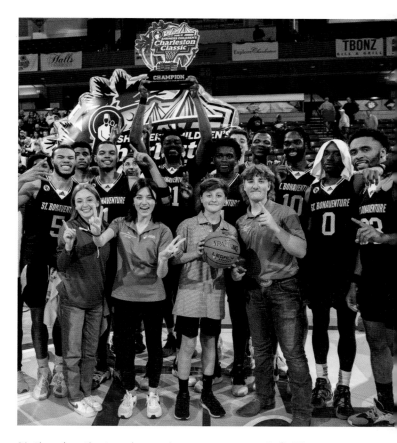

National patient ambassadors celebrate with the winning team from St. Bonaventure at the 2021 Charleston Classic.

127

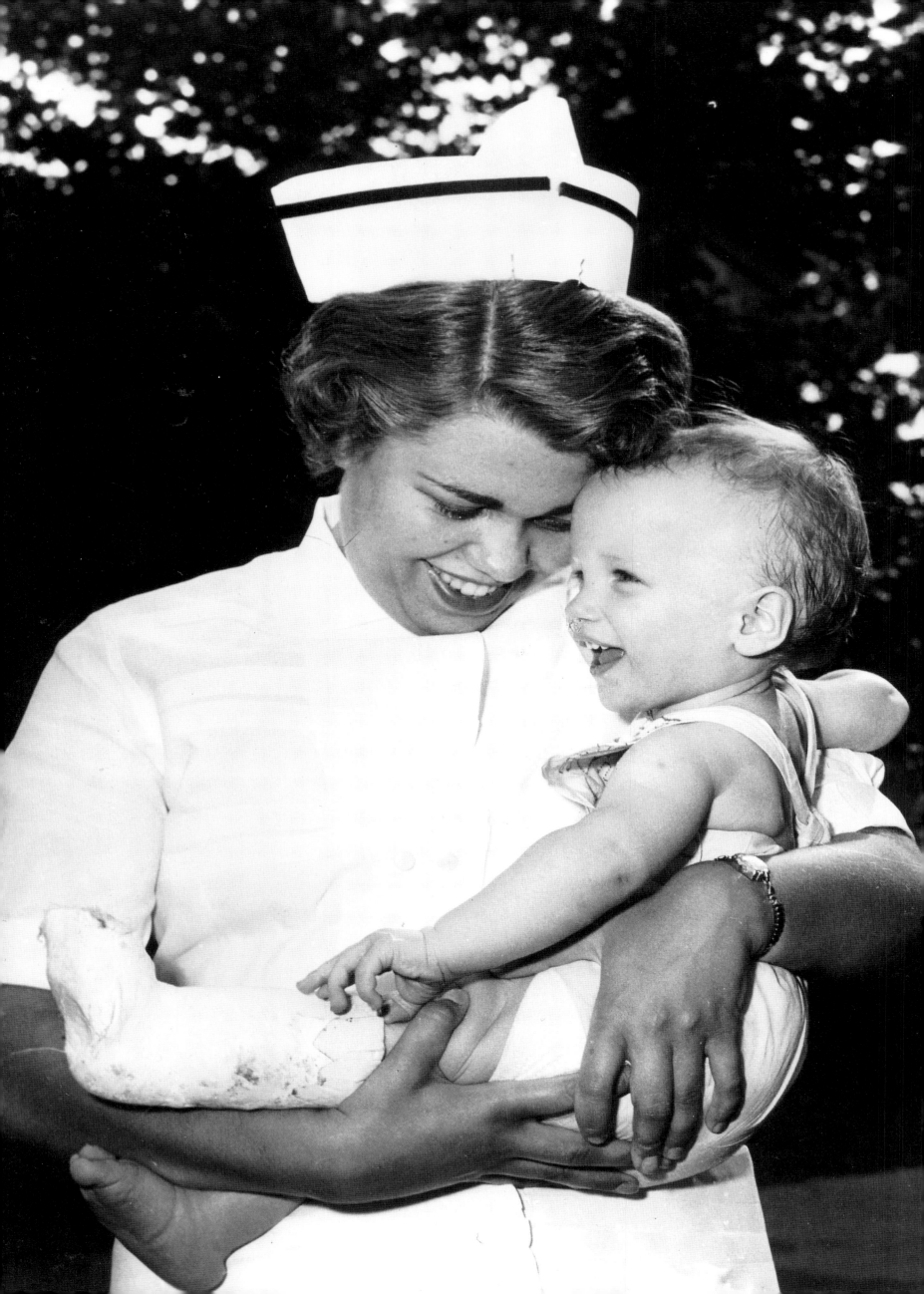

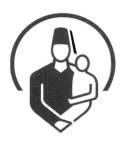

EVERYDAY MIRACLES

I N MODERN USAGE, THE WORD "MIRACLE" often suggests the divine. However, the term comes from the Latin word associated with wonder: a miracle is a manifestation or an act that inspires awe. For a century, the medical staff at Shriners Children's have inspired awe daily. From the beginning, the hospitals treated children with such severe conditions that they seemed beyond hope but restored their health. Children who could not stand up, walked. Children with limb deficiencies could catch a ball. Children with catastrophic burns not only survived but thrived. These awe-inspiring events at Shriners Children's have transpired every single day for 100 years.

The core mission of Shriners Children's has not changed significantly since 1922: to offer the best possible care to children with specialized medical conditions, regardless of their ability to pay or insurance status. The hospitals have always been inclusive in the broadest possible sense. In the earliest years, the hospitals ministered to patients with demonstrable economic need. They treated children "without regard to race, color, or religion" — a brave and bold move during a less enlightened age. Over the years, some of the parameters have changed. Originally, the age for treatment was capped at 14 years old; now it is 18. Treatment is still provided regardless of a family's ability to pay, but in 2011, the hospitals began accepting payments from insurance and government programs. The number and types of conditions Shriners Children's treats, while still focused, have expanded.

Over 1.5 million children worldwide have received treatment at Shriners Children's over the past 100 years.

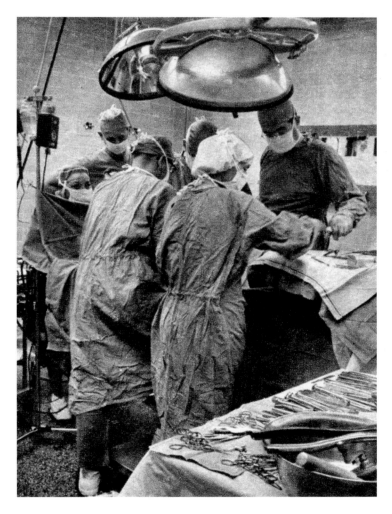

An operation at Shriners Children's St. Louis, 1963.

Facing page: A nurse at Shriners Children's Chicago and one of her patients, 1940s.

ORTHOPEDICS

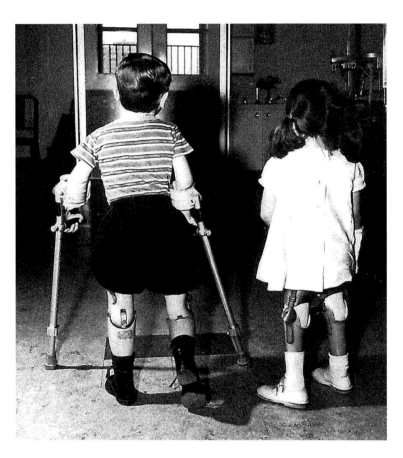

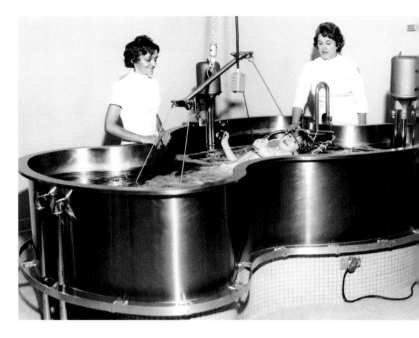

Before the conquest of polio, every Shriners Children's hospital had a Hubbard tank. Warm jets of water helped children with limited mobility to exercise their limbs in a playful environment.

Founded in response to the polio epidemic, medical care at Shriners Children's has always been centered on orthopedics – surgical interventions for disorders of the musculoskeletal system. Although polio has largely been eradicated, genetic factors continue to produce many of the conditions associated with the disease: malformations of the spine, hip and foot, limb length inequities and neuromuscular disorders. Today, the staff at Shriners Children's have a century of expertise to draw on, which they supplement with innovative research as they treat more than 100 orthopedic conditions.

Diagnosed with spinal tuberculosis in 1934, Noriyuki Morita was a patient at Shriners Children's Northern California until he was 11. Adopting the nickname "Pat," Morita became a celebrated actor best known for his role in The Karate Kid.

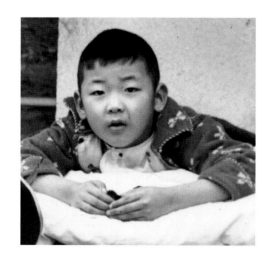

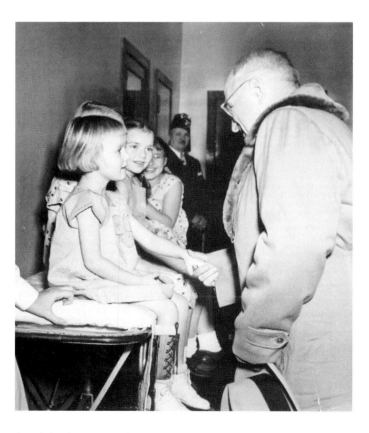

Patricia (in center, facing camera) shakes U.S. President Harry S. Truman's hand during his visit to Shriners Children's Twin Cities. Diagnosed with fibrous monostotic dysplasia, she underwent years of treatment. In 1989, she would become First Lady of Tangier Temple in Omaha, Nebraska.

ALTHOUGH MANY SHRINERS Children's patients have gone on to have distinguished careers, Louis James "Jimmie" Carrick was the first patient to enter the hospital as a celebrity. Diagnosed with spinal tuberculosis at the age of two, Jimmie knew little of the world outside of his home and hospitals. But in 1944, he saw *The Fighting Seabees*, a war film starring John Wayne. The film celebrated the courage of the Navy's combat battalion of construction engineers whose motto was "Can do!" Jimmie wrote encouraging letters to Seabees fighting in the Aleutians. When they saw that Jimmie was also a fighter, the Seabees awarded him the honorary rank of SM1c (Seabee Mascot First Class).

When Jimmie went to Shriners Children's Philadelphia for a series of surgeries, his treatment and recovery made national headlines. On April 14, 1947, shortly after his tenth birthday, Jimmie Carrick took his first step. Soon, he was making appearances as Shriners Children's first ambassador. Over the coming years, his health improved enough to play tennis, ride horses and raise a family of his own.

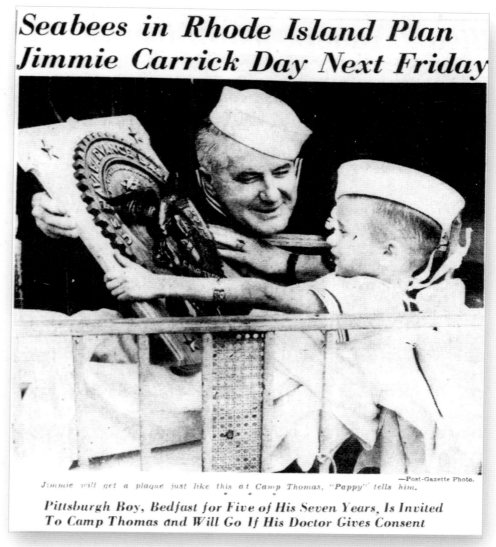

Seabees in Rhode Island Plan Jimmie Carrick Day Next Friday

—Post-Gazette Photo.

Jimmie will get a plaque just like this at Camp Thomas, "Pappy" tells him.

Pittsburgh Boy, Bedfast for Five of His Seven Years, Is Invited To Camp Thomas and Will Go If His Doctor Gives Consent

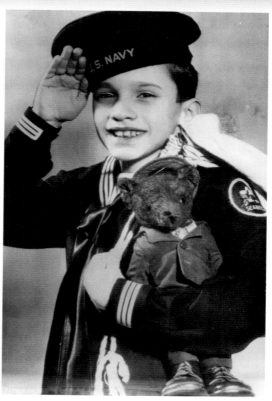

CLUBFOOT

Shriners Children's hospitals have been *treating* talipes equinovarus, *commonly known as clubfoot, for 100 years. The condition tends to run in families and may affect both feet (bilateral clubfoot) or just one foot. Clubfoot is treatable, and most patients enjoy fully-functioning use of the once-affected foot.*

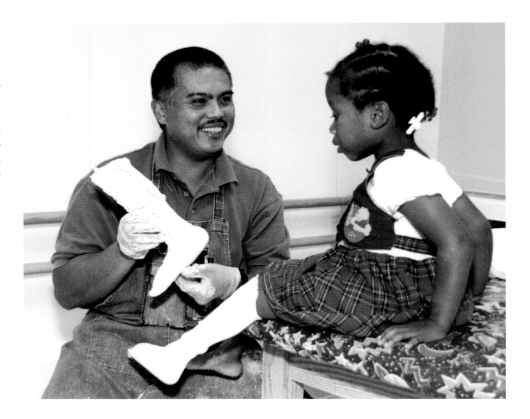

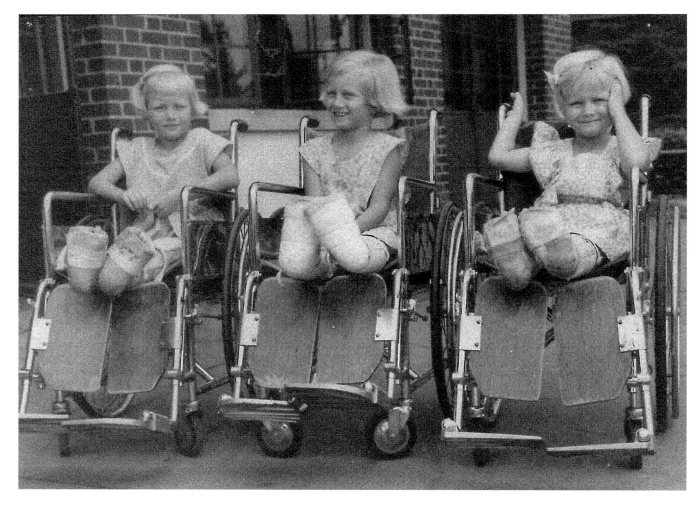

Triplets treated for clubfoot.

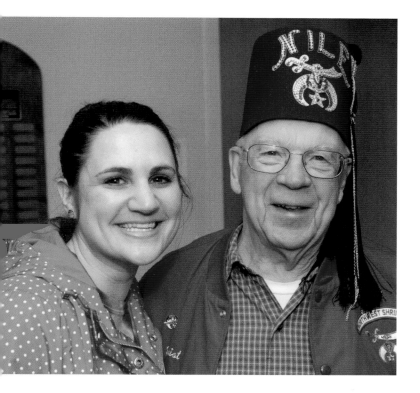

Born with clubfeet, Bill first came to Shriners Children's Twin Cities in 1934 when he was 6 months old. Two Shriners who worked with his father on the railroad in Proctor, Minnesota, had heard about his condition, and offered to help. Bill would return to the hospital for treatment every few months for about 7 years, riding the train from Duluth and walking to the hospital from the Franklin Avenue station. He is today an active member of Nile Temple in Mountlake Terrace, Washington.

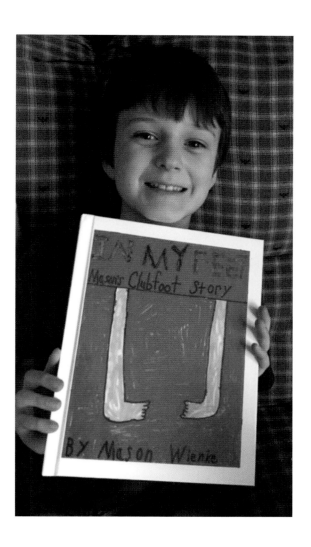

MASON, A PATIENT AT SHRINERS Children's Erie, has been receiving care for clubfeet since he was a baby. His case proved difficult, and he had several setbacks, but he made good use of his experience. After his third surgery, Mason wrote a book about his experiences. Published when he was 8, *In My Feet: Mason's Clubfoot Story*, is available on Amazon. He donates the proceeds to Shriners Children's and other organizations that have helped him along his journey.

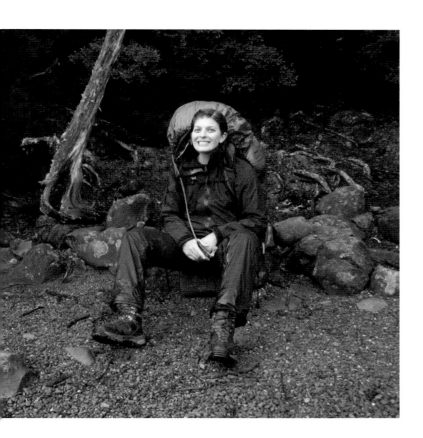

Born with bilateral club feet, Alyssa was expected never to walk. After surgery at Shriners Children's Northern California, she was required to wear leg and foot braces. "I had the same shoes as Forrest Gump until age 4 or 5. Then I wore leg braces up until about the 4th grade." Today, at age 40, she runs marathons and competes in triathalons.

SCOLIOSIS

In the 1940s and 1950s, severe curvatures were straightened by hanging from nets. This was uncomfortable but surprisingly effective.

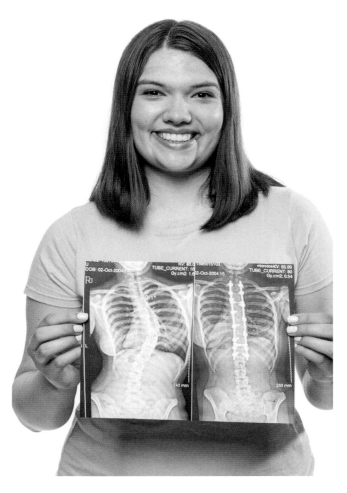

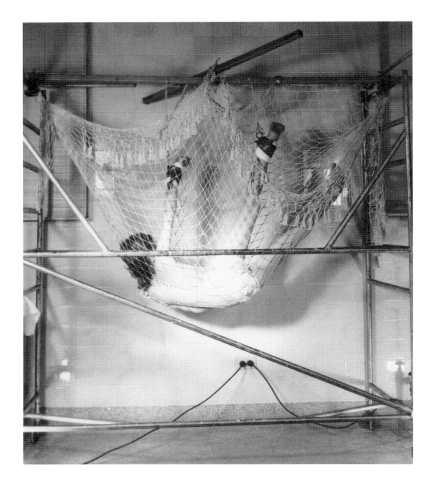

Chloe with X-rays of her spine before and after surgery. The physicians of Shriners Children's treat more than 10,000 children with scoliosis each year. In the United States, 2% to 5% of children develop scoliosis, where the spine curves to make a C shape or S shape, rather than growing in a straight line. Those with relatively mild cases can be treated with braces and exercise, but in some children, the curve is so severe that it interferes with the heart, lungs, and nervous system. Shriners Children's offers a range of treatment approaches, from physical therapy to advanced surgery.

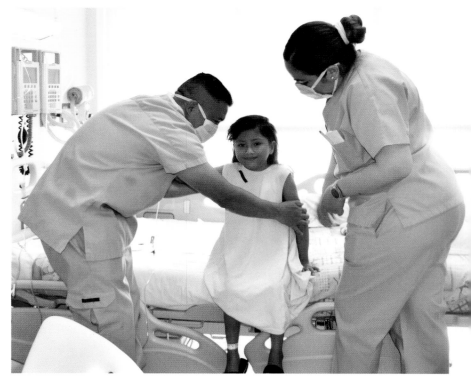

Before Ju Anne underwent surgery at Shriners Children's Mexico, doctors feared that her scoliosis was so severe that she would never be able to walk or speak. The staff at Shriners Children's proved the naysayers wrong.

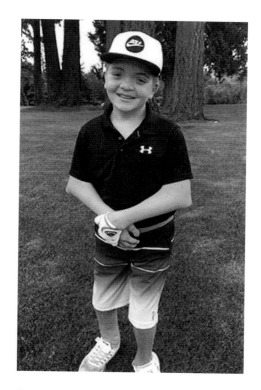

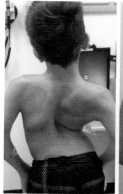 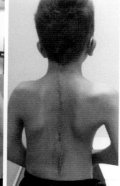

BORN IN 2004 WITH OTOPALATODIGITAL syndrome type II (OPD), Jake was not expected to live for six months. OPD comes with a wide range of symptoms, including clubbed feet, webbed fingers, dislocated joints, fused joints, an underdeveloped trachea, and severe scoliosis. By 2017, he had undergone 30 major surgeries.

"We had to deal with what was most important – kind of triage each thing along the way," said his mother, and other symptoms took priority. But by the time he was 12, it was time to deal with Jake's scoliosis, which worsened as he grew. The curvature was so severe that it was crushing his lungs, and he was hospitalized with pneumonia twice a year. So in 2014, doctors at Shriners Children's Portland inserted magnetic rods into his spine to straighten it and hold the vertebral column upright. The rod is expandable and has been lengthened gradually to keep pace with Jake's growth. Jake was born to a family of athletes. The surgery made it possible for him to play golf. He started in middle school. In 2021, his sophomore year in high school, he played his first varsity game.

Shameka, recovering from surgery at Shriners Children's Texas, 1989.

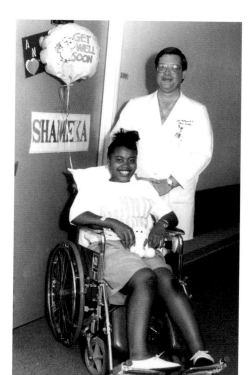

Halo traction is typically a first step in correcting severe scoliosis and other spine deformities. The treatment works by attaching a metal ring that surrounds the head — called a halo — to a pulley system. Children remain in the hospital the entire time they are in traction, typically three to eight weeks. After halo traction, children usually have spinal fusion surgery to permanently stabilize the spine. Halo traction reduces the risk of damaging the nerves or soft tissues that surround and support the spine during surgery.

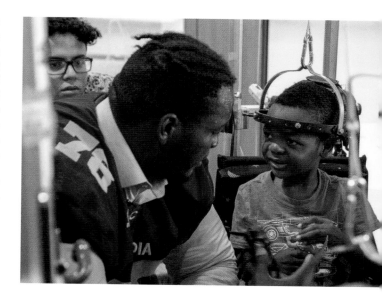

SPINAL CORD INJURIES

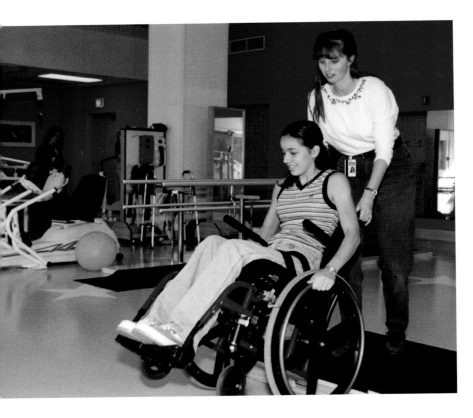

Left: In 1980, Shriners Children's Philadelphia established the first pediatric program in North America to address spinal cord injuries (SCI), which can be caused by infection, tumor, autoimmune conditions or trauma. Shriners offers care for a range of orthopedic spine conditions, some of which can be addressed by non-surgical interventions such as bracing or casting. SCI is more complex and can involve implants to enable severely injured children to breathe without a respirator and surgery to repair damage to tendons and nerves. Intensive rehabilitation is often required to restore function and sensation after spine trauma. The Shriners Children's SCI program expanded in 1984. A research project started at Shriners Children's Chicago in 1995 has tracked over 520 SCI patients to determine the long-range effects of these injuries and develop further treatments.

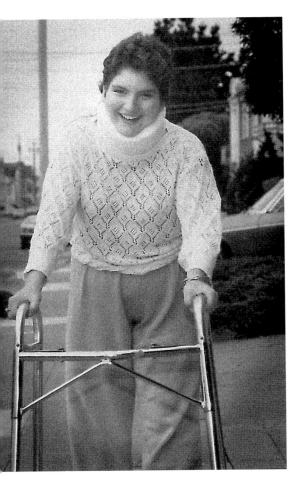

Left: June was 18 when she suffered a spinal cord injury in a car accident. When she was first brought to Shriners Children's Northern California, she had no motor function. But as this 1989 photograph demonstrates, she made remarkable progress.

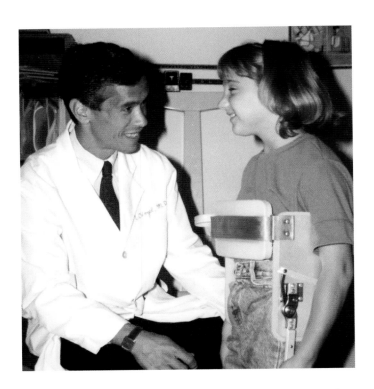

Dr. Lawrence Vogel with a patient, 1992. For 35 years, Dr. Vogel served as Medical Director for the pediatric spinal cord injury program at Shriners Children's Chicago.

Alyssa, a former SCI patient at Shriners Children's Northern California, won first place in the WCMX and Adaptive Skate World Competition in April 2020.

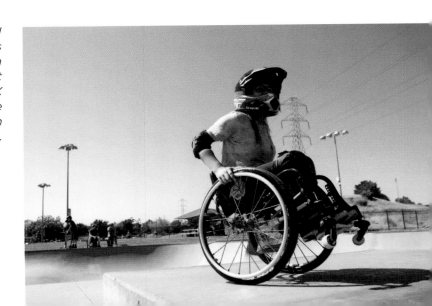

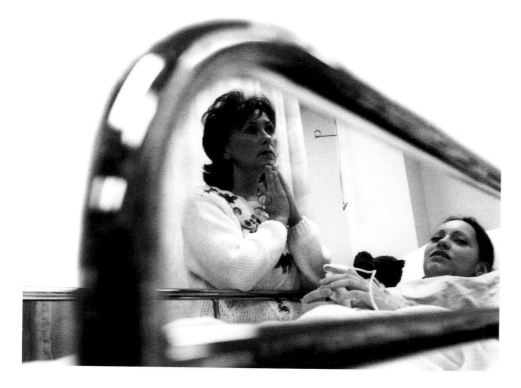

Ruta and her mother in the pre-op holding area of Shriners Children's Chicago in the last few moments before being wheeled into the operating room for spine surgery, 2001.

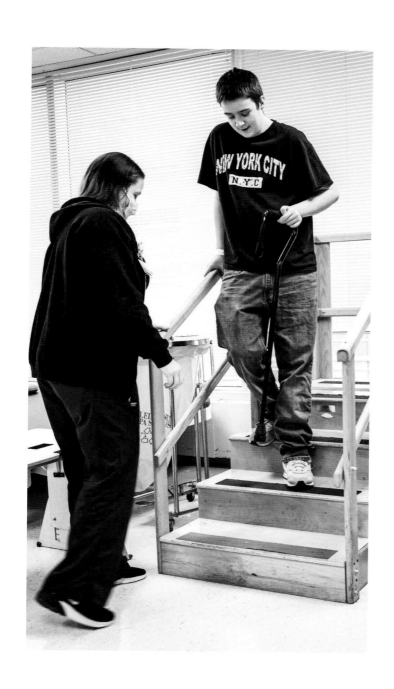

IN SPRING 2021, JESSE DOVE into a pool and broke his neck. The 14-year-old was airlifted to a local hospital for emergency care. Afterwards, he went to Shriners Children's Philadelphia for the hospital's specialized SCI intensive rehabilitation program. When he arrived, Jesse could barely move his left leg or toes. "I really didn't think I could walk again," he recalled. His care team created an inclusive plan to build up his ability, confidence and independence. As Jesse's mother noted, the team gave him the physical therapy he needed, but "they made sure we had emotional support as well," allowing him to decorate his room and bring articles from home. Less than two months later he had recovered enough to be discharged. "The amazing staff at Shriners Children's pushed me, believed in me and made me believe in myself," Jesse said. "And after about six weeks, I could walk again."

LIMB DEFICIENCIES

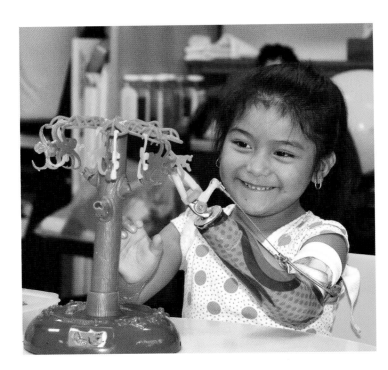

Limb deficiencies may be congenital, when part or all of a child's limb does not completely form during pregnancy. Every year, roughly four of every 10,000 babies is born with an upper limb deficiency, while two in every 10,000 is born with a lower limb deficiency. Some babies are born with both. The orthopedic team at Shriners Children's have long treated both common and rare conditions.

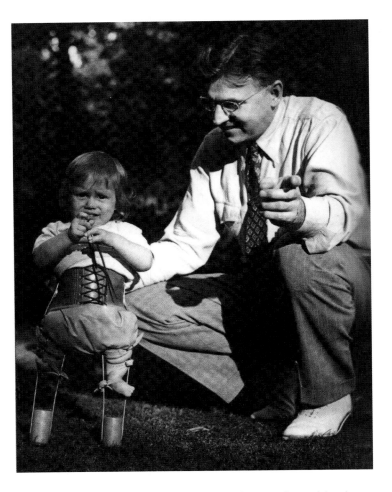

When Judith was born in 1945 with no legs and a webbed left hand, the doctor said, "Your daughter is going to live, I'm sorry to say." With the help of physicians at Shriners Children's, her parents saw that she would not only live but thrive. In 1991, she was one of three disabled Americans chosen to receive the Marian Pfister Anschutz Award for her public service.

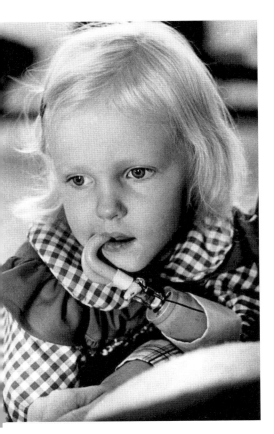

Born without legs and only one arm, Michelle was a poster child for Shriners Children's in the 1970s. Treated regularly at Shriners Children's Chicago, she was active in the Girl Scouts, graduated from the University of Northern Iowa, earned a graduate degree at Drake University and raised two children.

Bonnie, treated at Shriners Children's Southern California, was the second fastest woman in the world on one leg in 1984, when she won two bronze medals and a silver medal in the Winter Paralympics.

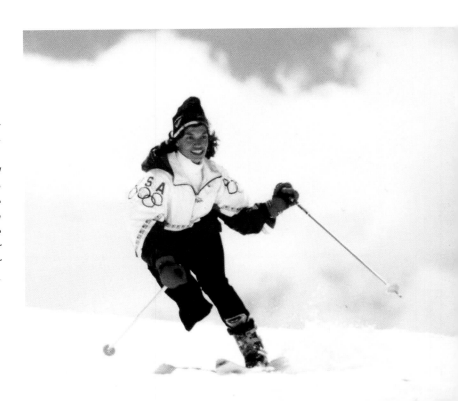

SEVEN-YEAR-OLD DIANE WAS ADMITTED TO Shriners Children's Twin Cities in 1982. She was born in Hickman, Nebraska, without a left hand or forearm. But that did not curtail her athletic ambitions. Over the next 10 years, she returned to be fitted for various custom attachments to her prosthesis that would allow her to play a range of sports. "For volleyball, I wear a cuplike hand that is made of rubber," she explained. "And for softball, I have one attachment that fits a fielder's glove and a different one for batting."

A star athlete at Norris High School, her volleyball team won the 1991 state championship, and she placed in both the high jump and the long jump at the state level. She credited the staff of Shriners Children's for making it possible. "Without them, I don't know if I'd be in athletics today," she said. After graduating high school with a 96.4 average, she studied education in college, where she lettered in volleyball and track. Today, she is the mother of two sons and teaches literature in middle school.

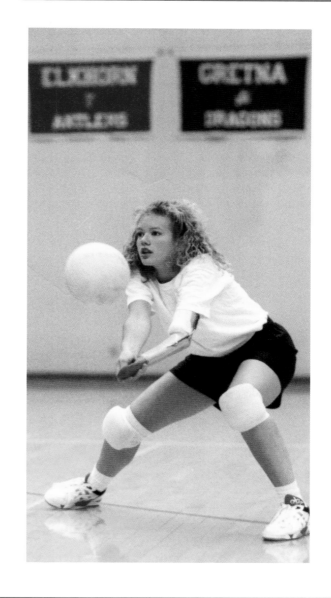

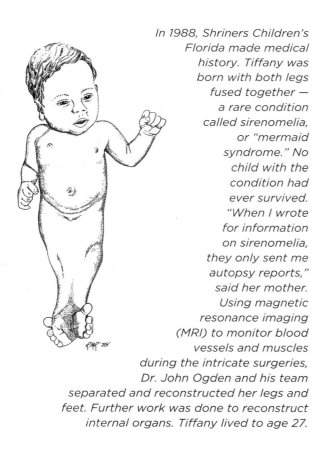

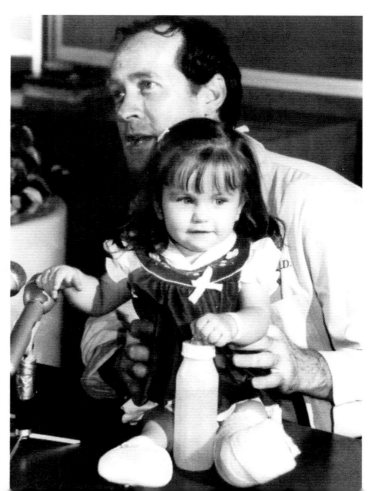

In 1988, Shriners Children's Florida made medical history. Tiffany was born with both legs fused together — a rare condition called sirenomelia, or "mermaid syndrome." No child with the condition had ever survived. "When I wrote for information on sirenomelia, they only sent me autopsy reports," said her mother. Using magnetic resonance imaging (MRI) to monitor blood vessels and muscles during the intricate surgeries, Dr. John Ogden and his team separated and reconstructed her legs and feet. Further work was done to reconstruct internal organs. Tiffany lived to age 27.

PEDIATRIC ORTHOTIC & PROSTHETIC SERVICES

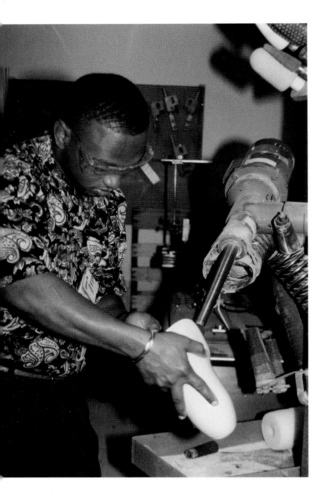

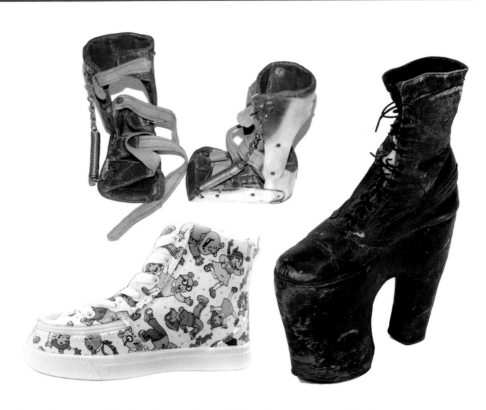

Fancy footwear: Early orthoses (top left); a boot to correct limb disparity (right); and a modern adaptive shoe (bottom left).

Shriners Children's has long provided custom-designed, expertly crafted orthotic and prosthetic devices to patients who need them, from entire limbs to small assistive devices. Today, Shriners Children's centers a streamlined Pediatric Orthotics and Prosthetic Services (POPS) operation in six regional fabrication centers with computer-assisted design capabilities, light scanners, laser carvers and other advanced technology to create devices precisely calibrated to the needs of each patient.

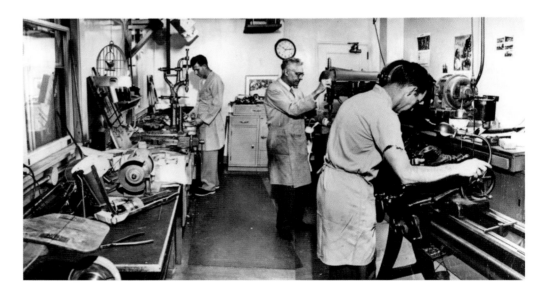

The Orthotics and Prosthetic (O&P) shop at Shriners Children's Portland in the 1950s.

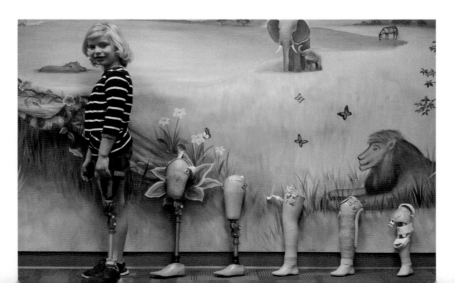

As children grow, they need new orthotics. Gianna, a patient at Shriners Children's Southern California, was 7 when she posed with the devices she had worn so far.

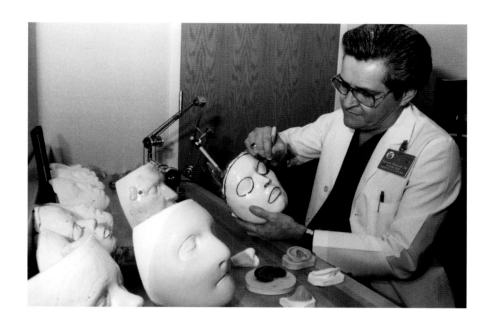

FOR 40 YEARS, ROLANDO MORALES SCULPTED PROSTHETIC BODY parts for burns patients at Shriners Children's Texas. These included noses, ears, and eyes fashioned of silicone used when surgical reconstruction was not possible. These protheses served important functions. For example, artificial ears directed sound to the auditory canal and helped support glasses. He colored the prostheses to match the patient's skin tone and added details — tiny lines to suggest blood vessels, for example — to make the devices as lifelike as possible. He also tailored face masks and pressure garments for individual patients to help reduce and soften scar tissue. Initially, medical sculptors worked by placing orthoplast (plastic sheets) directly on a patient's face, but Morales preferred to make plaster casts, which allowed him greater freedom to adjust the pressure at different points, as treatment required. Following Morales's death in 2021, his son, a plastic surgeon in Houston, Texas, established a charitable foundation in his honor.

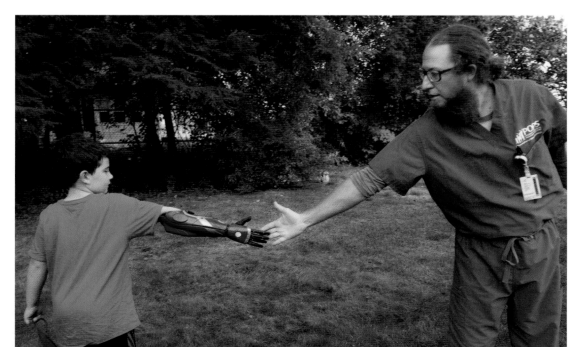

Sam reaches out with his new bionic hero arm to shake hands with Brock McConkey, CPO, manager of the POPS department at Shriners Children's New England.

SPORTS MEDICINE

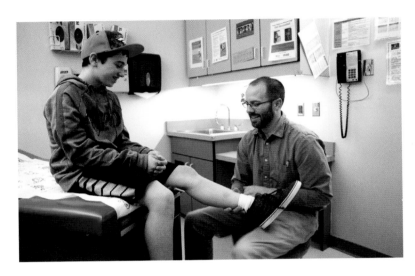

Whether playing sports, exercising, or having fun on the playground, sometimes children get hurt. At Shriners Children's, the medical team has 100 years of experience attending to children's bones, joints and muscles. They understand why injuries to growing bones and growth plates (the area where bones grow) need special attention. Working together, orthopedists, radiologists, occupational therapists, physical therapists, and other specialists create custom rehabilitation plans to help young athletes overcome their injuries.

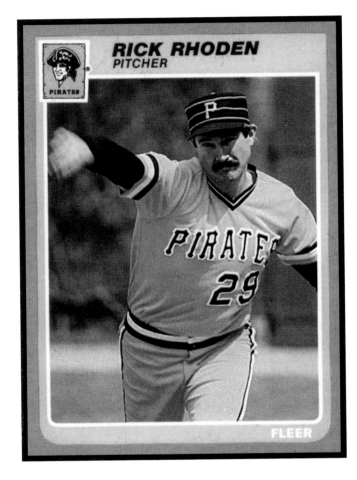

Rick Rhoden was 3 years old in 1961 when he slid down a water slide and landed knee-first on a pair of scissors. The wound became infected and developed into a case of osteomyelitis. Brought to Shriners Children's Greenville, he was fitted with a special brace and underwent multiple surgeries until he was 16. Rick overcame his injuries to pursue an athletic career, becoming a pitcher for the Los Angeles Dodgers, the Pittsburgh Pirates, the New York Yankees and the Houston Astros. Upon retiring from baseball, he became a professional golfer.

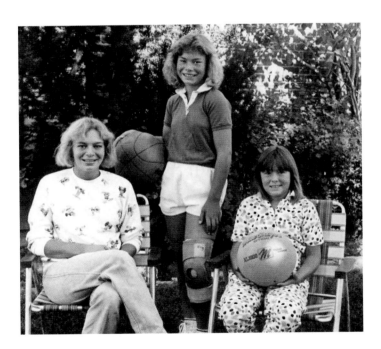

Amanda (center) injured her knee in a fall in September 1986. She was unable to walk without crutches. Several trips to local clinics could not pinpoint the problem and the swelling and pain continued. Doctors at Shriners Children's Spokane solved the mystery: a dislocated kneecap, torn muscles and ligaments. After being fitted with a special knee brace and undergoing 12 weeks of therapy, she was able to discard her crutches and pick up her basketball again.

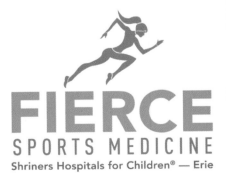

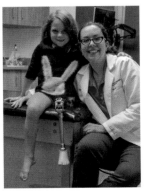

Female Initiative: Evaluation and Rehabilitation Care Excellence (FIERCE) is the brainchild of Dr. Corinna Franklin at Shriners Children's Erie. A specialized sports injury program, FIERCE focuses on the unique issues faced by female athletes and features an all-female care team. The hospital's highly advanced motion analysis center allows doctors to study the biometrics that can lead to distinctive injuries.

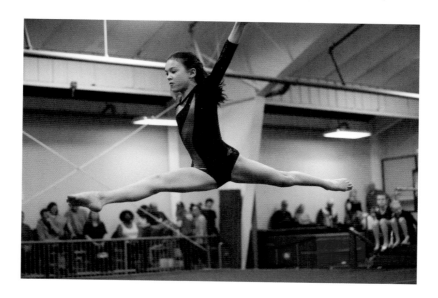

DURING THE FALL OF 2019, 13-YEAR-OLD MILA FROM GREENFIELD, Massachusetts, a cross-country runner and gymnast, began to experience pain in her right hip. Her primary care doctor referred her to the pediatric orthopaedic specialists at Shriners Children's New England. Dr. Ahmad F. Bayomy, medical director of the hospital's sports health and medicine program, diagnosed Mila with gluteus medius tendinopathy, which caused pain and decreased function in the muscle of her right hip. He referred Mila to physical therapy, where she began multiple sessions with physical therapist Megan Frazier. But then the COVID-19 pandemic hit. Unable to make in-person visits to the hospital, Mila continued her therapy sessions via the hospital's telehealth technology. With the further help of physical medicine and rehabilitation specialist Dr. Julio A. Martinez-Silvestrini, Mila is on her way back to a full recovery.

In final scrimmage on his last day of sports camp in summer 2019, 12-year-old Jaylen was tackled on his blind side just as he was pushing hard off his left leg. The blow tore his anterior cruciate ligament (ACL), the primary stabilizing ligament of the joint in his left knee. At Shriners Children's Northern California, orthopedic surgeon and sports medicine specialist Dr. Nicole Friel reconstructed Jaylen's ACL. After physical therapy, he had recovered full use of his knee and was able to return to the game he loves.

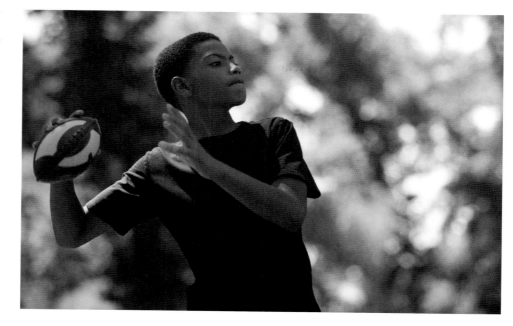

BURN INJURIES

Burn injuries have always been remarkably complex. Before the establishment of the first Shriners Burns Hospital in 1966, only half of the children admitted with extensive burns (defined then as 64% or more of total body surface area — or TBSA — affected) survived their injuries. Thanks to the extraordinary medical advances made by specialists at Shriners Children's, survival rates have soared. Now, 97% of burn patients survive, including half of the children with a TBSA of 98% or more. There have been tremendous advances in rehabilitation, with the development of new approaches to skin grafts, scar reduction and reconstructive surgery. Together with increased emphasis on the aftereffects of traumatic injury — including managing stress and reintegrating into social life — children treated at Shriners Children's not only survive but thrive.

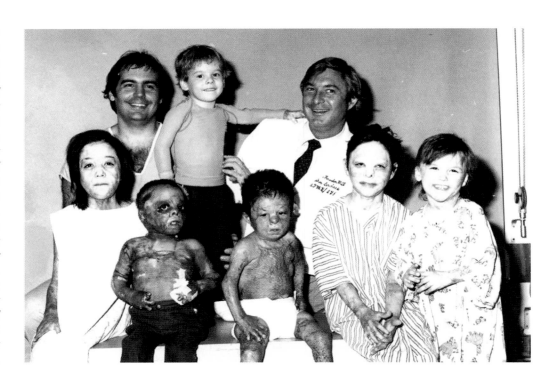

Right: Stephen was 9 years old when he was admitted to Shriners Children's Texas with burns over 73% of his body. Returning regularly for reconstructive surgery until he was 18, he was determined to become a doctor. As part of his training in medical school, he worked alongside the staff that had treated him as a patient. Today, he is a surgeon in Valdosta, Georgia.

A Shriner offers a balloon to a burns patient. Her compression garments are designed to reduce scarring.

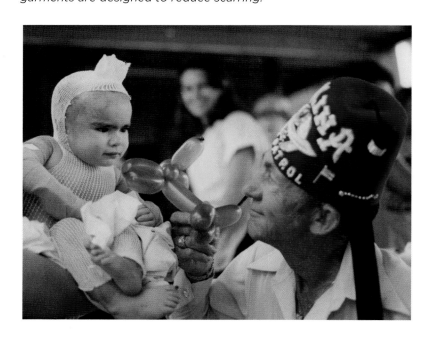

Shrine Patient Returns A Gift Of Love

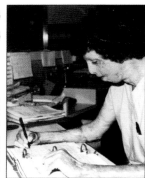

Since Shriners Burns Institutes were opened in the early 1960s, tremendous advancements have been made in the field of burns care. Today, children with burns over 90 percent or more of their bodies are surviving and going on to lead productive and challenging lives.

Stephen Zeigler was nine years old when he was admitted to the Galveston Unit in 1971 with burns over 73 percent of his body. Burned in a fire that started when spilt gasoline was ignited by a gas dryer, young Stephen was flown to the Galveston Unit, where he stayed for three months.

After Stephen went home, he returned to the hospital every six months for reconstructive surgery and other operations. The Galveston Unit became like a second home, said Stephen. The more time that he spent at the hospital, the more intrigued he became of what was being done there. Zeigler, now 25, knew early on that he would make a life of medicine.

"My experience at Shriners really led me into medicine," said Zeigler. "I was intrigued by what was going on there and the dedication of the staff."

More than just going into medicine, Zeigler had decided that he wanted to return to the Galveston Unit - this time on the other side of the table from his previous visits.

"I have seen a lot of hospitals, and I was really impressed by Shriners," said Zeigler, speaking from a physician's rather than a patient's viewpoint. "Shriners is one of the better run hospitals I've encountered – public or private. I wanted to get a large part of my education here, if possible."

In his first couple of years of medical school, Zeigler was able to spend several summers at the Galveston Unit in the research laboratories. He returned to the hospital in June of this year as part of a senior elective. In the fall, Zeigler will apply to the University of Texas Medical Branch in Galveston in hopes of obtaining a

residency in general surgery there, part of which will be spent in rotation through the Galveston Unit.

"I can't say enough about Shriners," said Zeigler. "The children here are very sick, and it takes a lot of strength and dedication to care for them. But everyone – janitors, secretaries, nurses – everyone has only one goal – to care for the children. Everyone really works together as a team. They are excellent at what they do because they take pride in their work."

Zeigler's return to the hospital as a physician was extremely gratifying to the staff members who cared for him when he was young. Foremost in the minds of staff members is first to save the children and then to help them achieve rewarding lives. When Zeigler returned to the hospital this year, he was able to work with the children and physicians. On one of his first days back in the hospital, the nurses who had cared for little Stephen watched as future Dr. Zeigler leaned across a table and cared for a child with 90 percent burns. Tears sprung to their eyes because they knew they had done their job, and done their job well.

Zeigler, who returned to the Galveston Unit in June as part of his medical training, was once a patient at Shriners.

Operating room nurses who helped prepare Stephen Zeigler for surgery as a patient were thrilled to help him prepare for surgery, 16 years later, as a future doctor.

July 1987

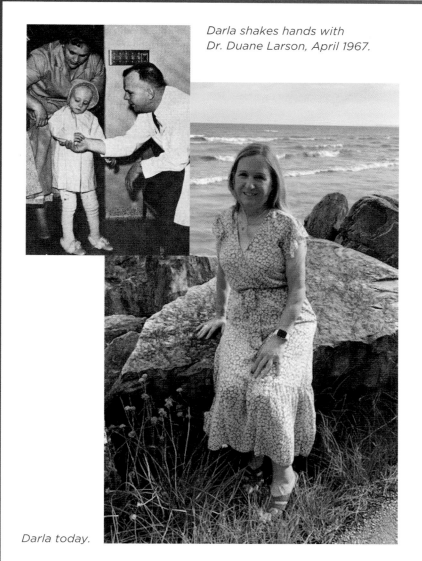

Darla shakes hands with
Dr. Duane Larson, April 1967.

Darla today.

DARLA IS ONE OF THE FIRST SUCCESSES of the Shriners Children's burns program. Born in Elk Horn, Iowa, Darla was injured in 1966 when her flannel nightgown burst into flames. More than 85% of her body was burned. After receiving emergency treatment locally, she was sent to the newly opened Shriners Children's hospital in Galveston. At the time, children typically did not survive such severe burns. Doctors gave her only a 5% chance of survival. Darla beat the odds. After 14 years of operations and skin grafts, Darla was able to pursue a full life. Working as a nurse and personal trainer, she is the mother of four children and two grandchildren. During off hours, she is a songwriter and storyteller. Darla recorded several CDs in Nashville with her band, Girls Nite Out, and today performs at local venues and the occasional Shriners convention.

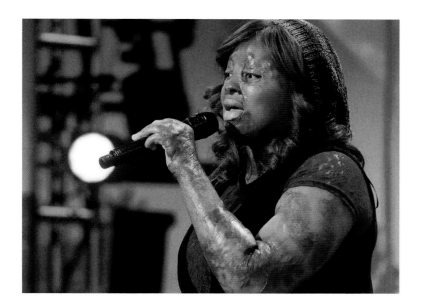

Kechi was severely burned in a plane crash in 2005 that killed all but two passengers. Her treatment at Shriners Children's Texas included music therapy. After her first singing performance at the hospital, she went on to become a finalist on America's Got Talent and a speaker at TEDx events.

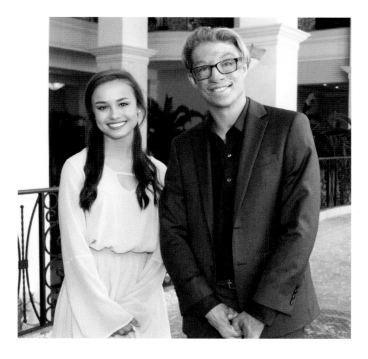

Marius (right) was 8 years old in 2007 when a house fire in his native Romania killed both of his parents and burned over 75% of his body, causing him to lose his fingers, nose and eyelids. He was adopted by an American family, who brought him to Shriners Children's Pasadena for treatment. Together with Karolina (left), another Shriners Children's patient, Marius served as National Patient Ambassador in 2016.

145

EMERGENCY RESPONSE

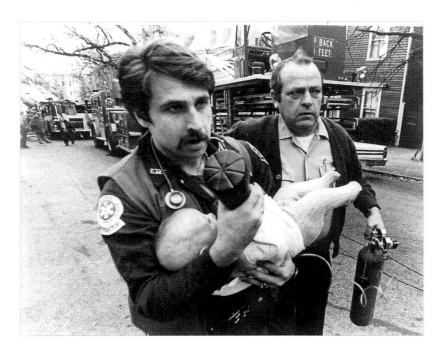

After the 1906 earthquake in San Francisco, Shriners International sent $25,000 to help the stricken city. In 1915, the fraternity contributed $10,000 for the relief of European war victims. When Shriners Children's was founded in 1922, its mission was to respond to the medical urgencies of children, wherever they might arise. Since then, the hospitals have developed procedures for responding rapidly to disasters both international and domestic.

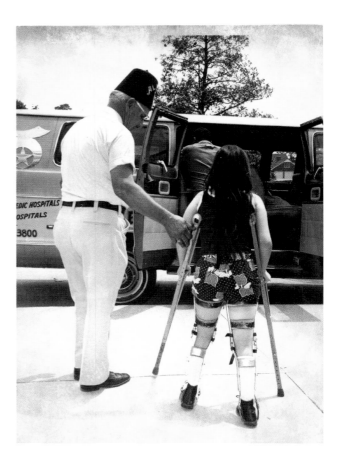

There is a long tradition among the Nobles of Shriners International of transporting patients to the hospitals for care. Many local temples have a vehicle — a car or a van — reserved for the purpose. Driven by volunteers, these transports set a precedent for more elaborate medical response.

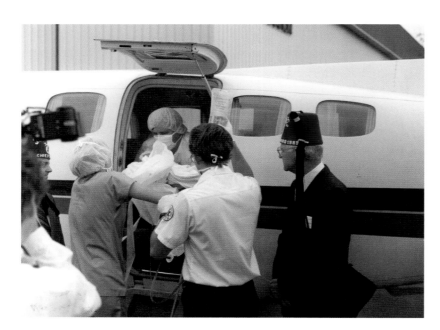

In February 1964, Shriners Children's established an air evacuation program for burns victims, receiving patients by both civilian and military aircraft. In 1990, an 8-year-old Russian child with third-degree burns over more than 30% of his body was flown from the Soviet Union, airlifted over the North Pole by a LifeGuard Alaska air ambulance, and then brought to Shriners Children's Texas for treatment.

In 1986, 15 children were flown to Shriner Children's facilities in Tampa and Boston for specialized treatment following a devastating earthquake in El Salvador. The hospitals also took in 28 children who lost limbs during the civil conflict in the country sent by the Amputee Referral Program regulated by Project HOPE.

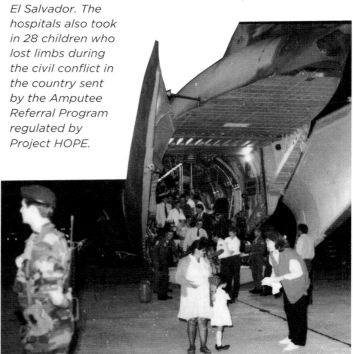

Normally focused on pediatric patients, the medical team at Shriners Children's have responded to extraordinary circumstances. Following the assault on the World Trade Center on September 11th, 2001, the Boston and Texas units sent medical professionals to New York to provide emergency burn care. Here Judy Wilkin, R. N. treats fire marshal Anthony DiFusco.

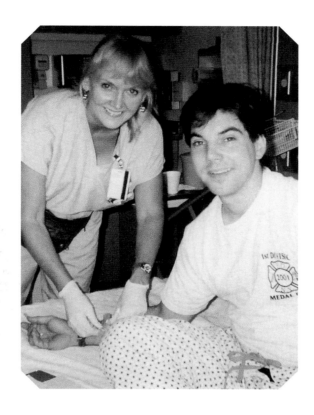

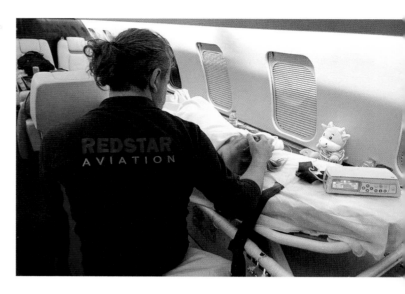

In April 2022, two children severely burned during the war in Ukraine were sent for highly specialized surgery and treatment at Shriners Children's Boston. The Shriners Children's healthcare system has provided medical help to Ukrainian children dating as far back as the 1990s for children affected by the Chernobyl disaster in 1986.

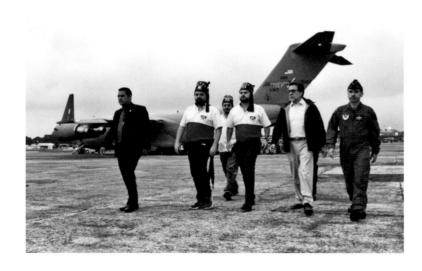

ON JUNE 3, 2018, GUATEMALA'S VOLCÁN DE FUEGO (Volcano of Fire) erupted, killing over 150 people and injuring many more, including children. The following day, Shriners Children's Texas dispatched burns specialists Dr. Jong Lee and Dr. Karel Capek, along with hospital administrator Mary Jaco. The two surgeons had done this before. They were part of a team that had traveled to Central America in 2016 and 2017 following earlier disasters. Met at the Guatemala City airport by local members of Shriners International, the emissaries from Shriners Children's visited local hospitals to help stabilize the victims.

Less than 48 hours after arriving in Guatemala, the Shriners team had identified the most acute pediatric cases. They escorted six patients and their families onto the U.S. Air Force's C-17 Globemaster III aircraft that the U.S. State Department had requested to use for transfer. The plane landed around 4:40 a.m. at Scholes International Airport in Galveston, where ambulances were waiting. "Once the wounds are closed, you move on to the rehabilitation phase," explained Dr. Steven Wolf, Chief of Staff at Shriners Children's Texas. "That really means getting them back to normal livelihood and activities. ... That's our mission. That's why we do this."

CLEFT LIP AND PALATE

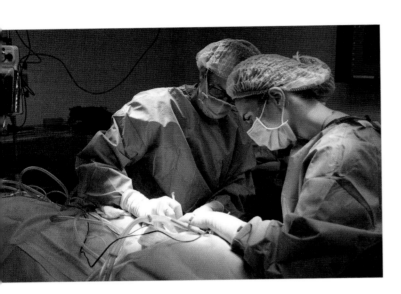

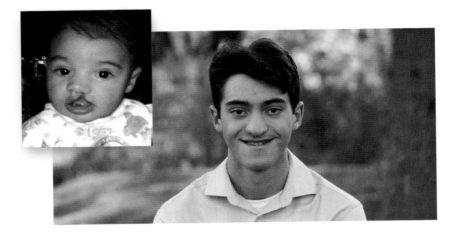

In 1970, Dr. Martin R. Sullivan first began offering cleft lip and palate repair surgery at Shriners Children's Chicago. Orofacial clefts are among the most common congenital disabilities. However, their consequences can run below the surface, affecting breathing, hearing, speaking and eating. It is common for self-esteem and emotional health to be impacted as well. By the early 1980s, Dr. Sullivan's initiative had developed into a well-coordinated program. The Chicago hospital's cleft lip and palate program became a model for other Shriners Children's facilities to follow. In 1998, Shriners Children's made a commitment to a full craniofacial surgery program. There are now board-certified plastic surgeons at nine of the system's medical facilities.

Griffin first went to Shriners Children's Boston for surgery on his cleft lip when he was was 4 months old and cleft palate surgery six months later. Further bone grafts and orthodontic care were required as he grew. Today, he is 19 years old and a student at the University of Florida in Gainesville. As his mother Jennifer says, it has been "an unbelievable journey."

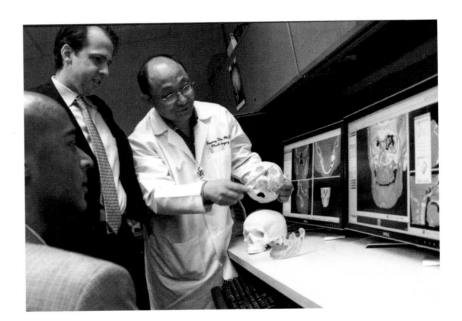

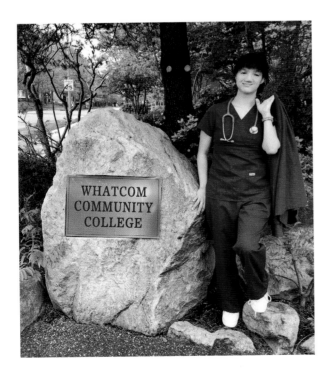

At Shriners Children's Chicago, biomedical engineer Dr. Linping Zhao (right) works with surgeons Dr. David Morris (center) and Dr. Marco Ellis (seated) to create a surgical plan for a patient who has cleft lip and palate. 3-D imaging allows for the production of custom implants and surgical templates before the operation. "Every day the technology is getting better and better," said Dr. Zhao.

Left: Born with a severe case of cleft lip and palate, as well as hemifacial dysplasia, a condition affecting the growth rate of the bones of her face, Megan was a patient of Shriners Children's for 16 years, beginning at the age of 5. "I was scared of doctors before I came to the Portland hospital and they helped me so I wasn't afraid anymore," said Megan. "I wouldn't be where I am today without the Shriners." Today, she is a registered nurse and a member of Daughters of the Nile, an affiliate of Shriners International. She is also the author of three children's books. She donates the proceeds from her book sales to Shriners Children's.

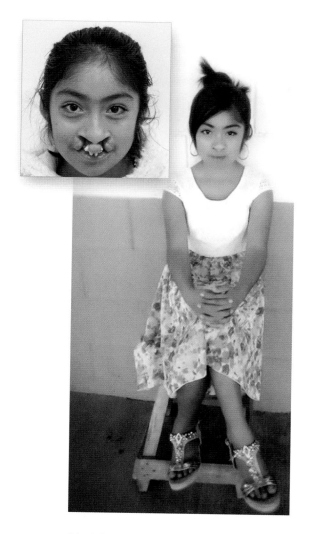

Mariela was 10 when she first underwent surgery to correct her congenital cleft lip and palate at Shriners Children's Southern California. "It is a great moment when, after the surgery, we give children like Mariela a mirror so they can see the change," said plastic Dr. Caroline Yao.

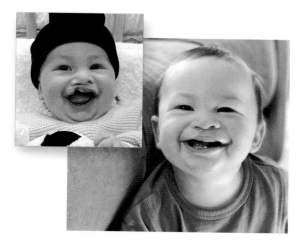

Saint, before and after his surgery at Shriners Children's Boston: different lip, same irresistible smile.

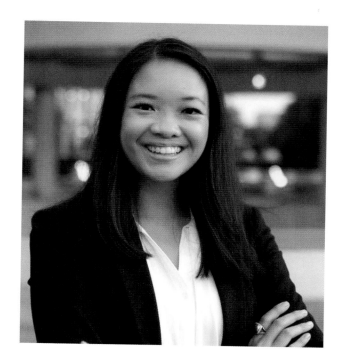

BORN WITH A CLEFT LIP AND CLEFT palate, Emma spent her first two years in an orphanage in Nanning, China, before coming to the United States in 1998 with her adoptive parents. Her condition affected her hearing and her speech, requiring multiple surgeries at Shriners Children's Texas, along with extensive therapy. As a 5th grader, Emma had surgery to harvest bone marrow from her hip to implant in her palate. During her senior year of high school, she received the first prosthetic tooth Shriners Children's ever implanted. The long and challenging years of treatment did not affect her achievement. Emma graduated from college magna cum laude. By the time she received her law degree from the University of Houston in 2021, she had won 19 awards and scholarships. Emma is now a practicing attorney in Houston, where she also volunteers at the Montrose Center and serves on the board of directors for the Texas Freedom Network and the Prism Foundation.

RHEUMATIC DISEASES

Pediatric rheumatologists treat a wide variety of conditions affecting children's joints, soft tissues, muscles and bones. Rheumatic diseases, which include autoimmune diseases and connective tissue disorders, can affect multiple parts of the body. The most commonly seen condition in the rheumatology clinics at Shriners Children's is juvenile idiopathic arthritis (JIA). Other conditions include dermatomyositis, fibromyalgia, lupus, lyme disease, mixed connective tissue disease, periodic fever syndrome, scleroderma, Sjogren's syndrome, spondyloarthropathy, and vasculitis. Some rheumatic diseases need attention right away and then fade away. Others are chronic and require lifelong care from a dedicated team.

To fill a void in the unmet health care needs of children in North America, Shriners Hospitals for Crippled Children has begun a comprehensive program of care for youngsters with juvenile rheumatoid arthritis (JRA).

In 1990, the Boards of Directors and Trustees of Shriners Hospitals approved the recommendation to move ahead on this major commitment.

In this era of cost containment, children with JRA and related disorders are finding it increasingly troublesome to get the care and treatment they need. For example, it is difficult for JRA patients with acute flare-ups of their arthritis to gain access to inpatient hospital treatment and intensive therapy, even if they have insurance. The primary reason is that insurance companies have placed undue prohibitions on this type of medical care. JRA patients also require complex coordinated multidisciplinary care, rarely found outside of children's children's medical center settings.

Specialists involved in the care of these patients include the pediatric rheumatologist, ophthalmologist, dentist, pediatric orthopaedic surgeon, nurse clinician, physical therapist, occupational therapist, psychologist, family services and orthotist. These disciplines need to be effectively coordinated and must be available for the care of such children in both inpatient and outpatient settings.

Though Shriners Hospitals has always cared for children with arthritis — and some of our units in the past have developed comprehensive programs of care, we are now taking the initiative to set up such treatment programs in all of our orthopaedic hospitals. As a result, Shriners Hospitals can serve as a community resource to pediatricians and pediatric rheumatol-

Shriners Hospitals take major step in treatment of juvenile rheumatoid arthritis

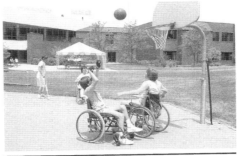

Juvenile rheumatoid arthritis patients can lead active lives, thanks to Shriners Hospitals for Crippled Children

By Newton C. McCollough III, M.D.
Director of Medical Affairs
Shriners Hospitals for Crippled Children

ogists for the care of their patients with JRA and related disorders. Our hospitals also can help to meet needs that are not now being addressed.

Of our 19 orthopaedic hospitals, 12 already have approved comprehensive programs for JRA patients. These include the Chicago, Erie, Honolulu, Houston, Lexington, Los Angeles, Montreal, Portland, St. Louis, Spokane, Springfield and Twin Cities units. Two other hospitals—San Francisco and Tampa—have pediatric rheumatologists on their medical staffs, but have not yet finalized their program organization. The remaining five hospitals are in the process of meeting the criteria for the start of their programs.

More than 800 patients with the diagnosis of juvenile rheumatoid arthritis are enrolled in our 19 orthopaedic hospitals. About 150 new JRA patients are seen annually.

Major research efforts on the possible causative factors in JRA are under way at the Montreal Unit's Center for Joint Disease Research. In addition, the Portland, Tampa and Honolulu units are conducting basic research in this area.

Shriners Hospitals for Crippled Children was instrumental in helping to develop the specialty of pediatric rheumatology by partial funding of its first national conference in 1976. In March 1991, "The World's Greatest Philanthropy" helped to fund a third major conference in pediatric rheumatology. More than 300 specialists — from the U.S., Canada and Mexico — attended.

We are very anxious to have all of our orthopaedic hospitals become involved in the care and treatment of JRA, because we know there are many children who are eagerly awaiting our help.

July 1991

Dr. Peter Blier, rheumatology specialist at Shriners Children's New England, with one of his patients.

Although arthritis is commonly thought of as a condition of old age, JIA affects nearly 300,000 children in the United States. However, "there are fewer than 400 pediatric rheumatologists in North America," notes Dr. Thomas G. Mason II of Shriners Children's Twin Cities. Many cases go undiagnosed.

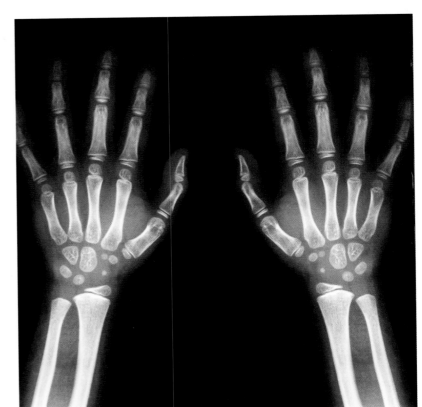

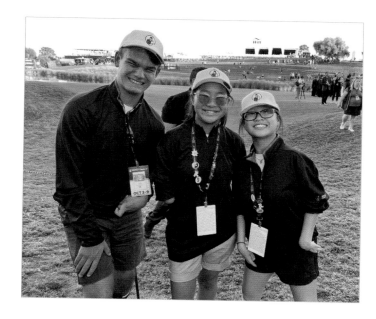

ISAAC (LEFT) WAS BORN SIX WEEKS EARLY with many medical complications, including juvenile arthritis. He suffered a stroke when he was one year old, causing hemiplegia on his left side, and has made his left arm and leg less functional. When it got to the point when he could no longer walk, his parents brought him to Shriners Children's Spokane. He was 6 years old.

Ten years later, Isaac is on the soccer field. Receiving care and medication not only helped him to walk again, but also connected him with a community of friends who are living with the same condition. He has grown to be a stronger, more confident young man. He still visits Shriners Children's regularly to improve the function of his left side. Dedicated as he is to the game, he aspires to become a soccer referee.

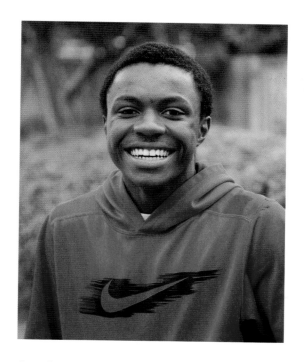

A nationally ranked runner with the attention of multiple college programs, Dominic was an active high school freshman with Olympic aspirations. When unexplainable pain in Dominic's legs began to affect his ability to walk without assistance, his family's search for answers led them to the Shriners Children's Shreveport, where Dr. Sarwat Umer provided something that had proven elusive for the better part of a year: a diagnosis, and a path to health. Nick is now back on track.

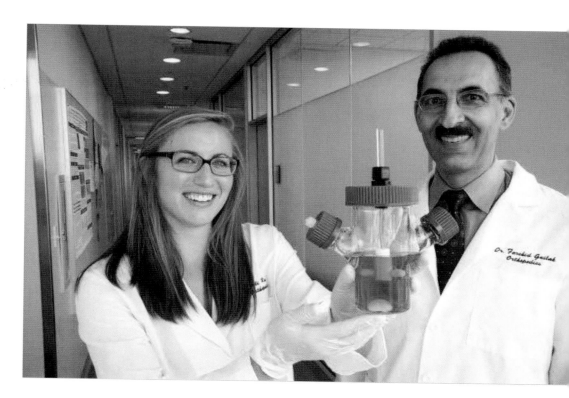

Dr. Farshid Guilak (right), a researcher at Shriners Children's Twin Cities, heads a lab focused on developing new molecular and cell-based therapies to address juvenile arthritis.

BRITTLE BONE DISEASE

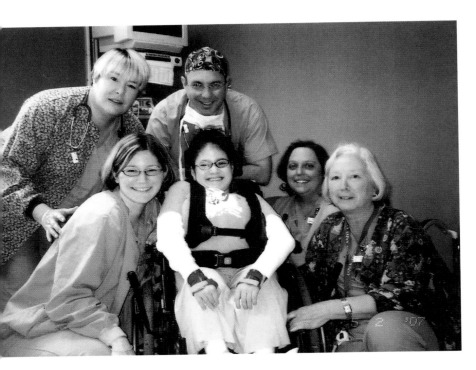

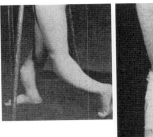
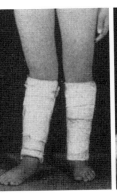
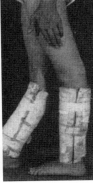

These pre- and post-surgery photographs document one of the first cases of osteogenesis imperfecta treated by Shriners Children's, back in 1925.

Affecting between 25,000 and 50,000 people in the United States, osteogenesis imperfecta (OI), or brittle bone disease, is a family of genetic disorders that prevent the formation of strong bones. Children with the condition are at risk for a wide range of additional problems, including weak teeth, hearing loss, respiratory difficulties and frequent fractures. In addition, because their leg bones cannot always support their weight, many children with OI require a wheelchair or other assistance. Doctors at Shriners Children's have been treating the condition since the 1920s, and the hospital's researchers — particularly in Montreal — have striven for decades to develop tools and therapies to improve the lives of children with OI.

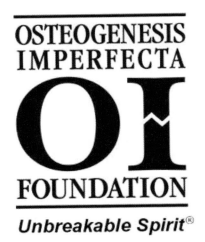

On April 22, 1970: Midge Peck, Gemma Geisman, Renee Gardner and Becky Keller organized a meeting at Shriners Children's Chicago to explore founding a national organization for OI families. With the help of Dr. Harold Sofield, Dr. Edward Milar, and nurse Frances Dubowski, they formed the Osteogenesis Imperfecta Foundation to sponsor OI research, support affected families and individuals, and raise awareness.

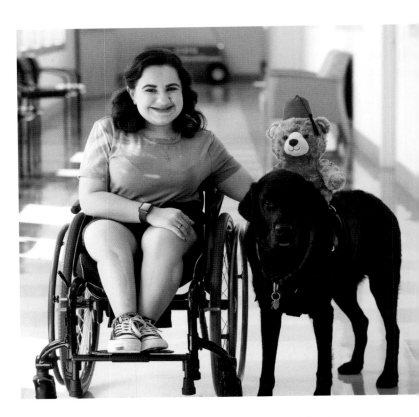

Leigh was registered as a patient at Shriners Children's Florida before she was born. At the age of 3, she adopted a practice of gratitude. Asked what she wanted for her birthday, the toddler replied that she was not interested in gifts; instead, she wanted people to donate to the hospital. By the time Leigh was 15, she had raised $1 million for Shriners Children's. In 2022, she graduated from the University of Tampa with a degree in nursing.

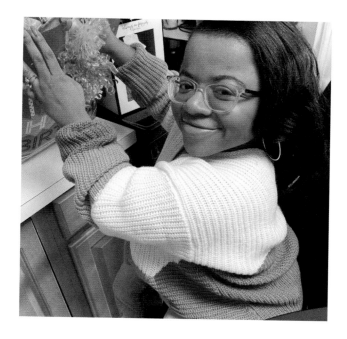

HANNAH HAS OVERCOME extraordinary odds to succeed. Born with OI, she was raised by her single mother in Maryland. Her condition causes her bones to fracture easily. A simple sneeze could break a rib. Hannah endured over 150 fractures by the time she was 15. Money was tight, and even though treatment at Shriners Hospitals for Children Canada, in Montreal, was available, there were many other expenses – such as a van to transport her safely in her wheelchair and a custom bed to reduce the possibility of falling. When Hannah was 8, the state stopped providing the nursing care she needed. Her mother had to quit her job to keep her safe, and the two faced eviction multiple times.

Despite her tremendous disadvantages, Hannah excelled, thanks in part to what everyone describes as her radiantly positive personality. When she was only 12, Hannah launched Goddiva Hannah, a YouTube channel to share beauty and lifestyle tips that has logged over 800,000 views to date. She graduated high school in 2018 with honors, receiving National Merit awards. In 2022, she received her bachelor of science, magna cum laude, from Stevenson University, where she majored in graphic design with a minor in entrepreneurship and business development. A proud member of Alpha Kappa Alpha Sorority, Inc., Hannah continues to achieve, never letting her physical limitations stop her from pursuing her dreams.

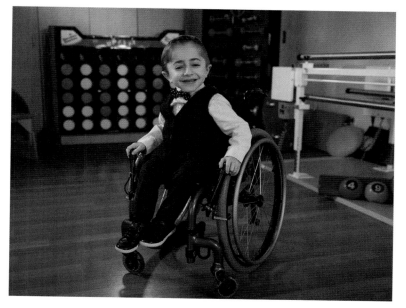

A medical team from Shriners Hospitals for Children Canada was on hand when Kaleb was born. Fourteen years, 11 surgeries and 200 fractures later, he still stays positive.

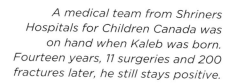

NEUROMUSCULAR DISORDERS

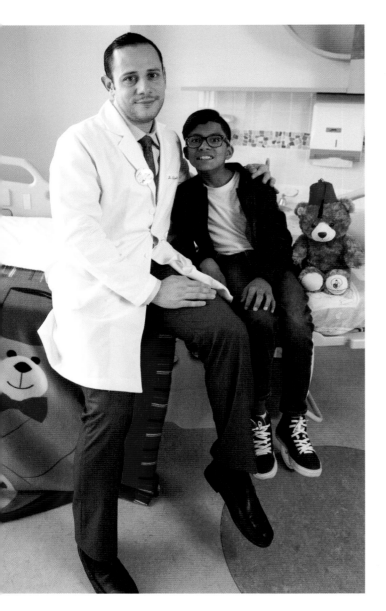

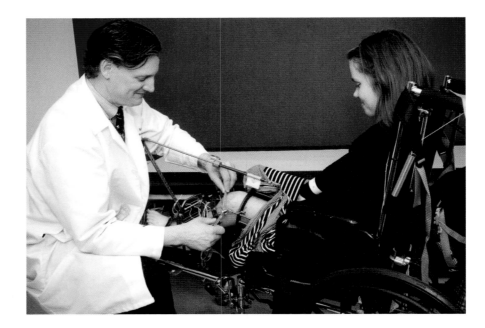

Olya, a patient at Shriners Children's Philadelphia, is affected with arthrogryposis multiplex congenita (AMC), a rare condition that curbs muscle development and affects the joints. Here, Dr. Harold van Bosse is adjusting an external fixator that is designed to rotate her knee gradually and pull it straight, reducing the number of surgical interventions.

Yael with Dr. Alejandro Dabaghi-Richerand, an orthopedic surgeon at Shriners Children's Mexico. Shriners Children's has long treated children with a wide range of neuromuscular conditions, including cerebral palsy, spina bifida, Marfan syndrome, muscular dystrophy, and arthrogryposis. These conditions range in complexity and severity, and they can appear in several ways, often evolving as a child grows. Because each case is different, staff at Shriners Children's work closely with each patient to develop an individualized treatment plan that meets his or her unique needs.

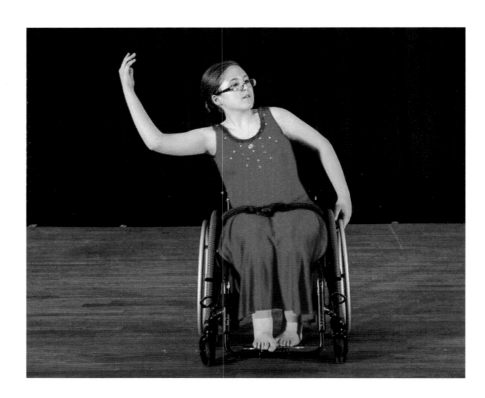

Jessie has been coming to Shriners Children's Florida since 2006. She was born with spina bifida, scoliosis, bilateral hip dysplasia and clubfoot, but that has not stopped her from pursuing her passions. At 15, she is actively involved in REVYouth, an all-ability dance group that meets weekly, and she has participated in dance marathon events at the University of South Florida. As a patient ambassador, she sets an example for younger patients who are overcoming similar challenges.

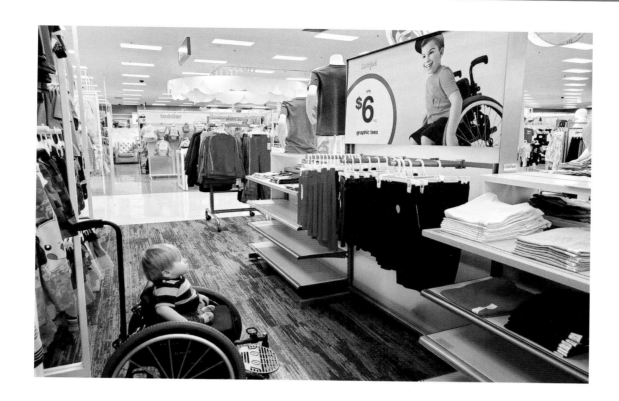

COLTON, BORN WITH SPINA BIFIDA, has been a patient at Shriners Children's New England since 2012 and a model since 2014, appearing in ads for Cat & Jack, Toys"R"Us, Tommy Hilfiger and Lands' End. He was the first child using a wheelchair to participate in New York Fashion Week. His public appearances are inspirational. In 2020, a mom named Demi posted on social media about the reaction of her 2-year-old son, a patient at Shriners Children's Salt Lake City with caudal regression syndrome: "Today Oliver stopped me dead in his tracks and turned back around to see this picture that he spotted! He just stared at it in awe! He recognized another boy like him, smiling and laughing on a display at Target. Oliver sees kids every day, but he never gets to see kids like him. This was amazing!"

Dr. Maya Evans, medical director of the spina bifida program at Shriners Children's Northern California, received national recognition from the Spina Bifida Association in 2020.

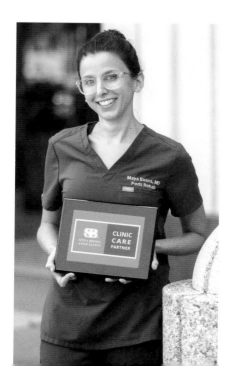

Nine-year-old Cooper, afflicted with Charcot-Marie-Tooth disease, a neuromuscular disorder, prepares to shoot some hoops with members of the 2019 rookie class of the Chicago Bears.

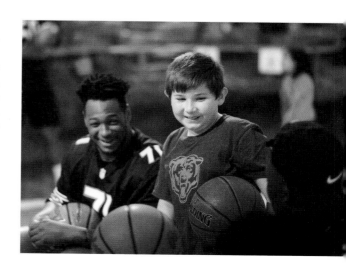

CEREBRAL PALSY

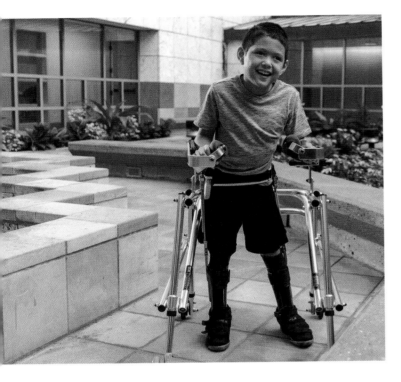

Left: Cerebral palsy is a general term applied to many conditions that can result from a disturbance to the developing brain. Cerebral palsy affects muscle tone, movement and coordination. This can make it difficult for a child to control the movement of their body. Common activities like speaking, standing or sitting can be challenging. Some children may have associated health conditions related to cognition, speech, vision, hearing, breathing issues or difficulty eating and swallowing. A definitive diagnosis may not be made until 24 to 30 months of age, as there can be other causes of these symptoms. Shriners Children's hospitals have multidisciplinary neuromuscular teams to maximize the function of children with cerebral palsy.

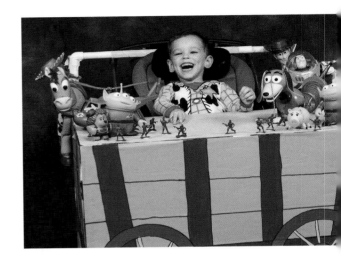

Above: Jaxson, diagnosed with cerebral palsy when he was 9 months old, first became a patient at Shriners Children's Greenville at age 2. "Before Shriners Children's, we felt like we were in the dark; we didn't know what he needed or the possibilities he could have," said his mother. Now, not only is Jaxson standing but he is also no longer in debilitating pain. "Jaxson has progressed so much, and the care he has received here is what made a difference."

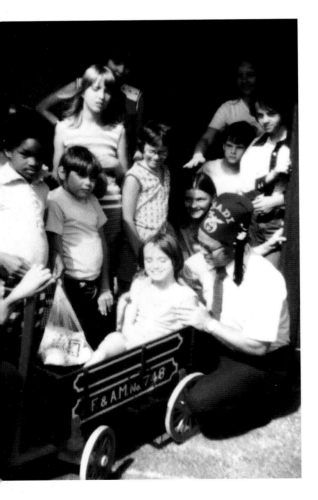

Of the thousands of children with cerebral palsy treated at Shriners Children's, the most iconic is Bobbi Jo. (left). When she began treatment at Shriners Children's St. Louis at age 5, she had difficulty walking or standing. Noble Albert L. Hortman of Hadi Temple. Evansville, Indiana, saw her struggling and gave her a hand (right). Captured by newspaper photographer Randy Dieter, the 1970 photograph known as "Editorial Without Words" was swiftly adopted as the Shriners Children's logo (below).

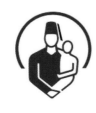

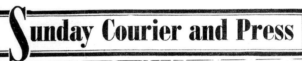

Sunday Courier and Press

VOL. 32, NO. 24   6 SECTIONS, SECTION A   EVANSVILLE, INDIANA, SUNDAY, JUNE 14, 1970   118 PAGES

Humphrey Launches Senate Bid

Special to The Washington Post

WAVERLY, Minn. — Former Vice President Hubert H. Humphrey Saturday began his long-expected bid for a political comeback, stressing his experience and bread-and-butter issues — and stirring new speculation about 1972.

He formally declared for the Senate seat his 1968 presidential contest nemesis, Sen. Eugene J. McCarthy (D-Minn.) is vacating with cryptic talk about a third party.

But Humphrey said he would not "turn away" from another presidential nomination "if it came my way."

Charging the Nixon administration was "devoid" of national objectives in a recession economy and in a "torn and divided" society, Humphrey added, however, that the war should not be a "partisan" issue.

He reiterated a call for troop withdrawal at accelerated pace "at the earliest possible date," while adding he's "encouraged" by congressional as well as presidential efforts for that objective. He is "irrevocably opposed" to further escalation, specifically in Cambodia.

So he's off and running again, coming on as an avowed member of the "Hubert & Muriel team" and against hard times and high prices.

Assured of party convention endorsement, he starts as the apparently well-in-front favorite in a contest against Rep. Clark MacGregor (R-Minn) the Nixon spokesman in Minnesota who owns the personal endorsement of Atty. Gen. John N. Mitchell and inferentially, therefore, of Mr. Nixon.

Humphrey declared he had heard "the true voice of our people" for leadership that "will stand calmly but firmly for reason and against chaos." MacGregory who says "HHH" is slipping in popularity opened a counter statement against Humphrey with the jab: "Old poli-

Nixon Na Campus I

By FRANK CORMIER

KEY BISCAYNE, Fla. ️— President Nixon appointed a special commission Saturday to seek causes and cures of campus unrest and violence. Four of the nine panel members are Negroes.

At the same time, Nixon's official spokesman said the White House has no intention of firing Secretary of Interior Walter J. Hickel, author of a "leaked" personal letter complaining to the President about the administration's attitude toward young people. There was speculation Hickel might soon resign or be dismissed.

Hickel, asked about the report after taking part in ceremonies near former President Lyndon B. Johnson's ranch in Texas, said, "I have no intention to resign. I am going to serve as long as I can be of service to the President."

Nixon signed an executive order creating what will be known formally as the President's Commission on Campus Unrest. The chairman is William W. Scranton, 52, former Republican governor of Pennsylvania.

Spurred by the shooting deaths of four students at Kent State University in Ohio and two youths at Jackson State College in Mississippi, Nixon directed the commission to "report to me before the beginning of the coming academic year." He will ask Congress to supply the body with subpoena powers and promised it would have access to the investigative facilities of the Federal Bureau of Investigation and other federal agencies.

Leaving the rest of the family in Washington, Nixon flew here Friday afternoon for a weekend in the sun, bringing with him H. R. "Bob" Haldeman, his chief of staff, and Robert H. Finch, secretary of health, education and

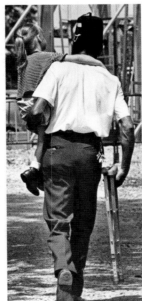

The "helping hand" of Hadi Shrine reached out and sent a group of local crippled children to Mesker Park for a day of summer fun and excitement last week. Here one of the Shriners who accompanied the happy group gives a lift to a youngster as she eagerly eyes one of the amusements.

North Viet Troops Flee Laotian City

SAIGON (UPI)—North Vietnamese forces were reported Saturday to have withdrawn under fire from Saravane, a strategic province capital in Southern Laos seized last Tuesday. In Cambodia the government said Communist troops were setting up hospitals and storehouses in the Angkor Temple ruins.

Communiques issued in the Cambodian capital of Phnom Penh told of government victories over Communist units in several sections of the countryside, including the breaking of a hold on the vital highway

tional Police for antigovernment activities.

Military sources in Vientiane, the capital of Laos, said a force of about 500 North Vietnamese troops who had seized Saravane last Tuesday withdrew from the city Friday night in the face of a counterattack by Laotian forces supported by air strikes.

The sources said U.S.-piloted planes pounded suspected enemy concentrations around Saravane, 375 miles southeast of Vientiane, while American-built T28 Fighter-bombers of the Laotian Air Force softened up the city itself in advance of the

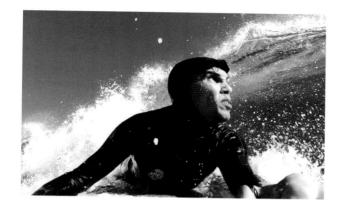

BORN WITH SPASTIC CEREBRAL PALSY, Jacob was 8 years old when he first went to Shriners Children's Northern California.

His time there shaped him into an individual capable of overcoming any challenge. "After a while, you start to feel like an experiment in hospitals, and it's depressing when you go because you're always told what's wrong with you," said Jacob. "Shriners Children's flipped that narrative and focused on possibilities – what I could do if I worked hard enough and who I could become." Today, he is a content creator, entrepreneur, model, professional surfer, and inspirational speaker based in Long Beach, California. "With surfing, a wave is very similar to life," he says. "It's going to keep coming at you and you have a choice. Either you go over it, under it, or you turn around and you catch that sucker!"

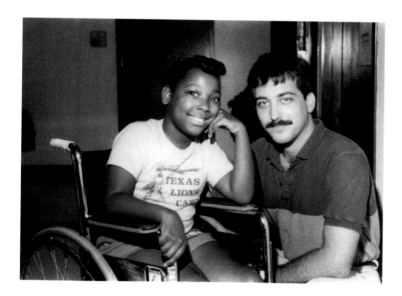

Jennifer was born in Wichita Falls, Texas, in May of 1979 just six weeks after a huge tornado devastated the area. She weighed only two pounds, five ounces at birth, and her weight dropped to one pound, nine ounces shortly thereafter. Doctors initially believed that she would have no long-term effects from the low birth weight. However, after nine months when she failed to develop early motor skills, the baby girl was sent to Fort Worth Children's Hospital, where doctors diagnosed cerebral palsy. She was soon referred to Shriners Children's Texas for specialized care, and the long process of helping Jennifer began.

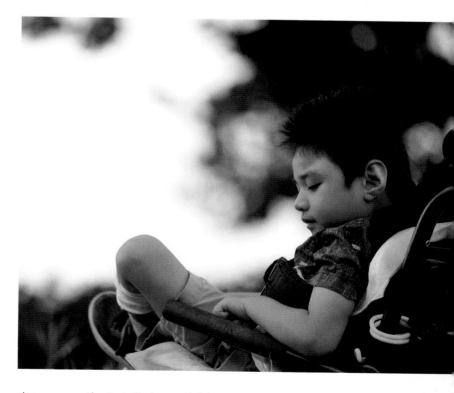

James, a patient at Shriners Children's Hawaii since 2013 and a classical music aficionado, follows a ketogenic diet to manage the seizures associated with his condition. "I really enjoy probiotic meals with fermented foods like natto, sauerkraut and poi because they are tasty," said James. "I am growing in all ways and am so grateful I have the equipment, doctors and therapists at Shriners Children's Hawaii to support me in my growth intellectually, emotionally and physically. I am enjoying life."

REHABILITATION AND THERAPY

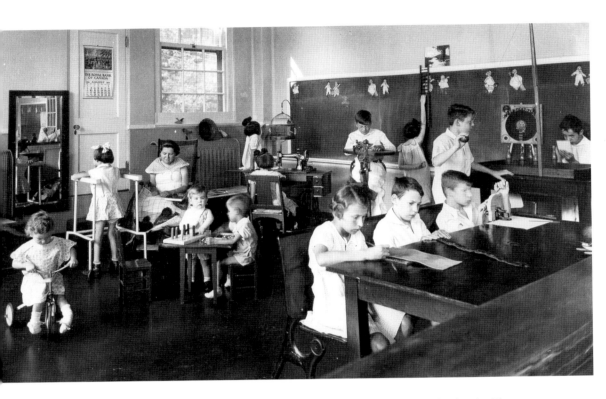

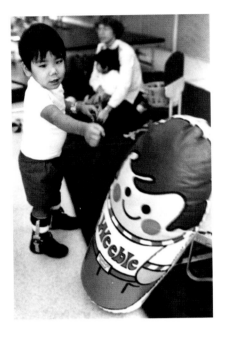

"Weebles wobble, but they don't fall down!" For this reason, they made useful tools for pediatric patients to practice balancing on new legs, as this young boxer has discovered.

Hospitals like Shriners Children's are foremost about healing the body. They also recognize that for pediatric patients especially, strengthening the spirit is equally important. Shriners Children's has long centered its mission on fostering a compassionate, family-centered and collaborative care environment. This happens in the hospitals with physical rehabilitation programs and counseling to help young patients manage the traumatic stress of their conditions. There are also programs to teach independent living skills and foster peer integration. A classroom at Shriners Hospitals for Children Canada in 1931 also served as a therapeutic space where recovering patients could work on their motor skills.

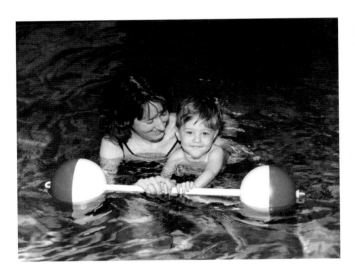

Doctors have long recognized the medical value of hydrotherapy for patients recovering from orthopedic surgery. Exercising in the water decreases pain, increases mobility, and builds strength. Pediatric patients have long recognized another value in hydrotherapy: playing in the pool is fun.

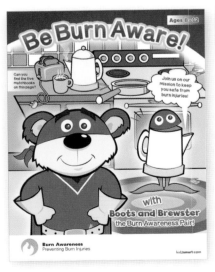

Beyond the care Shriners Children's lavishes on each patient individually, the network has long emphasized the importance of education more broadly. A nationwide burn prevention program launched in 1975 raised awareness and helped drive changes to make children safer.

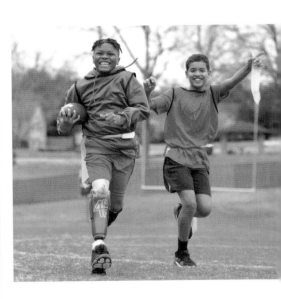

Tending to one's mental health is a vital part of physical recovery. Parker was an avid athlete when he lost his leg in a car accident at age 13. For months after the amputation, he struggled with severe depression and anxiety. Physical therapists, orthotists and other professionals at Shriners Children's Greenville helped Parker get back on the playing field and find his way back to joy. Today he shares his story to help others struggling with physical and emotional pain.

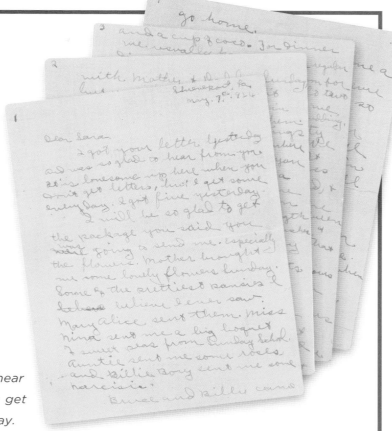

IN THE EARLY YEARS, THE ROAD TO recovery was long, and children could expect to stay in the hospital for months at a time. Corrie Lee was 13 and living on a farm just north of Grand Cane, Louisiana, when she broke her back when falling from a tree. Their local doctor sent her to Shriners Children's Shreveport for care. Her letter home, dated May 7, 1924, offers a wonderful glimpse of life in the hospital.

Dear Sara,

I got your letter yesterday and was so glad to hear from you. It is lonesome up here when you don't get letters, but I get some every day. I got five yesterday.

I will be so glad to get the package you said you was going to send me. Especially the flowers. Mother brought me some lovely flowers Sunday. Some of the prettiest pansies I believe I ever saw. Mary Alice sent them. Miss Nina sent me a big bouquet of sweet peas from Sunday School. Auntie sent me some roses, and Billie Boy sent me some narcisis [narcissus].

Bruce and Billy came with Mother and Daddy Sunday but you know they won't let children under a certain age in, so I didn't get to see them.

There are so many things to tell you I don't know where to begin. First I will tell you about my bed. It is about a yard wide and two and one half yards long. I am on a frame about the same length of the bed and about eleven inches wide. I am strapped at my shoulders and hips so I can't move my back. It gets so tiresome I don't know what to do sometimes.

Next I will tell you about the meals. For breakfast we usually have some kind of breakfast food, prunes, whole wheat bread toast, and a cup of coco[a]. For dinner [i.e. lunch] we usually have just a regular dinner. We have ice cream for dessert twice a week, & jello two or three times. Sometimes we have chocolate or rice pudding. At supper, it is what city people call tea, I suppose. We have it about 4:30 o'clock. It consists of a boiled egg, glass of milk, whole wheat bread, & canned apples, pears or some cereal. We have milk between breakfast and dinner, dinner & supper and after supper. That makes six glasses a day.

They have visiting hours twice a week. On Weds from 2:30 to 3:30. On Sun from 2:30 to 4:30. Ward round comes twice a week Mon and Sat. On ward round the doctors come around and look at you and tell you when you can go home.

Mother brought me a fountain pen Sun. I sure am proud of it. It writes so nice and easy.

As there is no other news I will close. Tell Aunt Alice and those in in your next letter, I will write to them when I find time. I have so many letters to answer I don't have much time.

Lots of love, write when you have time.

Your cousin,

Corrie Lee

A HOLISTIC APPROACH

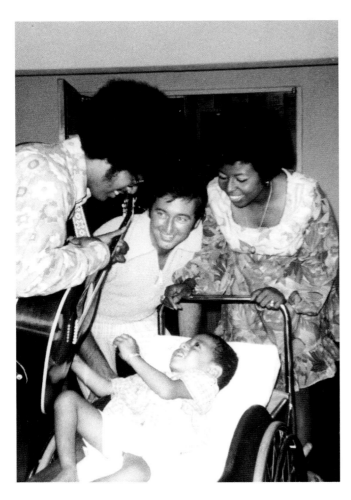

Over the years, hundreds of sports heroes and entertainment celebrities have volunteered their time to amplify the message, visiting hospitals to meet patients and appearing in public service announcements on behalf of Shriners Children's. Here, a patient at Shriners Children's Honolulu delights in the company of characters from Sesame Street including Bob (Bob McGrath) and Susan (Loretta Long).

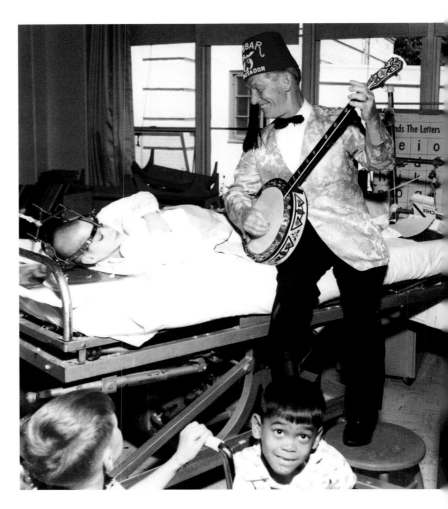

Banjo great Eddie Peabody, a member of Sabbar Temple in Tuscon, Arizona, serenades patients in Portland, Oregon. The Nobles of Shriners International have long taken it as their sacred duty to spread cheer. Some of the most famous and talented among them took on the special role of Ambassador, touring hospitals to entertain the children.

Patients at Shriners Children's Erie pose with local baseball stars, 1981. Assembled are Pittsburgh Pirates Bill Robinson (far left) and Rod Scurry (center). In plaid on the far right is sportscaster Lanny Frattare, the play-by-play radio announcer for the Pirates from 1976 to 2008.

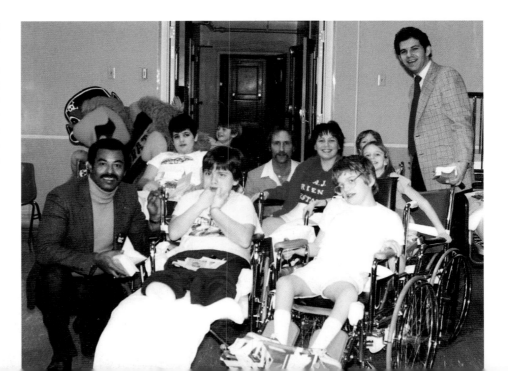

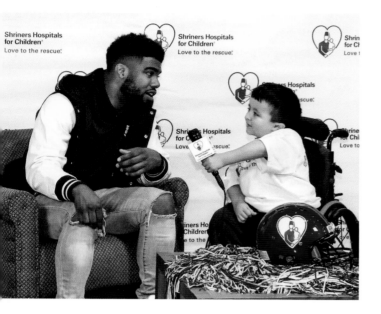

Alec began receiving treatment at Shriners Children's Chicago when he was 2 months old. An aspiring sportscaster, he has been the national face of the heathcare system since 2014. Here, he is interviewing future Dallas Cowboys running back Ezekiel Elliot in 2016.

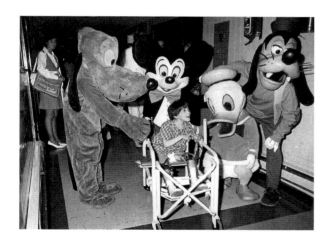

Disneyland figures admire a patient's ride at Shriners Children's Salt Lake City, 1970s.

Kelly Hansen with his new backup guitarist.

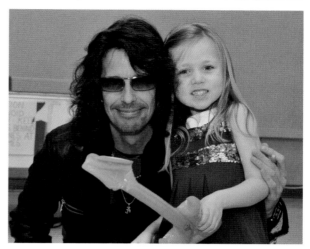

MICK JONES AND KELLY HANSEN of the band Foreigner have long supported the mission of Shriners Children's. In 2018, they made a priceless offer — they would record a new version of their #1 hit song "I Want to Know What Love Is" and donate all the proceeds. As the project unfolded, they upped the ante, recording a live version of their greatest hits to benefit Shriners Children's. Some patients even got the chance to sing backup vocals and appear in a Foreigner music video.

Seth, Sydney, Mia, and Connor, patient ambassadors for Shriners Children's, appear together at the 2021 Charleston Classic basketball tournament. Icons of hope and healing, these young role models demonstrate to the millions who have seen them on TV and social media that disability does not mean inability.

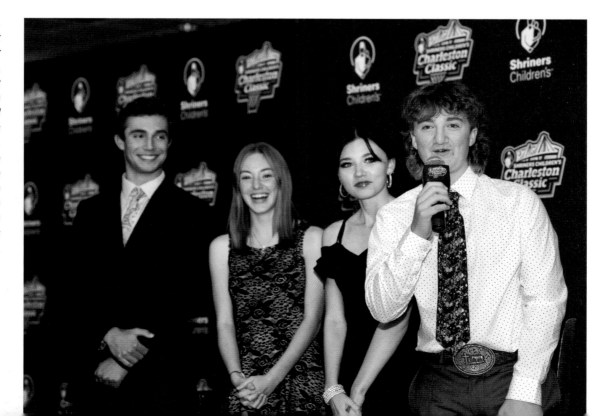

THE MIRACLE WORKERS

RUNNING A SINGLE PEDIATRIC HOSPITAL TAKES A SMALL ARMY, but for decades, Shriners Children's settled for platoons — small units of superbly trained and deeply dedicated men and women who over the past 100 years have devoted themselves to bringing children hope and healing. They include doctors and nurses, prosthetics engineers and artists, physical therapists and counselors, teachers and entertainers, van drivers and custodians and the thousands of volunteers who have donated their time to raise money, visit the wards, read stories, run programs, and ease the difficult passage to recovery. Their love brought joy to kids when they needed it the most.

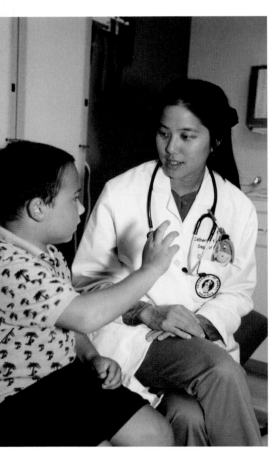
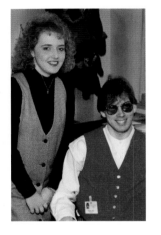
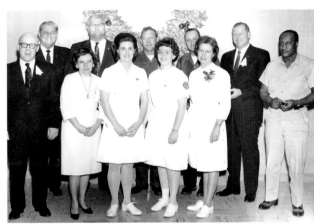
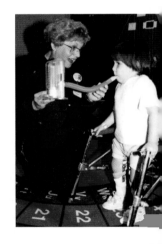
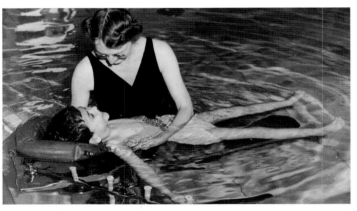
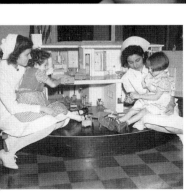
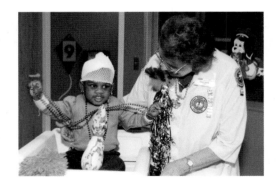
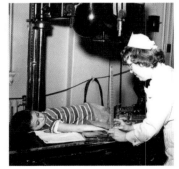
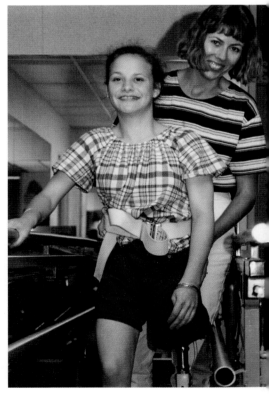

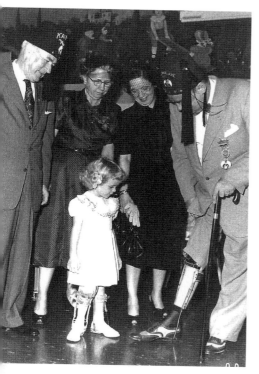
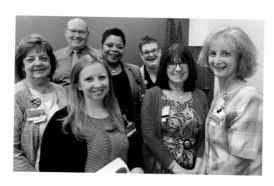
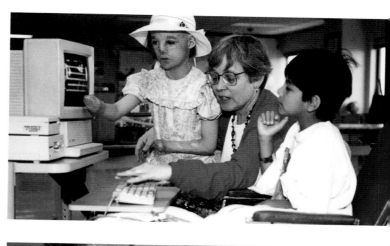
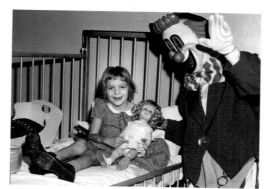
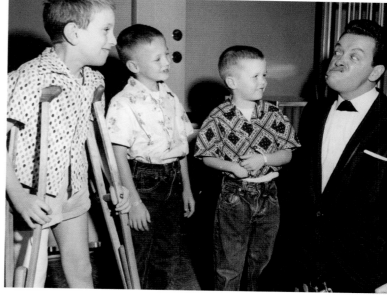
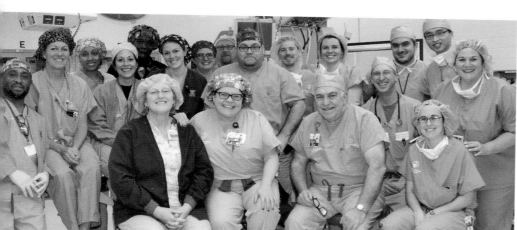
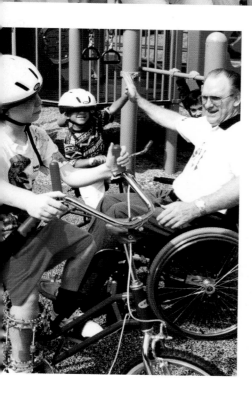
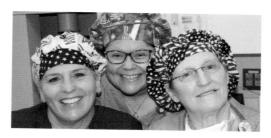
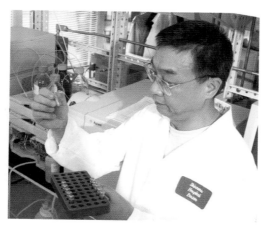
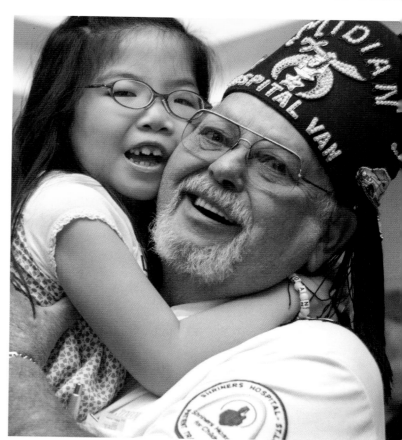

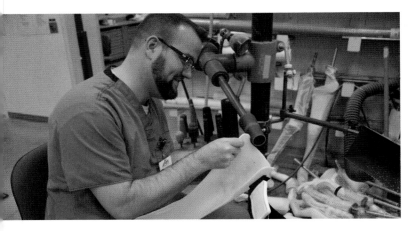

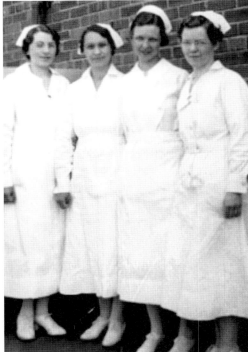

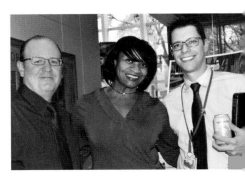

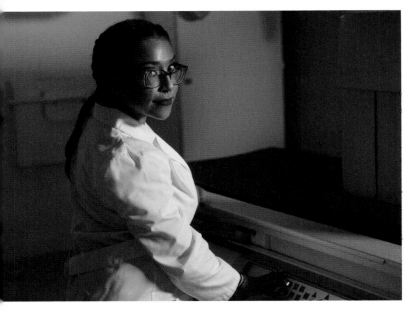

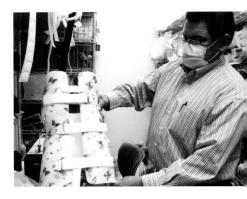

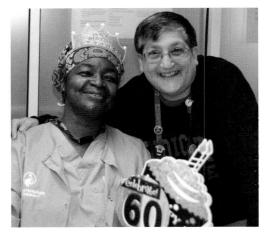

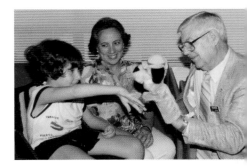

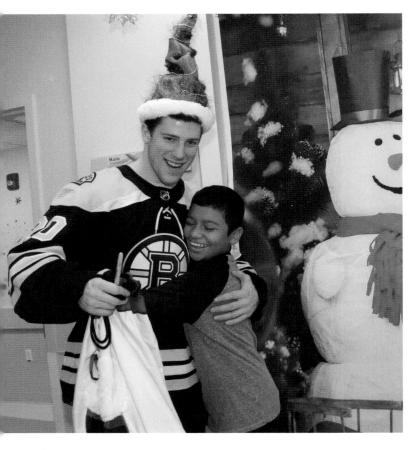

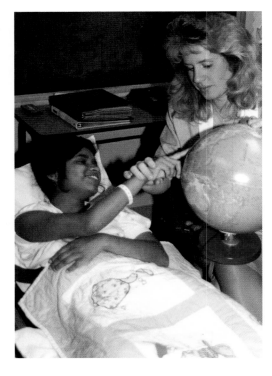

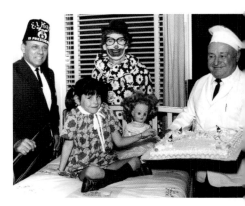

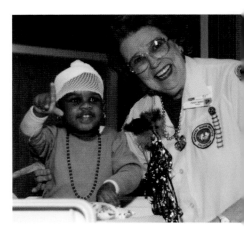

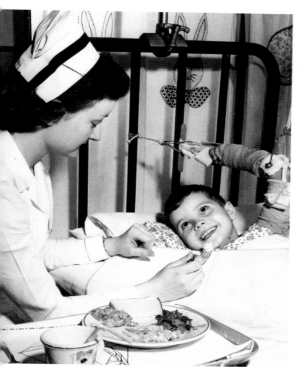
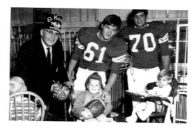
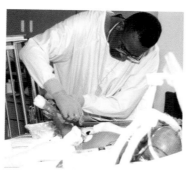
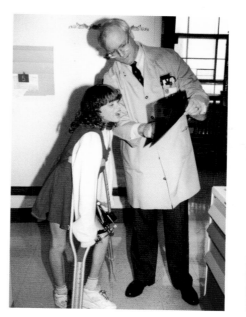
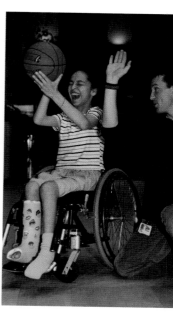
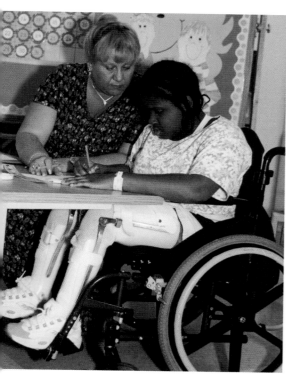
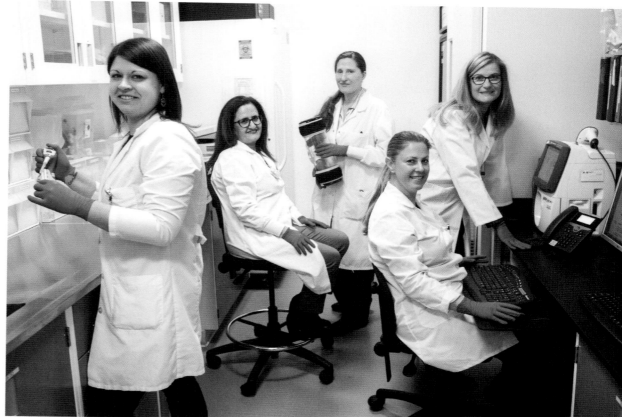
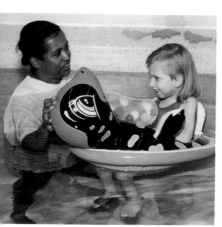
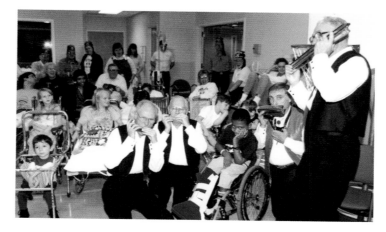
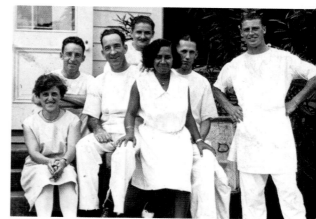

CELEBRITY ENCOUNTERS

OVER THE YEARS THOUSANDS OF PEOPLE HAVE GENEROUSLY volunteered their time to bring joy to the young patients of Shriners Children's. Among them have been hundreds of local and international celebrities, including presidents and beauty queens, actors and athletes, comedians and musicians. Here are a few of the luminaries who have graced our patients with their talents and time.

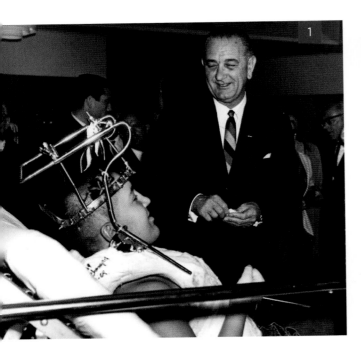

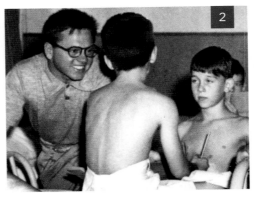

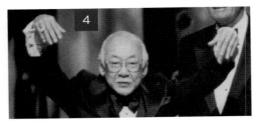

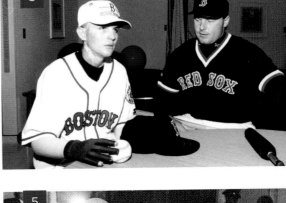

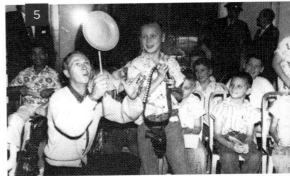

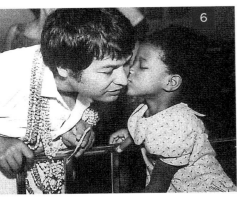

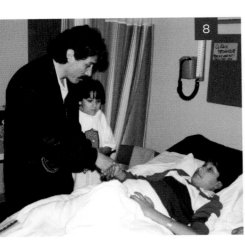

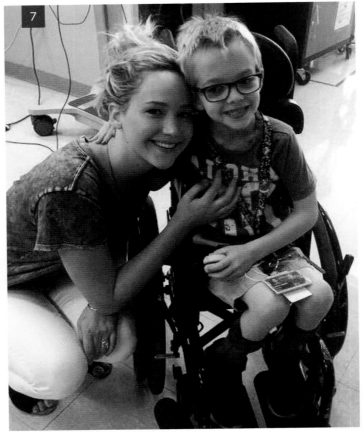

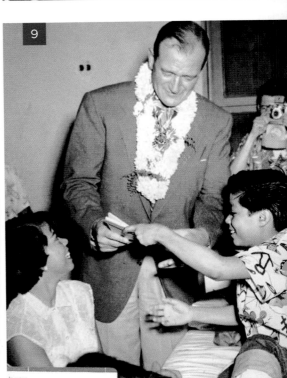

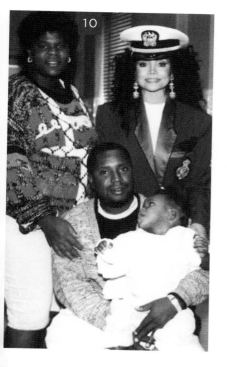

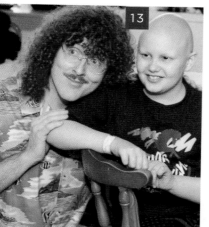

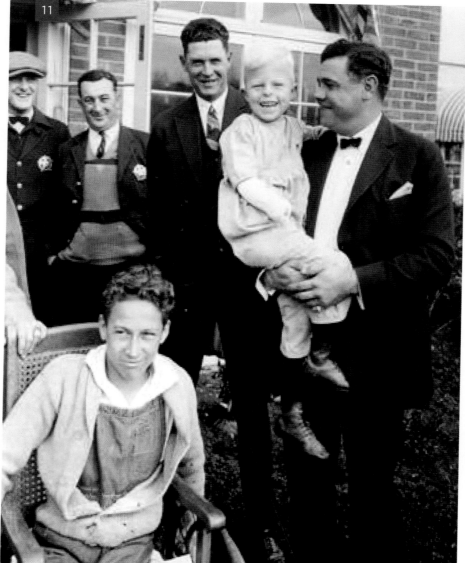

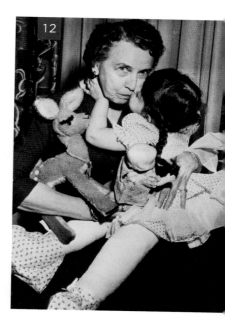

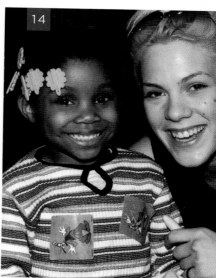

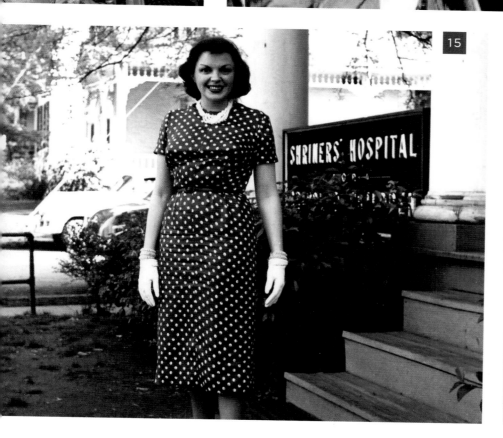

1. Lyndon B. Johnson, U.S. President
2. Mickey Rooney, actor
3. Roger Clemens, baseball player
4. Noriyuki "Pat" Morita, actor
5. Steve McQueen, actor
6. Don Ho, singer
7. Jennifer Lawrence, actress
8. Edward James Olmos, actor
9. John Wayne, actor
10. La Toya Jackson, singer
11. Babe Ruth, baseball player
12. Eleanor Roosevelt, humanitarian
13. Alfred "Weird Al" Yankovic, singer
14. Pink (Alecia Beth Moore Hart), singer
15. Judy Garland, singer

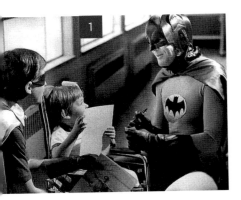

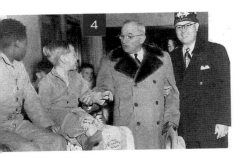

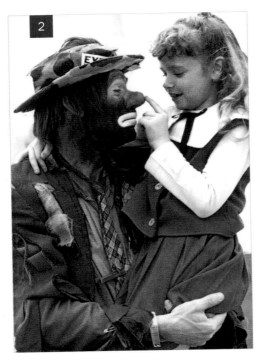

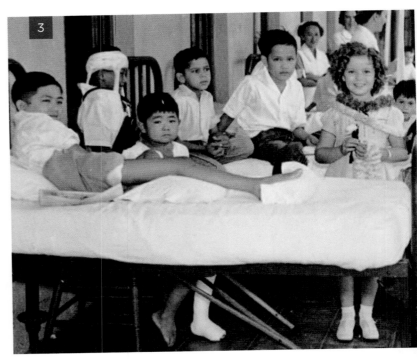

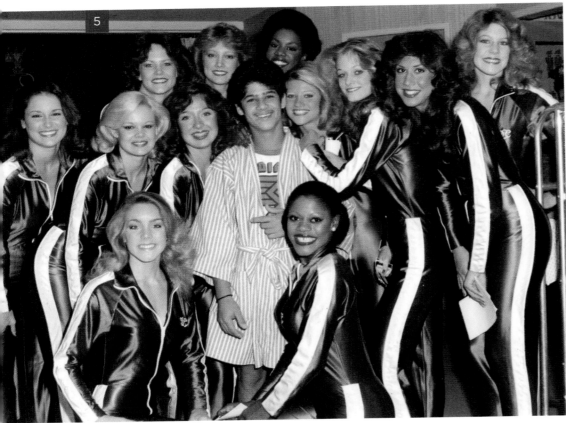

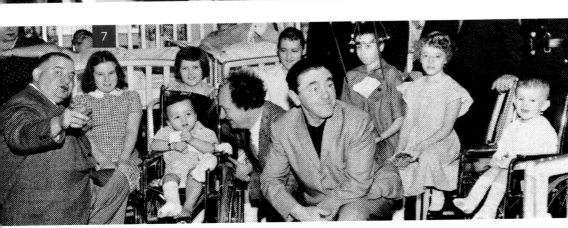

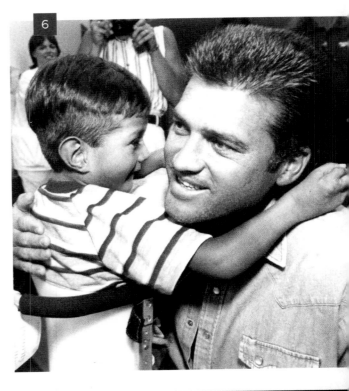

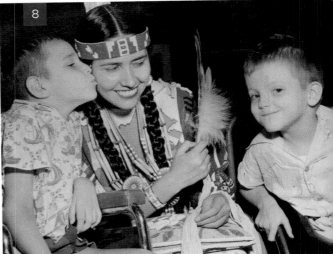

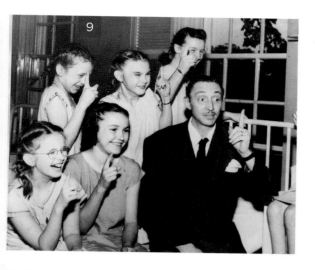

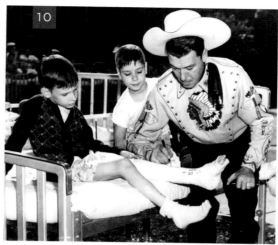

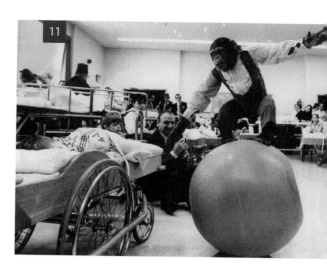

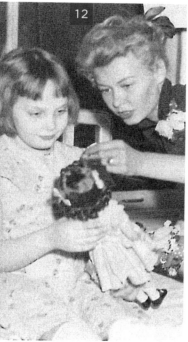

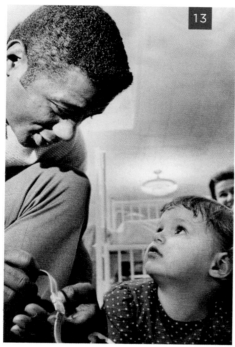

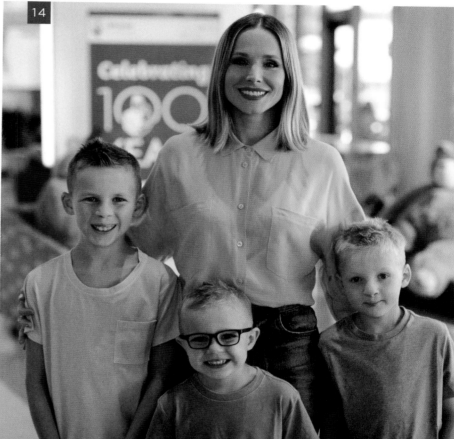

1. **Adam West and Burt Ward (Batman and Robin), actors**
2. **Emmett Kelly, clown**
3. **Shirley Temple (right, wearing lei), actress**
4. **Harry S. Truman, U.S. President**
5. **Dallas Cowboy Cheerleaders**
6. **Billy Ray Cyrus, singer**
7. **The Three Stooges, comedy team**
8. **Rita Ann McLaughlin, Miss Indian America III**
9. **Mischa Auer, comic actor**
10. **Dave Saunders (Red Ryder), actor**
11. **Medinah Shrine Circus**
12. **Vera-Ellen, dancer**
13. **Floyd Patterson, boxer**
14. **Kristen Bell, actress**
15. **Tiny Tim (Herbert Butros Khaury), singer**

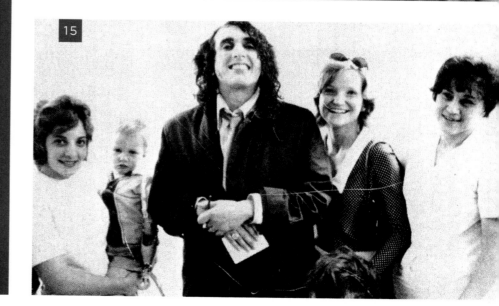

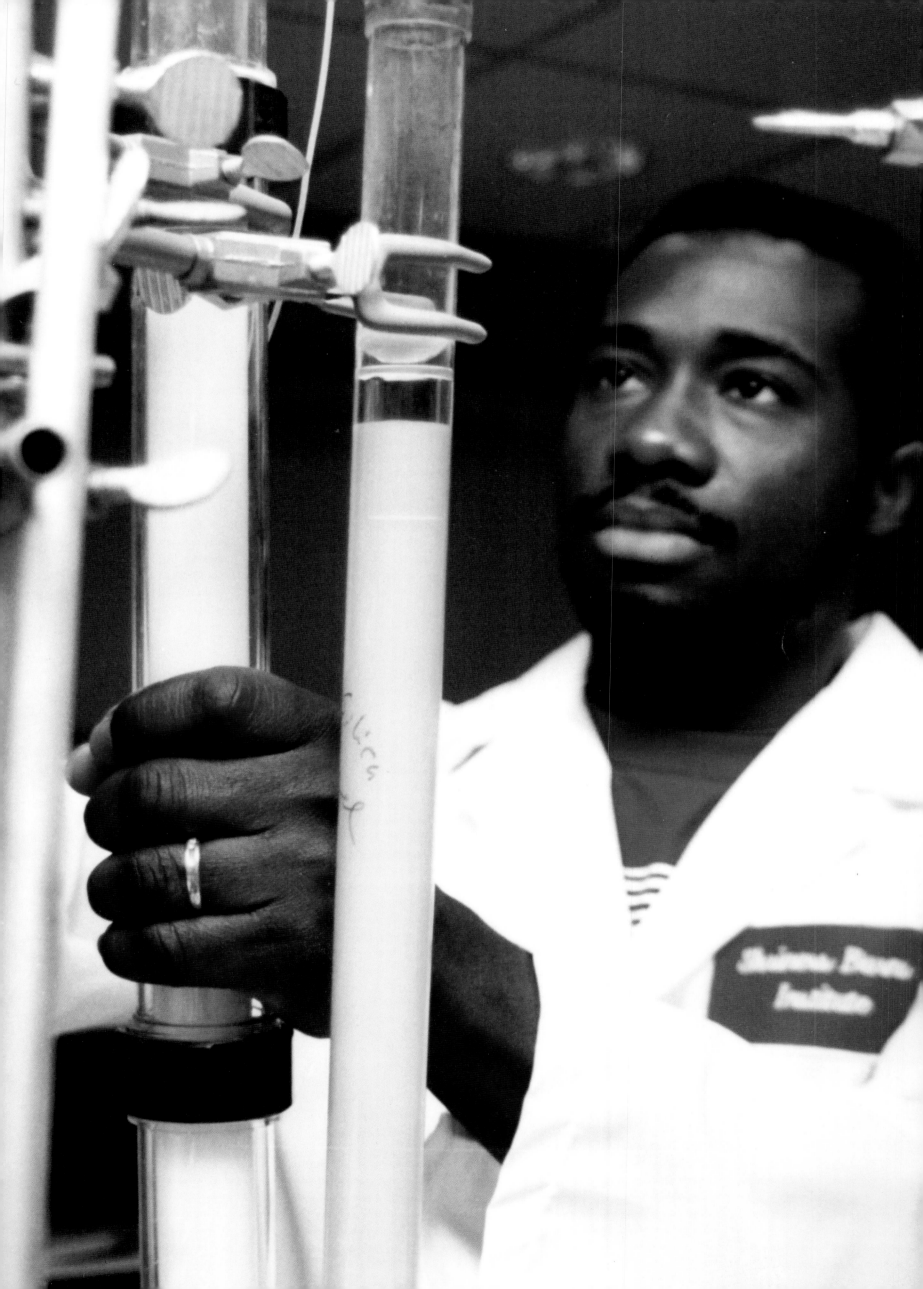

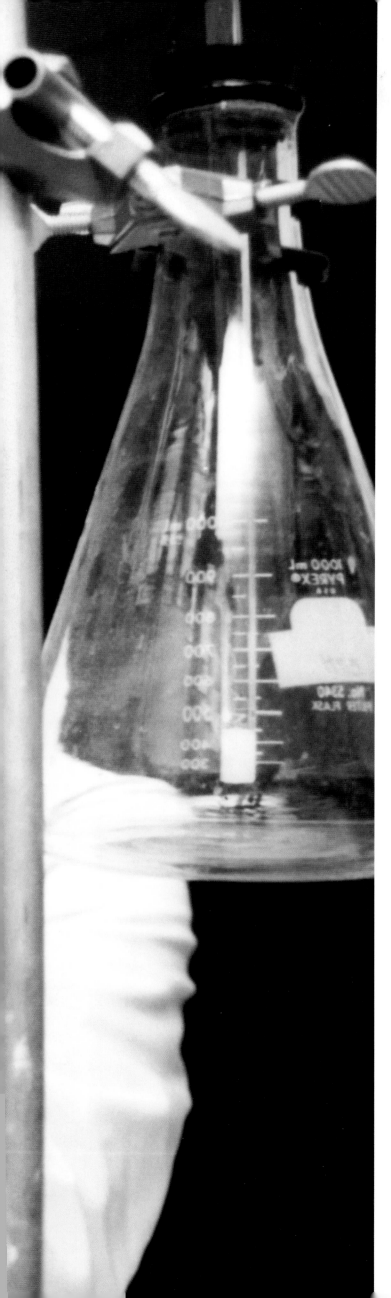

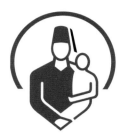

FURTHERING MEDICAL SCIENCE

SHRINERS CHILDREN'S WAS ORIGINALLY founded to provide healthcare, not to conduct medical research. The two turned out to be inseparable. There were good reasons for this. The hospitals specialized in fields that were still largely unknown. Splints and braces — the most basic apparatus in orthopedic treatment — were not developed until the late 1870s nor widely used before World War I. The first surgical approaches were developed at the turn of the century. In the 1920s, there were only a handful of doctors who had the requisite orthopedic training. So medical necessity became the mother of invention. A further factor was that the hospital network was overseen by a medical advisory board that took special care to appoint medical officers for each unit who were leaders in their fields. With top doctors on staff working on the frontiers of pediatric medicine, every Shriners hospital was also fundamentally a research hospital. Every year since the early 1920s, physicians at Shriners Children's have published clinical papers on their medical work. In the past 100 years, work at the hospitals has generated thousands of research articles.

Laboratory studies were first funded at Shriners Children's St. Louis in 1924, under the direction of Dr. J. Albert Key, whose research focused on arthritis. The research program expanded dramatically with the opening of the three original burns hospitals, each of which was planned with research facilities. In 1972, Shriners Children's founded a new research department to support the hospital's long history of clinical invention with a seed grant of $12,000. By 1977, the research budget was $233,000. By 1980, it was more than $2 million. Today, Shriners Children's allocates over $38 million to research annually in an effort that has generated major medical breakthroughs and promises to yield many more.

As a postdoctoral fellow at Shriners Children's Boston in the early 1990s, Dr. Howard Matthew focused his research on cultivating cells for tissue applications. He is working here with a perfused culture system – one in which cells are grown in continuously flowing liquid rather than on a petri dish.

171

RESEARCH: THE FIRST DECADES

In 1924, Dr. John Albert Key at Shriners Children's St. Louis was appointed the first director of research for the hospitals. He earned his early experience in the Army Medical Corps during World War I, stationed in a field hospital in Bazoilles-sur-Meuse. After the war, he underwent graduate training at Children's Hospital and Massachusetts General Hospital in Boston. At Shriners Children's, he balanced his surgical duties with teaching at the Washington University School of Medicine and conducting fundamental research. Among his many publications is the standard textbook, The Management of Fractures, Dislocations, and Sprains (1934), co-written with Hugh Earle Conwell. A portrait of Dr. Key, shown here at its unveiling, was presented to the University following his death in 1955.

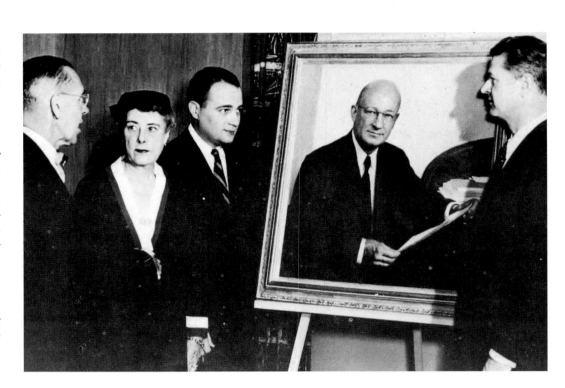

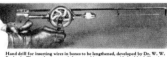

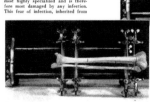

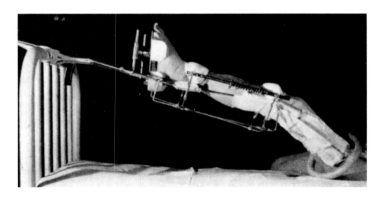

In 1924, Dr. LeRoy C. Abbott was appointed the first Chief Surgeon of Shriners Children's St. Louis. Like most orthopedic surgeons of his generation, he had honed his skills in military field hospitals during World War I, but polio presented a new set of challenges. Abbott had never encountered a case of uneven limb development before, but this condition was relatively common among children with the disease. Necessity moved him to invent a new technique for lengthening the tibia and fibula. Abbott's basic process still forms the foundation for leg lengthening procedures today. In 2022, Dr. J. Eric Gordon, also an orthopedic surgeon at Shriners Children's St. Louis, performed a new procedure for limb lengthening — an internal rod where the Ellipse Nail is on the outside of the bone instead of inside the center of the bone. Only a handful of hospitals in the world offer this procedure.

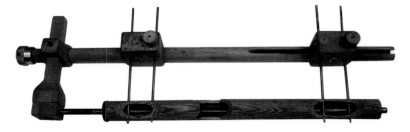

A leg lengthening apparatus based on Dr. Abbott's technique. This example was used at the Shriners Children's hospital in Shreveport, Louisiana.

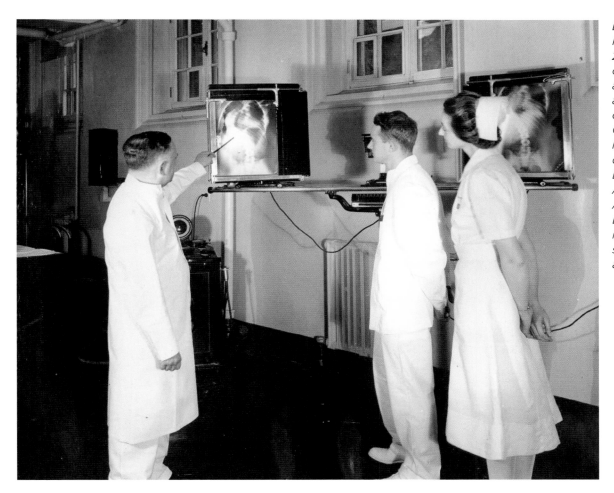

Dr. Alexander Mackenzie Forbes (left) had a 20-year career in pediatric orthopedics before he was appointed in 1924 to serve as the first Chief Surgeon of Shriners Hospitals for Children Canada, a position he held until his premature death in 1929 at age 54. Elected president of the American Orthopedic Association in 1928, Dr. Forbes published a number of papers on scoliosis, poliomyelitis, and spinal tuberculosis.

Nurses and other professionals at Shriners Children's were working in territory that was largely uncharted. Early publications by staff include articles by Directors of nursing Florence Potts and Gertrude Folendorf, superintendent Louise M. Dickson (Montreal), and occupational therapist Jean Perigoe (Montreal).

RESEARCH: EARLY BREAKTHROUGHS

A CURIOUS CONGENITAL ANOMALY OF THE SPINE *

RICHARD B. DILLEHUNT, M.D., AND ROBBIN E. FISHER, M.D.,
PORTLAND, ORE.

A boy, aged 5, pre
proportion between tl
ties. Study revealed
overgrowth of the sp

Anesthesia and Analgesia—March-April, 1929

ton theory is incomplete in that it
leaves out of consideration the influence
of the electric ionization.

shall continue this work as much as
possible and would appreciate any help
or cooperation. A continuation of these

AN ANALYSIS OF THE CASES OF INFANTILE PARALYSIS
TREATED AT THE SHRINERS' HOSPITAL FOR
CRIPPLED CHILDREN, SPRINGFIELD,
MASS., DURING 1925

BY R. NELSON HATT, M.D.,* AND GARRY DE N. HOUGH, JR., M.D.*

THIS study consists of an analysis of 116 cases
of anterior poliomyelitis in children, treated

and eastern New York, with a few of this series
from farther South.

XCIII. THE SIGNIFICANCE OF THE NON-
FERMENTABLE REDUCING SUBSTANCES
OF THE BLOOD IN DIABETES.

BY ISRAEL MORDECAI RABINOWITCH.

From the Department of Metabolism, The Montreal General Hospital, and the
Henry J. Elliott Laboratory of The Shriners' Hospital, Montreal, Canada.

(Received April 14th, 1928.)

FOLIN has recently demonstrated that the hyperglycaemia of diabetic blood
is not all due to accumulation of glucose. From 15 to 25 % of the sugar
in such blood may be represented by other fermentable substances which
this author groups under the term of "non-glucose fermentable sugars." The
reaction of these sugars to insulin was similar to that of glucose, at least in
so far as their concentrations in blood were concerned. These findings renew
interest in all the non-glucose reducing substances of blood, very little of
which can be accounted for, in the absence of nephritis, by nitrogenous
materials.

The greatest difficulties, heretofore, in studying the metabolism of these
substances, were due to the technical methods involved in their estimation,
since the methods commonly in use for estimating the sugar of human blood
measure not glucose alone, but also other reducing substances which are now
generally known to be found in blood. Some are fermentable whilst others
are not.

The commonest and most logical, theoretically, of older methods of estimating the concentrations of the non-fermentable reducing substances of
blood, depended upon measuring the total reducing substances before and
after alcoholic fermentation, and with proper precautions it is now possible,
with a reasonable degree of accuracy, to estimate the true contents of non-
fermentable reducing substances.

Hiller, Linder and Van Slyke [1925] have shown that it is possible to
reduce the fermentation period to 20 minutes. At a later date Folin and
Svedberg [1926] found that it was possible to reduce still further the fermentation period. More recently Somogyi [1927] has shown that it is unnecessary
to incubate blood with yeast even for the brief periods mentioned above.
Sugar may be completely removed, at room temperature, in the course of the
Folin-Wu precipitation of the blood-proteins, if the water for dilution and
laking of the blood is replaced by a 10 % (moist weight) yeast suspension.

In order to study the significance of these non-fermentable reducing substances in diabetes, it was considered advisable, firstly, to obtain standards

*Working on the cutting edge
of pediatric medicine, doctors
from Shriners Children's regularly
published articles on unusual
cases they encountered and novel
treatments they developed. In the
first decade, these included articles
by Dr. R. Nelson Hatt and
Dr. Gerry de N. Hough, Jr. (Springfield),
Dr. Richard Dillehunt and
Dr. Robbin E. Fisher (Portland),
Dr. Alfred L. Craig (Honolulu),
Dr. Israel Mordecai Rabinowitch
and Dr. W. J. Patterson (Montreal),
Dr. John R. Moore (Philadelphia),
and Dr. Emma Buckley (San Francisco).*

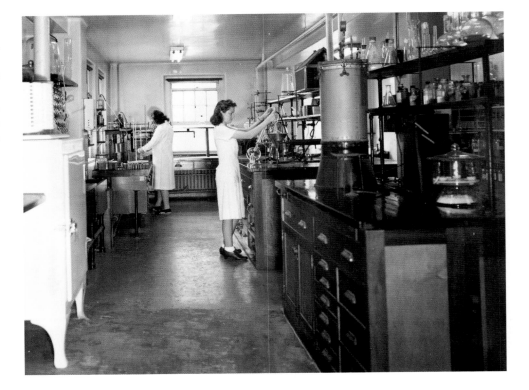

*While the directors
of medical research
during the early years
were invariably men,
they relied on skilled
scientists of both sexes.
These two biochemists
are working at the
laboratory at the
hospital in Montreal,
late 1940s.*

In the 1940s, Dr. Harold A. Sofield of Shriners Children's Chicago, pictured here with one of his patients, began experimenting with a radical technique for treating the genetic disease osteogenesis imperfecta (OI). Brittle bones result in repeated fractures. With his colleague Dr. Edward A. Millar, Dr. Sofield discovered that if one removed a broken leg bone, slipped the pieces onto a stainless-steel rod, and replaced them, the leg would heal straight and strong.

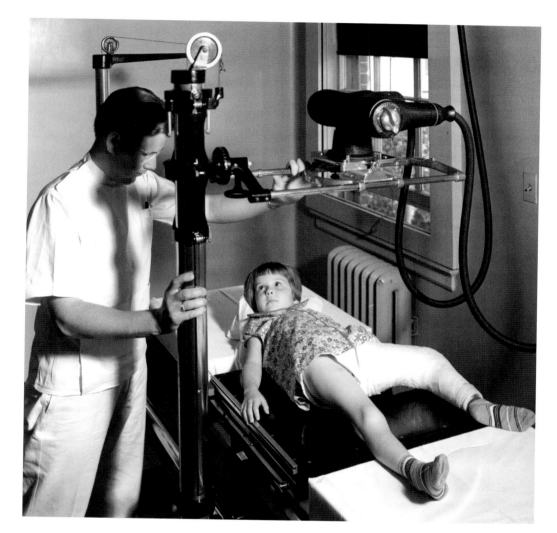

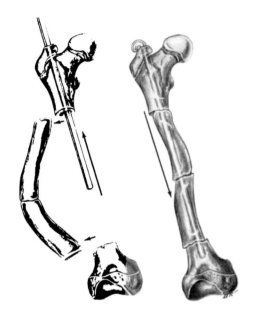

Above: An illustration of the Sofield-Millar operation from their 1959 article in The Journal of Bone and Joint Surgery. Modified over the years, the Sofield–Millar operation is fundamental to the treatment of OI and other orthopedic conditions today.

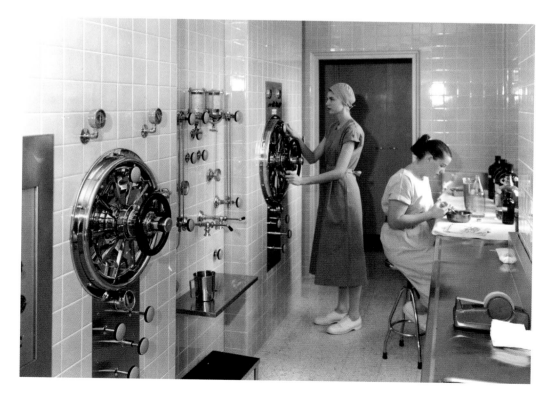

Sterile instruments were crucial for both medical research and patient care. Every Shriners Children's hospital featured autoclave systems, which used steam at high pressure to eliminate microscopic contaminants. This photo is from the facility in Chicago.

175

RESEARCH: THE 1960s

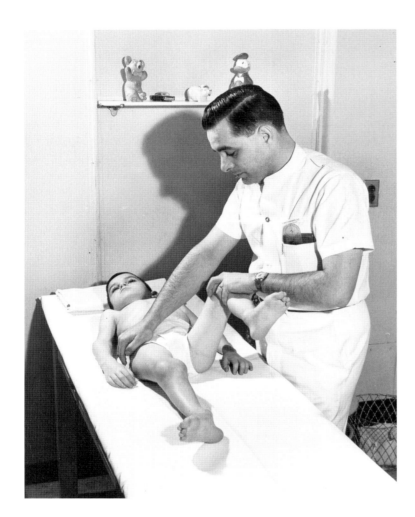

Dr. J. Gordon Petrie, Chief Surgeon of Shriners Hospitals for Children Canada from 1946 to 1968, with one of his patients. Legg-Calve–Perthes disease is a hip condition of unknown origin that usually affects children between the ages of 4 and 10. To treat it, Dr. Petrie invented a post-operative treatment now known as the Petrie cast.

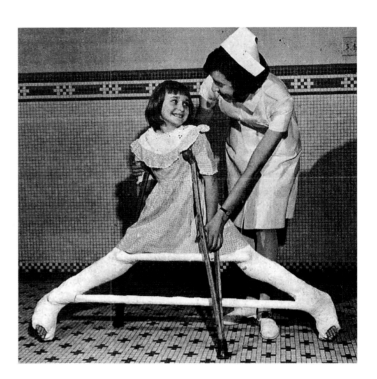

An illustration of the cast from Dr. Petrie's article, "The abduction weight-bearing treatment in Legg–Perthes' disease." The cast is designed to keep the ball of the femur in the hip socket during a period of recovery that usually lasts four to six weeks. A plaster cast covers the thighs and lower legs of the patient but leaves the hips exposed. A bar placed around the shin keeps the legs spread wide. This simple but effective treatment is easily replicated without the need for special equipment. Some doctors in severely underserved areas around the world have reported fabricating bars from broom handles.

When the Shriners Burns Institutes were founded in the mid-1960s, they had a dual mission. First, to provide care for pediatric patients who had suffered major injuries. Second, to advance medical knowledge in a field that was still in its infancy. The early years saw major advances in burn shock and wound closure. In 1969, doctors at Shriners Children's Boston reported the first cases of children surviving the massive trauma of full-thickness burns covering over 70% of the body.

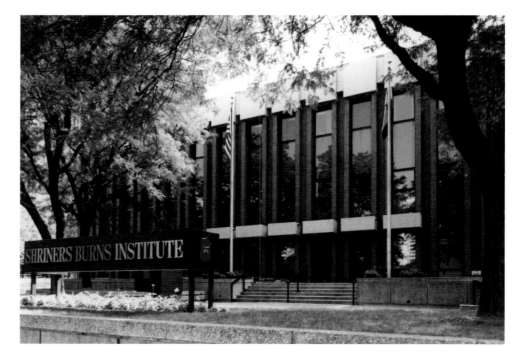

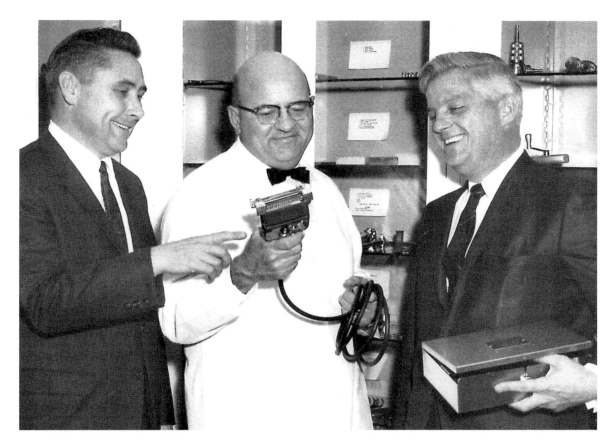

Dr. Bruce G. MacMillan (center), first Chief of Staff of Shriners Children's Ohio, examines the hospital's new Brown Air-Dermatone, a new invention to facilitate skin grafts for patients with severe burns, 1967. With him are two representatives of the Zimmer Company, which produced the instrument. The apparatus, which Dr. MacMillan helped develop, was capable of removing a layer of healthy skin one ten-thousandth of an inch thick for replacement on areas where skin was lost.

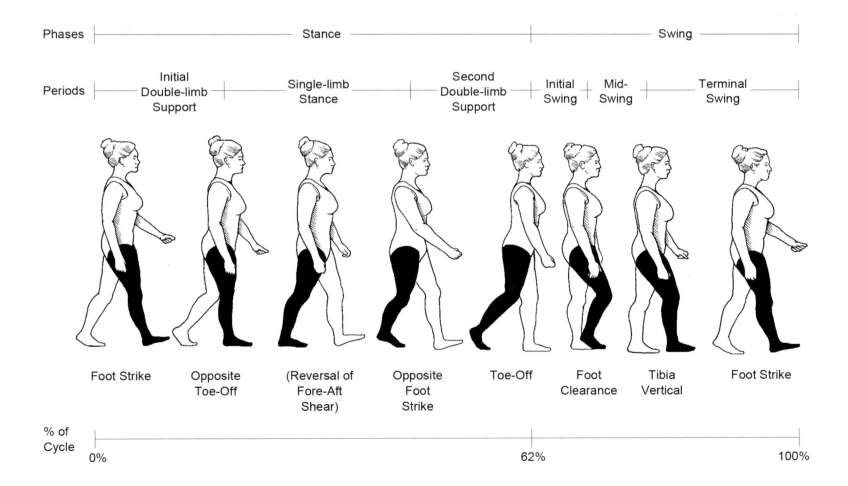

Phases	Stance				Swing		
Periods	Initial Double-limb Support	Single-limb Stance	Second Double-limb Support	Initial Swing	Mid-Swing		Terminal Swing

| Foot Strike | Opposite Toe-Off | (Reversal of Fore-Aft Shear) | Opposite Foot Strike | Toe-Off | Foot Clearance | Tibia Vertical | Foot Strike |

% of Cycle

0%   62%   100%

In 1965, Dr. David H. Sutherland, an orthopedist at Shriners Children's Northern California, hit upon the idea of measuring rotational abnormalities in patients with cerebral palsy by filming them with high-speed cameras. Working with two engineers from Lockheed, he developed the first processes for gait analysis. His work was quickly taken up by his colleagues at other Shriners Children's hospitals. Today, motion analysis is used as an essential diagnostic tool for a range of orthopedic and neuromuscular conditions.

RESEARCH: THE 1970s

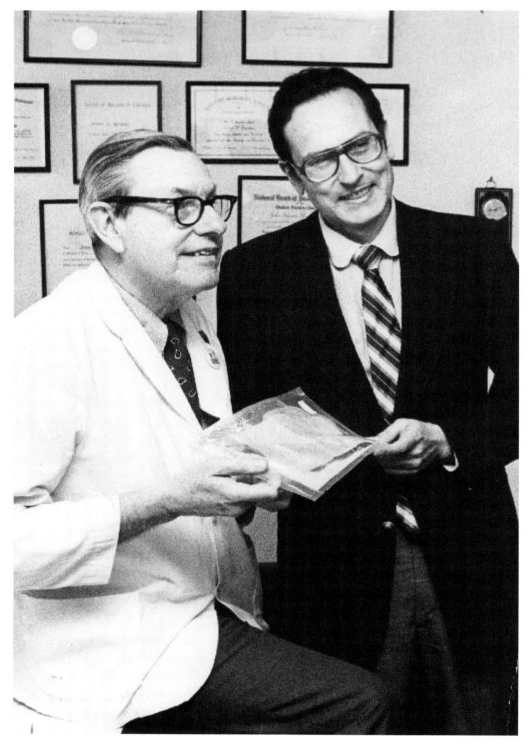

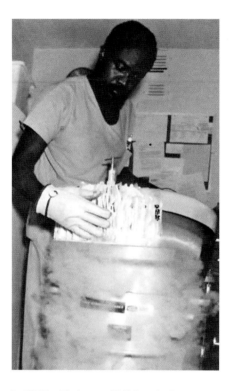

In 1969, Shriners Children's Boston opened the world's first skin bank, long curated by Philemon Walters, pictured here in 1983. When someone is burned over 40% of his or her skin, there is a tremendous strain put on all the other vital organs, which can often cause death. The bank supplies the surgeon with human skin collected from organ donors. The skin was kept frozen in liquid nitrogen at 292 degrees below zero until needed for grafting over burn wounds. The solution offered by donated skin is temporary only, because the body ultimately will reject it, but it allows time to develop grafts of the patient's healthy skin.

At the same time the hospital was inaugurating its skin bank, two researchers, Dr. John F. Burke, Chief of Staff at Shriners Children's Boston, and Dr. Ioannis Yannas, a professor of polymer science and engineering at the Massachusetts Institute of Technology, developed a process for growing skin — long thought to be an impossibility. They prepared a material composed of two layers: a synthetic coating of silicone over an organic scaffolding made from cow tendons and shark cartilage. This artificial skin performed double duty, serving as a bandage to protect wounds while allowing new skin cells to grow. It was the first example of organ regeneration in human adults.

In 1972, Shriners Hospital for Children Canada hired Dr. Francis Glorieux as the director of a newly established research program. As a specialist in congenital bone diseases, he built a multidisciplinary group drawing on genetic analysis, bone histomorphometry, molecular diagnosis, and other approaches. Over the years, their many breakthroughs, particularly with respect to the treatment of familial rickets and osteogenesis imperfecta, have redefined standards of care around the world. In 2004, Dr. Glorieux was made an officer of the Order of Canada, the country's highest honor for lifetime achievement.

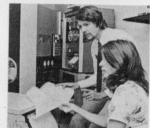

L'hôpital Shriners se dote d'un centre de recherche en génétique

L'hôpital Shriners pour enfants infirmes vient de se doter d'un centre de recherche génétique pour étudier les maladies métaboliques des os. Situé à Montréal, ce nouveau laboratoire est le seul au monde à se consacrer à ce type de recherche pédiatrique. Il fera partie du réseau québecois de médecine génétique, qui comprend déjà des centres à Montréal, Sherbrooke et Québec.

Le chirurgien en chef et directeur des services professionnels de l'hôpital, le docteur Richard Cruess, a déclaré que les projets de recherche seront limités à deux ou trois au plus.

Actuellement, deux projets sont en cours. Le premier se rapporte au rachitisme fam[...] réditaires de [...] d'exister et l[...] parvient pas [...] après un cert[...]

Le docteu[...] teur de la [...] expliqué que [...] ble donner [...] longue échéa[...] de cette mal[...] ments de pl[...] celui qui est [...] par les reins. [...] Shriners étu[...] blème du tr[...] phosphore. I [...] niveau des [...] Les études o[...] rénaux laisse[...] puisque le ta[...] ne des enfa[...] héréditaire e[...] dans celui d[...]

Selon le d[...]

bable que les suppléments de phosphore pourront être discontinués une fois que la croissance de ces enfants sera terminée.

Le deuxième projet d'envergure se rapporte directement à la matière osseuse. Il porte sur les enzymes lysosomiaux. Dans chacune des conditions de déficience génétique des ces enzymes, la substance s'accumule dans la cellule pour finalement la détruire. Les maladies reliées à cette déficience affectent sérieusement le développement et la fonction des os et de plusieurs organes.

Les chercheurs du nouveau centre de recherche ont mis sur pied onze essais de laboratoire pour parvenir à détecter si les enzymes lysosomiques sont présents ou non. Il n'existe pas de moyen de corriger cette déficience, mais un diagnostic de la maladie durant la grossesse permettra à la mère d'obtenir un avortement thérapeutique, si elle l[...]

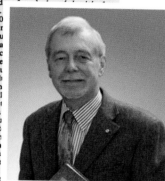

Le docteur Francis Glorieux et Mlle Rose Travers, technicienne au centre de recherche, examinent les données de l'ordinateur surnommé "le petit génie".

Le centre de recherche a pu être mis sur pied [...] Shriners. [...] $500,000 [...] toire d'in[...] ordinateu[...] Cet appa[...] aminés c[...] de sang e[...] la structu[...]

En pl[...] des Shri[...] demi-mill[...] les proje[...] tion sera [...] temps qu[...] rentabilit[...] présenten[...] rique du [...] et trois i[...] brûlures. [...] projets g[...] des memores, aux dons et aux legs qui leur sont faits. Ils retirent également des profits de certaines activités sociales, comme celle du cirque Shriners.

L. DE G.

L/NOVEMBER 16, 1974/VOL. 111 **1155**

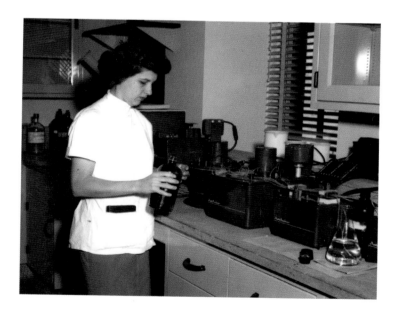

Born in the small town of Refugio, Texas, Sally Abston earned her medical degree at the University of Texas Medical Branch Galveston in 1962. She was the first woman surgical resident there and joined the burns unit at Shriners Children's Texas shortly after its founding. At Galveston, she helped develop compression garments to improve the healing of burn scars, pioneered the use of ketamine anesthesia, and identified the utility of a milk diet in helping to maintain body weight and prevent catastrophic ulcers in burn victims. After her death in 2008, the Association of Women Surgeons established an annual award in her honor.

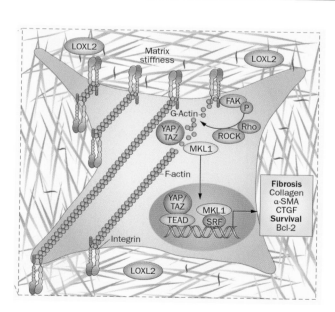

Working with Duane Larson and others at Shriners Children's Texas, electron microscopist Paul S. Baur, Jr. first reported the presence of myofibroblasts in hypertrophic (thickened) scars in 1975. Myofibroblasts, which were first discovered in 1971, are specialized cells that play an important role in the contraction and closure of wounds in soft tissues. Understanding their role led to a revolution in the understanding of scar formation and remodeling after surgery. The image of a myofibroblast here is from a 2016 article by Yuen Yee Ho of Shriners Hospital for Children Canada and her colleagues.

RESEARCH: THE 1980s

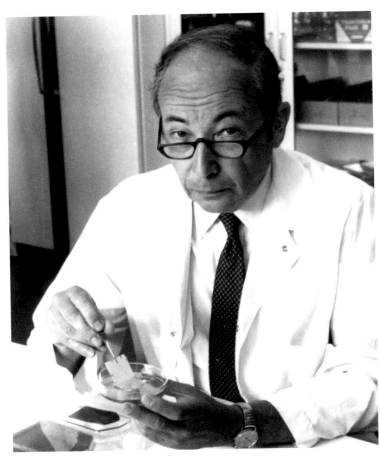

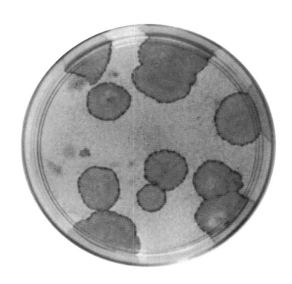

Left: In 1983, three young boys in Wyoming who had been playing with paint covered themselves with solvent to get rid of the evidence. Then, someone lit a match. One died in the flames; the other two, 5-year-old Jamie and his 7-year-old brother Glen, sustained third-degree burns over 97% of their bodies. They were rushed to burn specialists in Denver, who said their only hope was in new research being done at Shriners Children's Boston. A traditional skin graft — taking skin from one area of the body to cover a burned area — was impossible: the only unburnt areas were their armpits, the soles of their feet and the creases of their thighs. So Dr. Howard Green tried something desperate. He removed postage stamp-sized samples of healthy skin from each boy and cultivated the cells until he grew several square yards of epidermal tissue that his team could graft onto their bodies. It took a year, but finally, the boys were able to go back home. This was the first use of stem cells for medical treatment. His success inspired subsequent research in the field of stem cells. In 2016, Mrs. Rosine Kauffman Green gave Shriners Children's Boston a $3 million gift to establish the Howard Green Center for Children's Skin Health and Research to honor Dr. Green's memory.

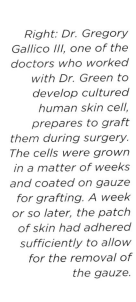

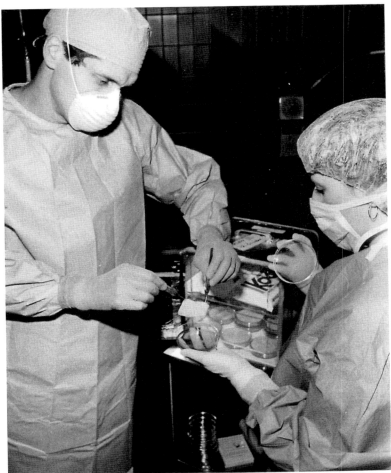

Right: Dr. Gregory Gallico III, one of the doctors who worked with Dr. Green to develop cultured human skin cell, prepares to graft them during surgery. The cells were grown in a matter of weeks and coated on gauze for grafting. A week or so later, the patch of skin had adhered sufficiently to allow for the removal of the gauze.

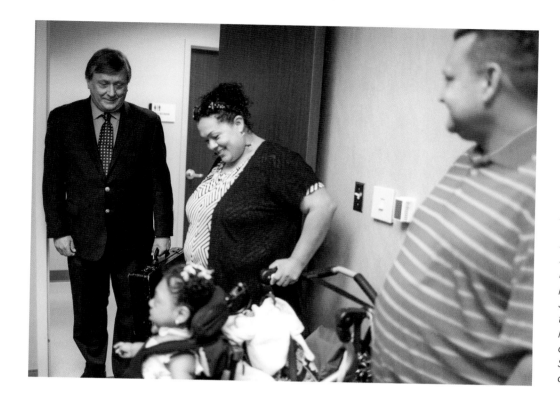

In 1983, Dr. Michael P. Whyte founded the Center for Metabolic Bone Disease and Molecular Research at Shriners Children's St. Louis to study the genetics of skeletal disorders. Over the past four decades, the Center has identified etiologies, diagnostics and treatments for more than 100 rare metabolic bone diseases. Contributing foundational knowledge on inborn disorders of skeletal metabolism and skeletal dysplasias, the Center's work has provided the basis for the development of new therapies for such genetically based bone disorders as osteogenesis imperfecta, hypophosphatasia and hypophosphatemic rickets. In this picture, Whyte (left) visits 6-year-old Janelly, born without bones. Doctors at the Vanderbilt Children's Hospital treated her with an experimental drug therapy developed by Whyte and his team at Shriners Children's to stimulate bone development.

In 1986, researchers at Shriners Children's Philadelphia began a project to develop computer-controlled apparatus to simulate the muscles of paralyzed patients. In 1998, the long years of research bore fruit when Robert, a 14-year-old from Shawboro, North Carolina, became the world's first child to receive a totally implanted functional electrical stimulation (FES) system. When he was 2, Robert sustained a spinal cord injury in an automobile accident that left him paralyzed from the waist down. The FES system allowed him to stand upright and walk around without a wheelchair.

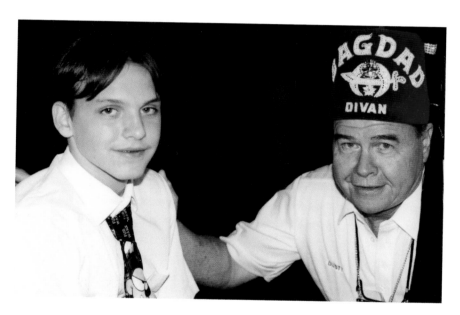

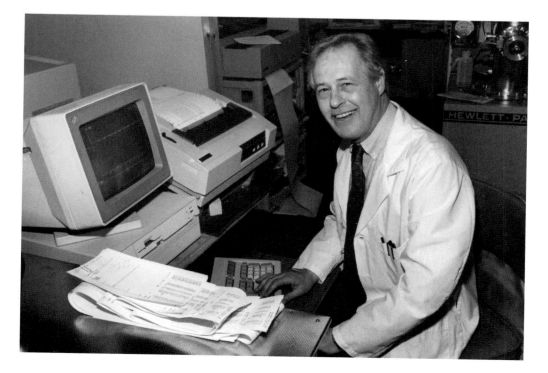

In 1989, Dr. Vernon Young, director of research at the Shriners Children's Boston, was awarded the J. Arthur Rank Prize by the Royal Society in London for "his signal contributions to our knowledge of the metabolism of protein and amino acides in man and of human protein requirements." Dr. Young was only the third American scientist to receive the Rank Prize since it was established in 1972.

RESEARCH: THE 1990s

Together with their colleagues at Shriners Children's Portland, Dr. Lynn Sakai (center) and Dr. M. Peter Marinkovich (right) discovered a number of tissue proteins, including fibrillin, which is associated with Marfan syndrome, and kalinin, used as a biological glue for skin grafting. Their work was conducted by using antibodies in techniques such as affinity chromatography, immunofluorescence, and immunoelectron microscopy. At left is Senator Mark Hatfield from Oregon, who sponsored legislation to support research on Epidermolysis Bullosa at the hospital.

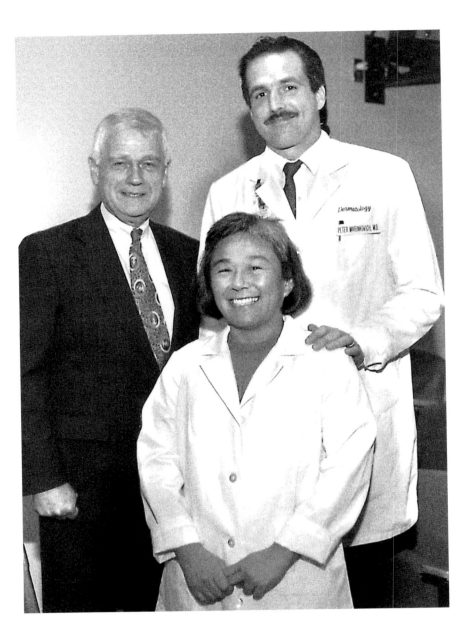

Microimagining specialist Douglas R. Keene of Shriners Children's Portland produced this image of a section of human tendon, which shows type III collagen fibrils. Researchers at the unit were the first to demonstrate that this protein, which plays an important role in early wound healing, is also a significant component of tendon. The banding pattern on the collagen fibrils is caused by overlapping molecules.

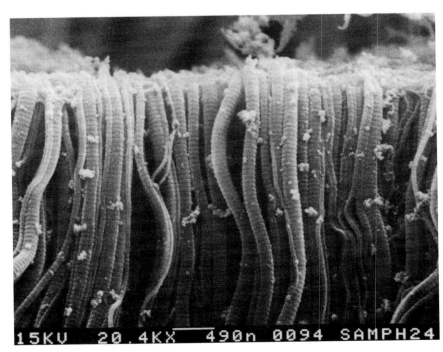

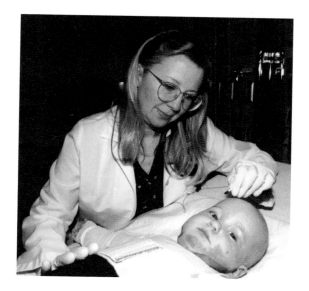

Dr. Michele Gottschlich, director of nutritional services at Shriners Children's Ohio, won the American Burn Association's 1994 Clinical Research Award for her first study of sleep patterns in pediatric burn patients. Measuring brain waves, eye movements, and other indicators, she has documented the vital role that uninterrupted sleep plays in recovery.

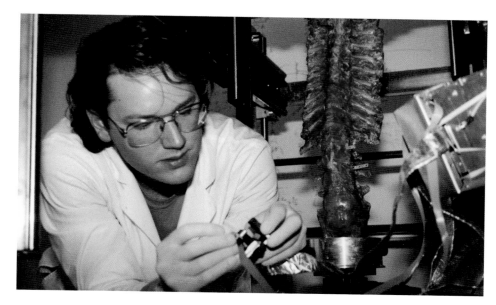

In this 1992 photograph, a researcher at Shriners Children's Salt Lake City tests instrumentation systems on spines. Doctors agreed that spine implants for children were too bulky and stiff. The goal was to develop a lighter and more flexible system. Such efforts would lead to major advances in the treatment of scoliosis in the coming decades.

In 1994, a research team led by Dr. Jennifer T. Hecht of Shriners Children's Texas discovered the genetic link to pseudoachondroplasia, a form of dwarfism that limits average adult height to four feet and causes a number of problems related to bone development. Dr. Hecht and her team identified a mutation of the cartilage oligomeric matrix protein (COMP) that leads to the disorder. Because pseudoachondroplasia is heritable, identifying the gene is the crucial first step for understanding and treating the condition.

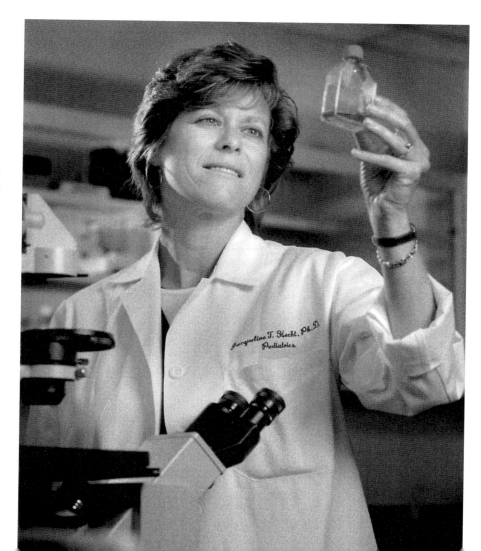

183

RESEARCH: ENTERING THE NEW MILLENNIUM

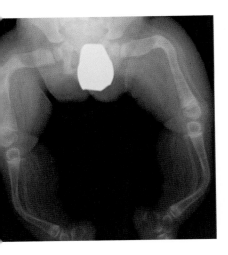 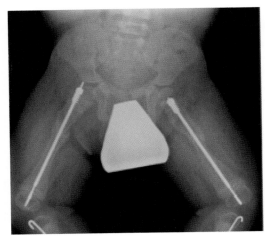 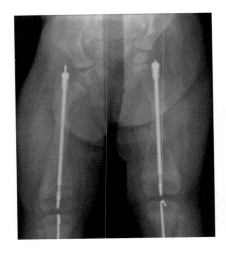 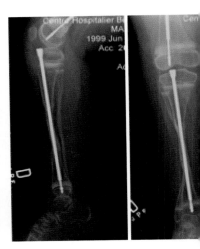

Above: One of the many discoveries and innovations to emerge from Shriners Hospital for Children Canada is the telescoping rod invented by Dr. François Fassier and Dr. Pierre Duval in 2001. Used in the surgical procedure pioneered by Harold A. Sofield and Edward A. Millar of Shriners Children's Chicago, the Fassier–Duval rod is a leg implant that extends as the child grows, offering maximum stability with minimal surgical intervention. As these X-rays show, rods placed in the femur (thighbone) and tibia (shinbone) of a 2-year-old child with osteogenesis imperfecta generated dramatic results only two years later.

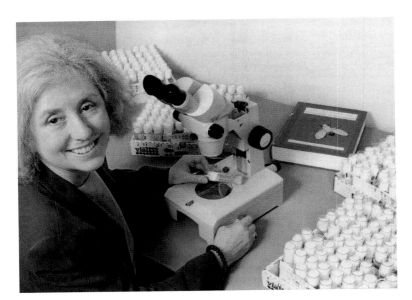

Left: When Shriners Children's Northern California moved its hospital from San Francisco to Sacramento, Dr. Linda Hall was brought on board to establish a new state-of-the-art research facility.

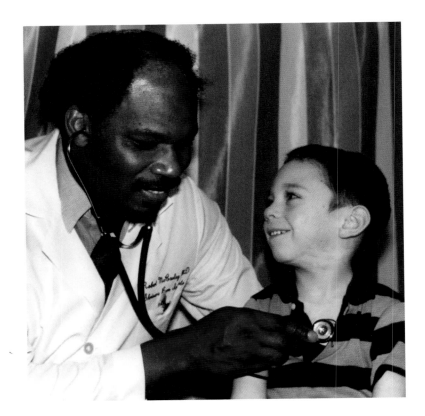

Left: Dr. Robert L. McCauley of Shriners Children's Texas has written or contributed to over 30 research papers based on his clinical work. He was part of the team awarded the 1991 Lindberg Award from the American Burn Association and in 2000 published a detailed analysis of reconstruction of the pediatric burned hand.

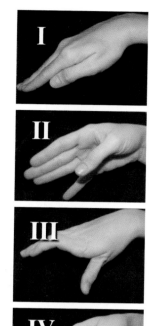

Table 1: Indications for upper extremity surgical procedures.					
Procedure	Physical Examination	Radiographic Examination	SHUEE		
			SFA	DPA	GRA
Thumb MCP Arthrodesis	Thumb MCP hyperextension instability	AP Hand: skeletal age 10 or greater	-	Thumb segment: closed or in palm	-
Thumb MCP Sesamoid Capsulodesis	Thumb MCP hyperextension instability	AP Hand: skeletal age less than 10	-	Thumb segment: closed or in palm	-
Thumb Web Release	Limited thumb passive palmar extension/ abduction	-	-	Thumb segment: closed or in palm	-
EPL Rerouting	Ability to selective active EPL	-	-	Thumb segment: closed or in palm	-

In 2006, Dr. Jon R. Davids and his colleagues at Shriners Children's Northern California developed a new assessment tool for assessing the upper limb function of children with cerebral palsy. The Shriners Hospital Upper Extremity Evaluation (SHUEE) uses video to capture patients performing a series of simple tasks. The results are used to plan surgical interventions and evaluate their outcomes. SHUEE has been used as a tool for other medical conditions as well — rheumatic diseases, for example.

Since 1995, researchers at Shriners Children's Chicago have managed a study of long-term outcomes and life satisfaction of individuals with pediatric-onset spinal cord injury (SCI). The study was initiated in 1995 by Dr. Lawrence C. Vogel and is still ongoing today, under the direction of Dr. Kathy Zebracki, with over 500 current and former patients participating. "There is no comparable study," said Dr. Zebracki. "Knowledge of psychosocial outcomes, such as attainment of employment, is critical to developing targeted state-of-the-art interventions addressing the current needs of aging adults living with SCI, as well as creating effective evidence-based rehabilitation and educational/prevention programs for those newly injured."

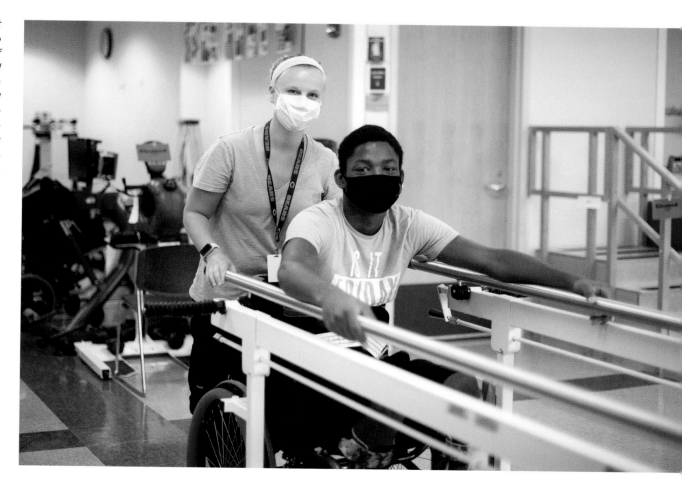

RESEARCH: RECENT BREAKTHROUGHS

In 2012, Dr. Amer F. Samdani and his colleagues at Shriners Children's Philadelphia developed a new treatment for certain patients with idiopathic scoliosis called vertebral body tethering (VBT). During the procedure, surgeons fix a strong, flexible cord to pull gently on the outside curve of the spine, causing it to straighten. VBT is far less invasive than spinal fusion, which was for decades, the leading option for treating scoliosis. The cord is flexible, allowing it to continue to correct spine curvature as the child grows without needing further surgery. In 2019, the VBT cord that the medical staff at Shriners designed was approved by the FDA.

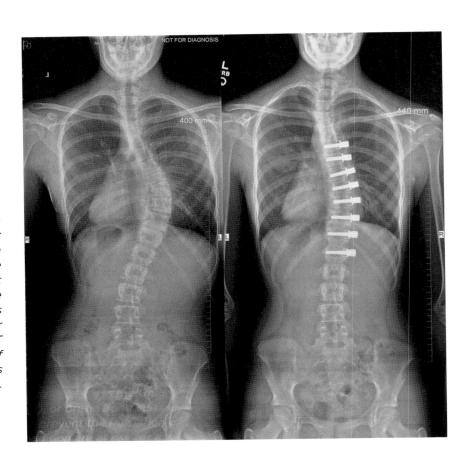

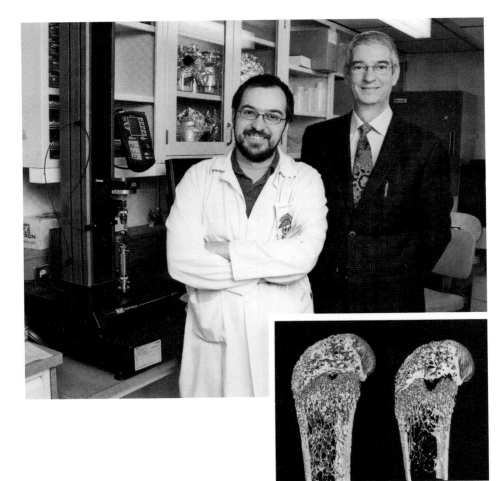

In 2014, Dr. René St-Anaud (right), Dr. Martin Pellicelli (left), and their colleagues at Shriners Hospital for Children Canada studied the effects of a drug used to increase the bone mass of pediatric patients with orthopedic conditions. They discovered that when the drug binds to bone cells, it activates signals that sent the protein alphaNAC to the nucleus of the cells. In turn, the nuclear alphaNAC protein regulates the bone-forming activity of the cells. Establishing the type and sequence of signals opens the door for further study and the development of new treatments.

Figure

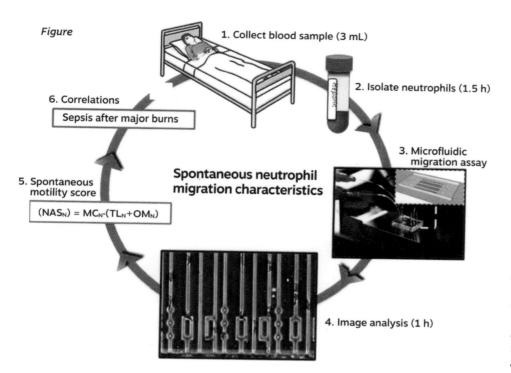

1. Collect blood sample (3 mL)

2. Isolate neutrophils (1.5 h)

3. Microfluidic migration assay

Spontaneous neutrophil migration characteristics

4. Image analysis (1 h)

5. Spontaneous motility score

$(NAS_N) = MC_N \cdot (TL_N + OM_N)$

6. Correlations

Sepsis after major burns

Sepsis is a severe and persistent inflammatory response to infection that can lead to tissue damage. It occurs in 50 percent of patients with major burns and is a risk for all patients in critical condition. A major issue with sepsis, especially for children with burn injuries, is diagnosis. Almost all patients have some clinical indicators such as elevated heart rate and temperature, and, therefore, infection has to be diagnosed by standard tests that take three or more days. At the Shriners Children's Boston, Dr. Daniel Irimia and his colleagues developed a new point-of-care test that instead looks at the behavior of the patient's immune cells. The group has noted that changes in migration patterns of neutrophils (a type of white blood cell) can predict sepsis in patients with major burns two days in advance. This is likely to enable early use of antibiotics with increased survival. They also demonstrated that using drugs to restore altered white blood cell behavior back to the healthy state prevents liver damage after burns and infection, and further reduces fatality from sepsis. The investigators are currently pursuing efforts to both develop a patient-side diagnostic device that can produce results within a few hours and develop a new drug to restore immune cell activity to avoid systemic infections.

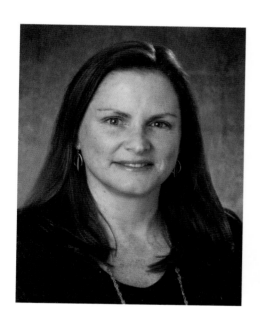

Dr. Heather Russell, licensed clinical pediatric psychologist at Shriners Children's Philadelphia, was awarded the 2019 Essie Morgan Lectureship Award in recognition of her leadership and scholarly work in the psychosocial rehabilitation of persons with spinal cord injuries. Her lecture was titled, "Pint-Sized Pearls of Wisdom: What Kids Can Teach Us about Working with Adults."

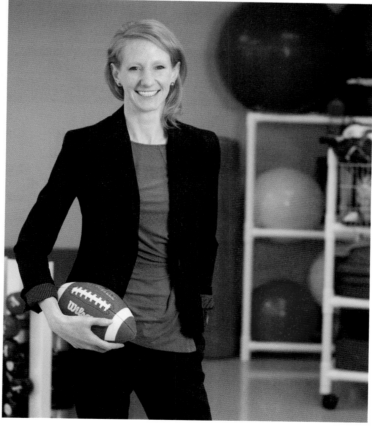

Dr. Nicole Friel, a sports medicine orthopedic surgeon at Shriners Children's Northern California, is one of a group of sports medicine professionals who come together in the Shriners Consortium for Outcomes, Research and Education in Sports (SCORES). The consortium pools the expertise of surgeons, physical therapists, engineers and research coordinators from 10 Shriners Children's sites to share current findings and plan future initiatives. Among current efforts is a project launched in collaboration with biomedical engineers at Georgia Tech and Emory University to build a comprehensive data registry. The registry will aggregate clinical information gathered across the Shriners Children's network, providing researchers with the data they need to answer large-scale questions in pediatric sports medicine.

CONTINUING INNOVATION

When Dr. Marc Lalande (right), joined Shriners Children's in 2017 as Vice President of Research Programs, one of his first projects was to found the Genomics Institute. With Dr. Kamran Shazand (left) at its helm, the Institute conducts fundamental research on gene sequencing and stem cell therapeutics.

By analyzing the data from the DNA of patients and their families, Shriners Children's scientists can better understand the roots of genetic disorders and develop therapies for addressing them. "The fundamental knowledge is so rich that you can spin it in different ways, whether it's diagnostics, treatment, prognostic tools, so this can do all of it logically depending on the nature of the genes on one side and the nature of symptoms and the disorder on the other side," says Dr. Shazand. "I really enjoy as a father imagining that someday our hard work will pay off for these kids."

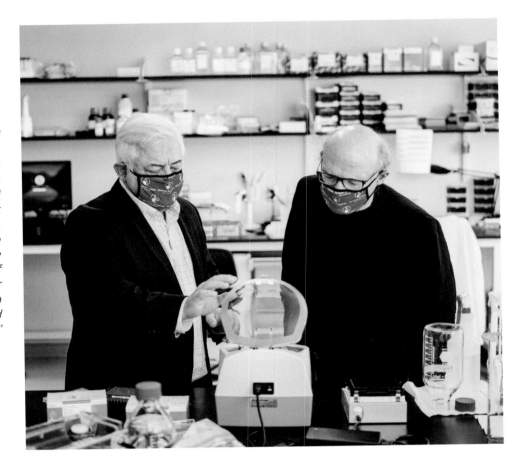

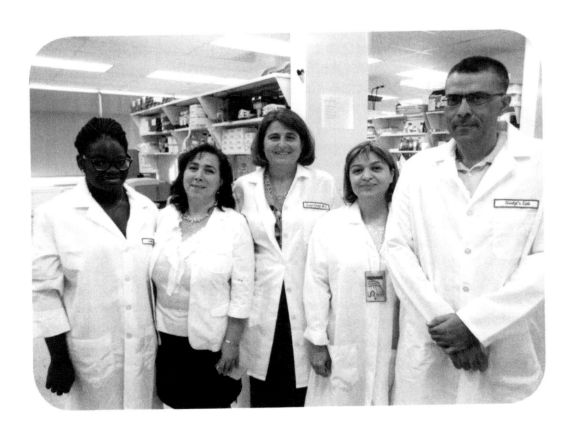

Dr. Laura Goetzl (center) is an OB-GYN specialist at the Center for Neural Repair and Rehabilitation at Shriners Children's Philadelphia. She and her team are researching the maternal factors that cross the placenta and cause the fetus to develop cerebral palsy. With a grant from the National Institutes of Health and a prestigious Challenge Grant from the Bill and Melinda Gates Foundation, Dr. Goetzl is isolating molecules that are released from the fetal brain, cross the placenta and can be detected in the mother's blood. Once fully developed, her tests can be used to pinpoint the timing of in-utero brain injury that leads to cerebral palsy, and potentially to monitor the effects of in-utero treatments to reduce brain injury.

Below: Muscle atrophy, a common result of burn injuries, can have mental, social, and physical health consequences that diminish quality of life and increase the risk of additional medical complications. At Shriners Children's Boston, scientific investigator Dr. Masao Kaneki (left) and Dr. J. A. Jeevendra Martyn (right), Chief of Anesthesiology, have recently identified the role that specific proteins play in the regulation of skeletal muscle mass and strength. Identifying these proteins, called sestrins, is the first step toward developing new strategies for preventing or even reversing muscle loss.

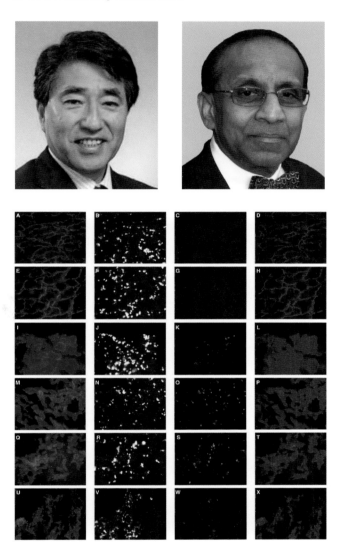

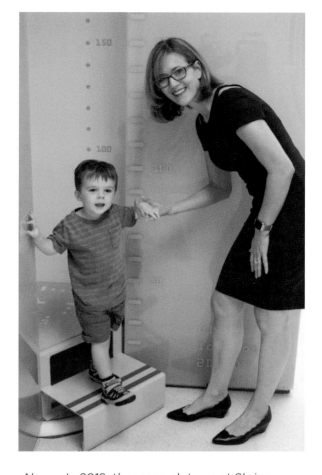

Above: In 2019, the research team at Shriners Children's Portland, led by Dr. William Horton, made an innovative discovery impacting the way physicians track a child's growth rate. Through a simple finger-prick blood test, the team discovered a protein (biomarker CXM) that mirrors a child's rate of bone growth. Since the discovery, Dr. Michelle Welborn (right), a pediatric orthopedic surgeon at the hospital, has analyzed how this blood test could help her improve care for patients with scoliosis and other spine conditions. "Assessing a patient's growth is a vital factor in determining the treatment for patients with scoliosis," said Dr. Welborn. "By determining the rate of growth in real time, we can make sure that we are bracing patients for the correct amount of time and that we are performing surgery at the optimal time. The utilization of biomarker CXM will enable us to improve treatment plans, and it can minimize the number of surgeries needed." In the summer of 2019, the Scoliosis Research Society awarded Dr. Welborn the Thomas E. Whitecloud Award for her work.

Dr. Robert Bernstein, Chief of Staff of Shriners Children's Portland, models a new 3D-printed, hard-shell N95 mask for medical use. Designed by anesthesiologist Dr. Lee Taylor, using face-scanning technology, the mask has two parts: a hard outer shell and an inner medical-grade silicone liner, which provides the fit and comfort. The pediatric orthotics and prosthetics (POPS) staff at the hospital have worked on construction of the mask prototype with a personalized fit, an important feature when wearing a mask during long medical procedures. Dr. Taylor and Dr. Bernstein are collaborating with a consortium that includes staff of the Georgia Institute of Technology to identify filter materials to increase the protective efficiency of the mask.

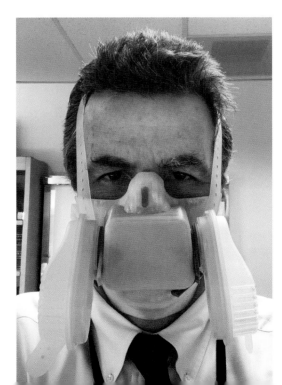

CURRENT PROJECTS

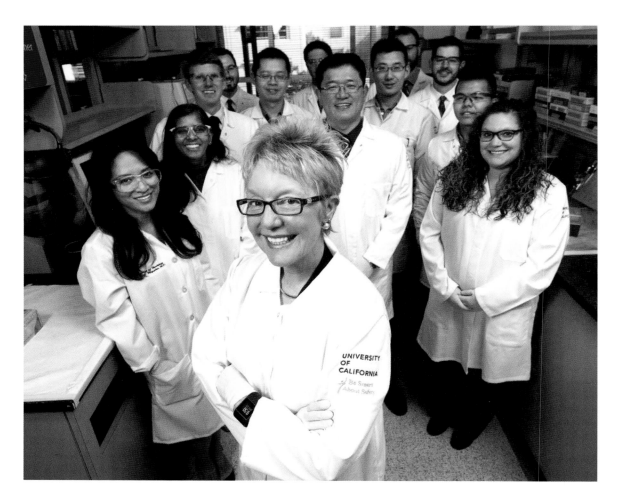

Dr. Diana L. Farmer (front), a surgeon at Shriners Children's Northern California, is only the second American woman ever to be elected to the UK's Royal College of Surgeons. This is only one of her many honors. She is best known as a pioneer in fetal surgery – repairing congenital defects while children are still in the womb. Working with Dr. Aijun Wang (second row, centr) and other colleagues, Dr. Farmer's research is focused on developing a stem cell therapy to repair in utero the most severe form of spina bifida. "There is no doubt that my mission in life is to have these kids with spina bifida walk," she says. "We're going to solve this problem, and I'd like to solve it soon, because I can't retire until it's done."

Dr. Farshid Guilak (front), Director of Research at Shriners Children's St. Louis, has thrice been awarded the Kappa Delta Award from the American Academy of Orthopaedic Surgeons — the field's equivalent of the Nobel Prize. His most recent award, in 2021, was for developing a method for regenerating cartilage in patients with osteoarthritis and other degenerative joint diseases. "Through mechanogenetics, we can engineer cartilage cells to respond to the mechanical loading of the joint," Dr. Guilak explains. "Every time cells are under that stress, they produce an anti-inflammatory, biologic drug to reduce inflammation and limit arthritis-related damage."

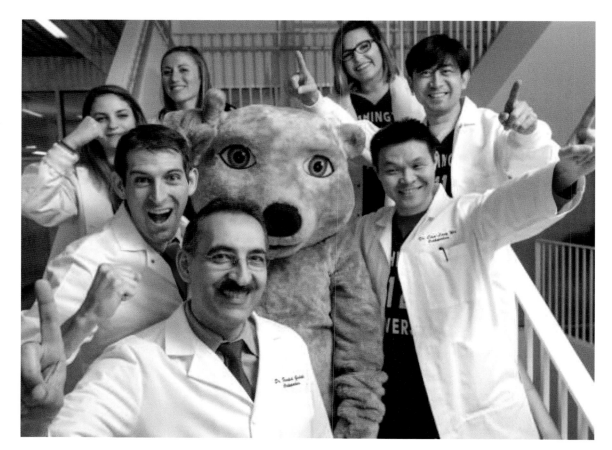

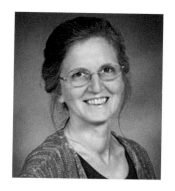

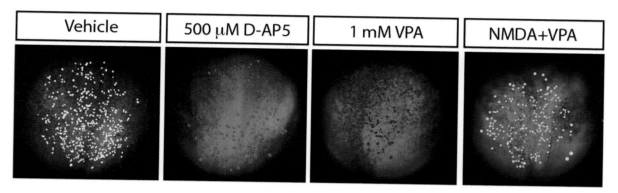

Vehicle	500 µM D-AP5	1 mM VPA	NMDA+VPA

Dr. Laura Borodinsky (above), a principal investigator at the Institute of Pediatric Regenerative Medicine (IPRM) at Shriners Children's Northern California, has discovered that valproic acid, a drug widely used to treat epileptic seizures, may lead to birth defects if used during pregnancy. Her research found that the drug compromises the formation of the neural tube, a major factor in spina bifida and other congenital malformations. "The findings uncovered in Dr. Borodinsky's lab bring us one step closer to preventing a disabling birth defect," said Dr. David Pleasure, Director of Research at the Northern California Shriners Hospital. "They also may lead to the development of new and safer medications to treat epilepsy."

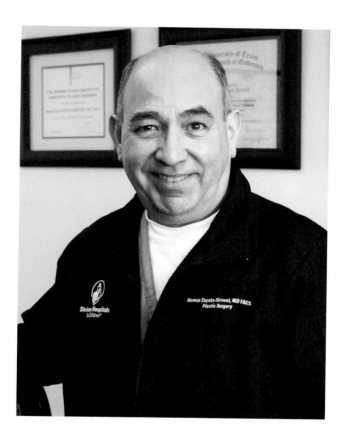

An accomplished plastic surgeon, leader and educator at Shriners Children's Texas, Dr. Ramon Zapata-Sirvent (left) is the author of eight books on burn care and plastic surgery and hundreds of papers specific to reconstructive care. Born and raised in Caracas, Venezuela, Dr. Zapata-Sirvent became known in Venezuela and across Latin America as a medical leader, working to improve burn care in a country with a large oil and gas industry (which can involve dangers that lead to burn injuries) and later founding the Venezuelan Burn Association. Dr. Zapata-Sirvent also served as president of the Venezuelan Society of Plastic, Reconstructive, Aesthetic and Maxillofacial Surgery and is currently a member of the board of directors of the Ibero-Latinoamerican Federation of Plastic Surgery.

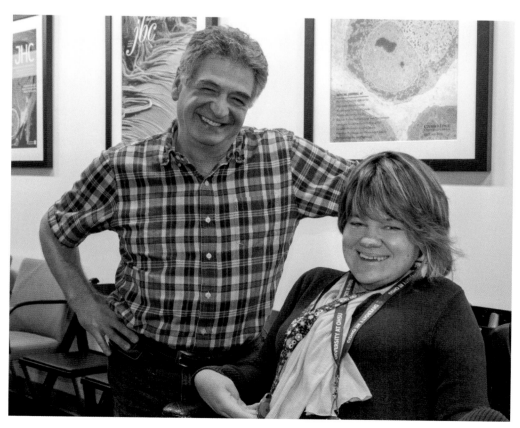

Jennifer (right), who is studying bioinformatics and computational biomedicine at Oregon Health and Science University, was born with arthrogryposis multiplex congenita (AMC). She has joined the research team at Shriners Children's Portland as a student researcher and will be studying this condition with Dr. Ronen Schweitzer (left), whose research focuses on tendon development. "I was really struck by Jennifer's positive energy and how fiercely independent she is," said Dr. Schweitzer. As for Jennifer, she is thrilled to be part of the Shriners Hospitals family. "As someone who understands this condition on both a scientific level and a personal level, my hope in joining Shriners Hospitals is to be able to bridge the scientific community and the patient community as we work toward the goal of developing treatments," she said.

LOVE TO THE RESCUE

ONE HUNDRED YEARS AGO, EVERY MEMBER OF SHRINERS INTERNATIONAL PLEDGED to contribute at least $2 annually to provide medical care to children in need. What they founded would become the world's largest pediatric specialty hospital system, which has never wavered in its mission to provide the best possible patient care, regardless of a family's ability to pay. Everything that the doctors and staff at Shriners Children's have achieved over the past century has been made possible thanks to the selfless generosity of supporters. Every gift has helped, no matter how small. Together, the individuals, communities, foundations, and corporations who have contributed to Shriners Children's have built a network of love that has healed over 1.5 million children worldwide.

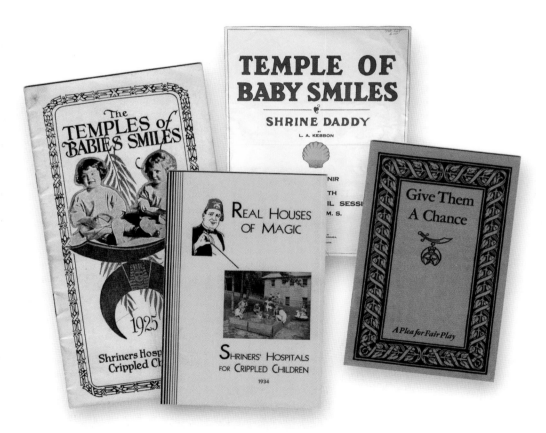

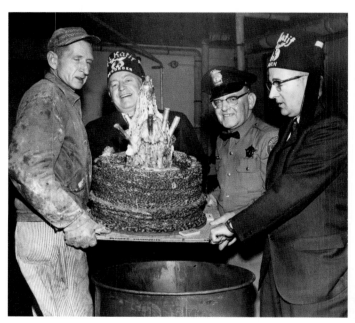

Every cent helps. In 1957, a couple who operated a diner in Sumner, Washington, placed a burning candle near the cash register and invited patrons to press coins into the soft tallow to raise funds for Shriners Children's Spokane. As one candle burned down, they added another. Five years later, the mass of wax and money, which included over 21,000 pennies, exceeded 200 pounds. The amount of money generated was not large in ultimate terms — $335.15 — but the spirit of community generosity the measure generated for the hospital was incalculable.

Promotional campaigns and reports from the first decades of the hospitals emphasized the role of medicine in restoring joy to children afflicted by polio and other orthopedic conditions.

In 1935, in the depths of the Great Depression, Shriners Children's began a program of offering lifetime membership certificates to those who contributed the equivalent of 30 years of dues to the hospital fund. At the time, this amounted to $60 — over $1300 in 2022 dollars. Each certificate was signed by W. Freeland Kendrick, the founding spirit of the hospitals.

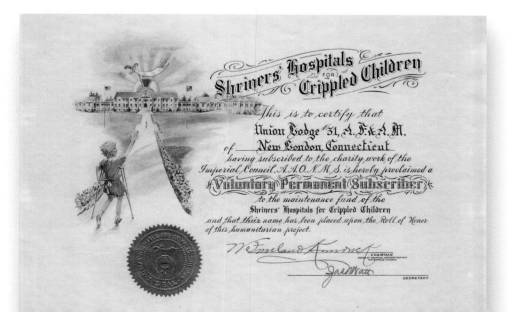

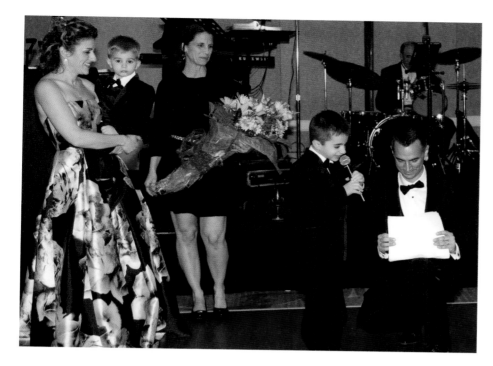

Above: Adam and Danielle Yenish of Warren, New Jersey, wanted to give something back to Shriners Children's Philadelphia. Their son, Anthony ("A.J."), was born with arthrogryposis, a rare orthopedic condition. Physicians worked with him weekly, splinting his hands and casting his feet to help them become positioned correctly. To express their gratitude and help other children in need, the Yenish family with the help of their local community established the Raise Your Glass Foundation. With a slogan of "Toasting Those Who Make the Impossible, Possible," the foundation has held annual fundraisers, including cocktail parties, silent auctions, and golf tournaments. Their inaugural event in 2013 raised $45,000 for Shriners Children's Philadelphia, and cumulative totals to date exceed $445,000.

Below: Since 2015, Shriners Children's hospitals have hosted annual Walk for LOVE™ fundraisers. Offered in 1-mile or 5K varieties, the walks have and raised millions of dollars in small donations and helped thousands of participants nationwide to show their support for the kids Shriners Children's serves.

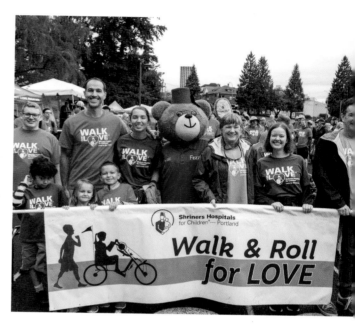

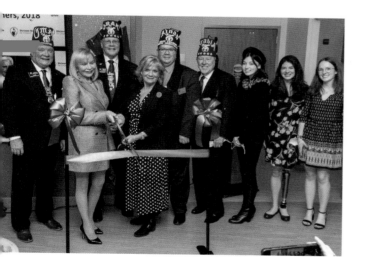

In 2022, Marcia Billhartz of Collinsville, Illinois (second from left) found the perfect way to honor her brother, Edward D. Allan. A longtime member of Ainad Shriners in Southern Illinois, Allan has spent decades working on behalf of Shiners Children's St. Louis. Billhartz matched his commitment by donating a very generous $2 million in his name. "I am so proud of my brother and his dedication to this mission – that he would volunteer nearly a decade of his life ... to make a difference in the life of children," she said. Billhartz's donation is the largest single gift ever received by the St. Louis hospital. It leaves a lasting legacy that will help kids for years to come.

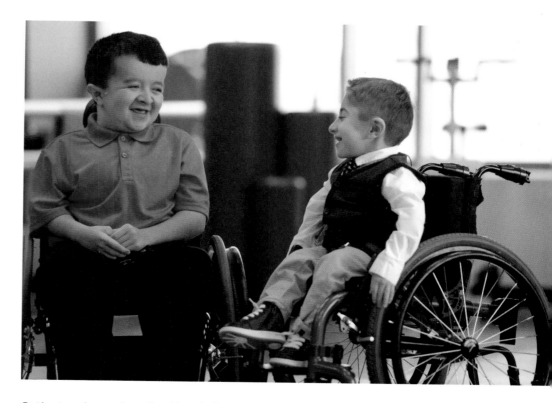

Patient ambassadors like Alec (left) and Kaleb (right) represent Shriners Children's at local, national, and media events. Their public service announcements have inspired millions of viewers. Through their example, these young spokespeople have served as vital fundraisers to further the mission of Shriners Children's.

193

THE NEXT HUNDRED YEARS

MEDICINE PROGRESSES BY QUANTUM LEAPS. THE MIRACLES EFFECTED TODAY WERE inconceivable in 1922 – who then could have imagined a genetic test? A single breakthrough has the power to change the entire healthcare landscape. Shriners Children's was only one of a host of institutions founded to cope with the scourge of polio, and many of these dissolved once the disease was eradicated in the United States. With advances in medicine, models of patient care have also changed. When Shriners Children's was founded, a hospital served primarily as a convalescent home. Patients stayed for months on end, and with only a limited number of beds, the waiting lists could be very long. Today, hospitals serve primarily as medical clinics that offer the most advanced care to the greatest number of patients through outpatient services.

For 100 years, Shriners Children's has adapted to changes in medicine. After the polio vaccine reduced the number of polio cases, the healthcare system expanded its mission to meet other pressing needs in pediatric care. Of the first 15 hospitals founded between 1922 and 1927, one-third were embedded in larger medical complexes. For the breadth of a century, Shriners Children's has been recognized worldwide as a leader in not just one, but many fields of specialized medicine.

No one knows what the future holds. What we take for granted today would seem miraculous in 1922, and it is possible that the practice of pediatric medicine in 2122 will unfold in dimensions that now seem impossible. However, one thing is certain: by staying true to its fundamental mission, Shriners Children's will continue to lead the way.

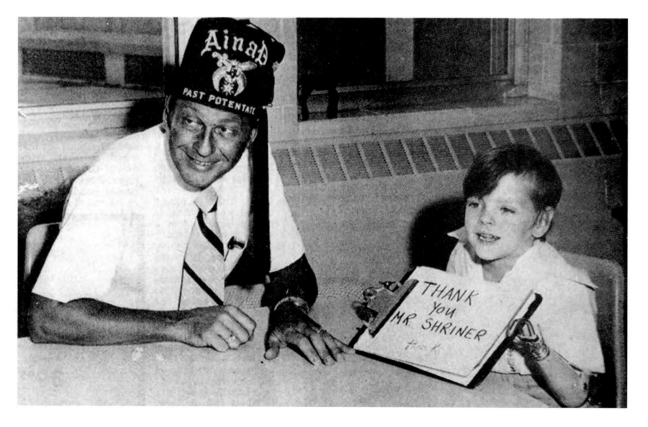

Noble Bill Walker, former pitcher for the St. Louis Cardinals and the New York Giants, and Past Potentate of Ainad Temple, visits a grateful patient at Shriners Children's Chicago, early 1960s.

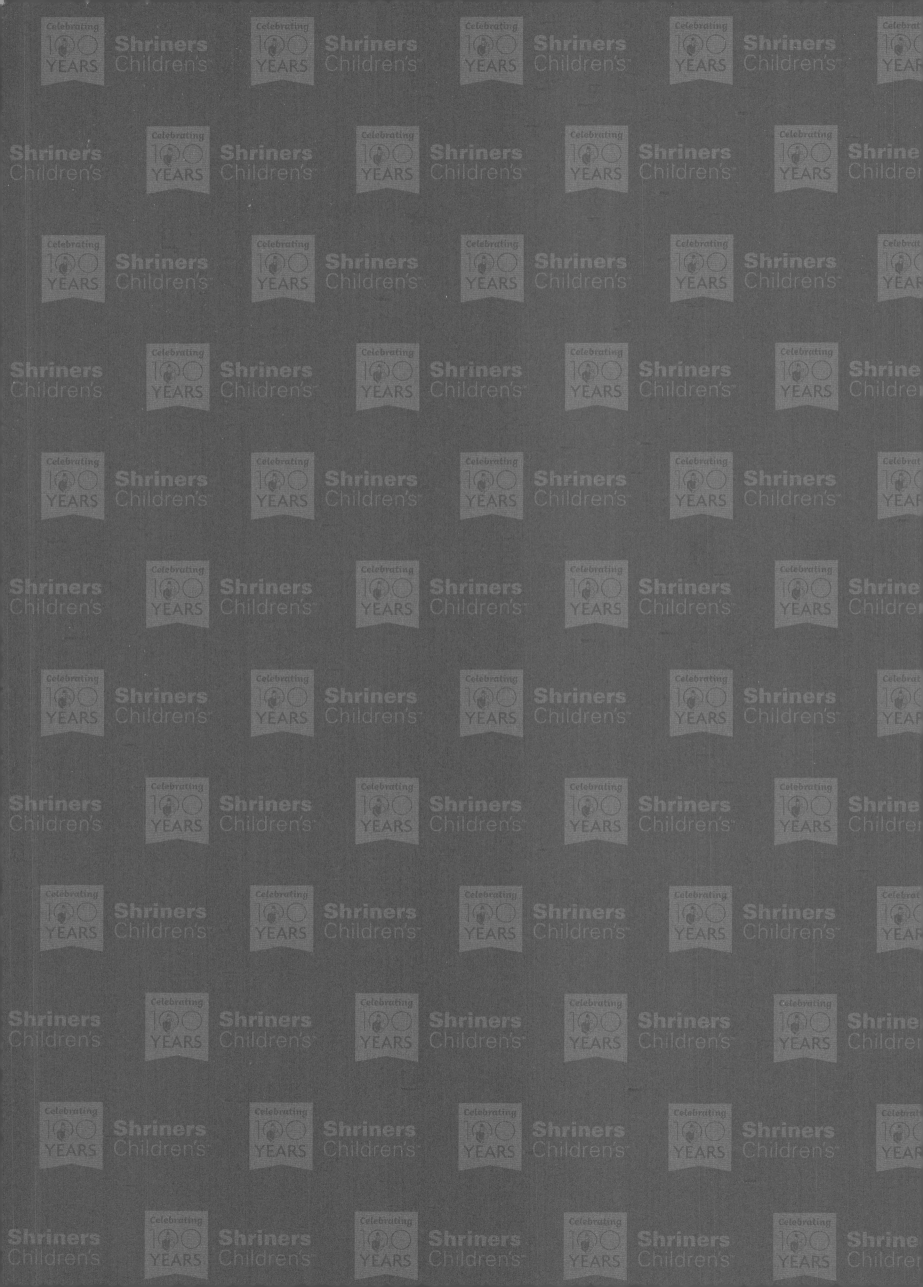